THE Allergy BIBLE

The Conventional and Alternative Guide to Understanding, Avoiding, and Treating Allergies

THE
All**e**rgy
BIBLE

LINDA GAMLIN

CONSULTANT: **PROFESSOR JONATHAN BROSTOFF**

The Reader's Digest Association, Inc.
Pleasantville, New York/Montreal

A Reader's Digest Book
Edited and designed by
Quadrille Publishing Limited

Editorial Director: Jane O'Shea
Creative Director: Mary Evans
Art Director: Helen Lewis
Project Editor: Hilary Mandleberg
Art Editor: Sue Storey
Production: Julie Hadingham
Picture Research: Nadine Bazar
Picture Assistant: Sarah Airey

NOTE TO READERS

The information in this book should not be substituted for, nor
used to alter, medical therapy without your doctor's advice. For
a specific health problem, consult your physician for guidance.

READER'S DIGEST PROJECT STAFF

Project Editors: Anita Winterberg, Marianne Wait
Project Art Director: John McGuffie
Copy Editor: Gilles Humbert
Medical Consultant: Antony J. Ham Pong, MD, FRCPC
Pharmaceutical Consultant: Gerald N. Rotenberg,
B.Sc.Phm., FACA

READER'S DIGEST ILLUSTRATED REFERENCE BOOKS

Editor-in-Chief: Christopher Cavanaugh
Art Director: Joan Mazzeo
Director, Trade Publishing: Christopher T. Reggio
Senior Design Director, Trade: Elizabeth L. Tunnicliffe
Editorial Director, Trade: Susan Randol

Library of Congress Cataloging in Publication Data
Gamlin, Linda.
  The allergy bible : the conventional and alternative guide to
  understanding, avoiding, and treating allergies / by Linda
  Gamlin; consultant, Jonathan Brostoff.
     p. cm.
  ISBN 0-7621-0293-4
  1. Allergy—Popular works. I. Brostoff, Jonathan. II. Title.

RC585 .G36 2001
616.97—dc21   00-062582

Printed in Italy

contents

Chapter 1
what is allergy?

Words matter, particularly in medicine. Using the same words to mean different things is a major difficulty for patients when discussing allergies with a doctor. Unfortunately, few patients realize this, and doctors are frequently too busy to give detailed information about the meanings of words. The result can be a great deal of misunderstanding, confusion, and irritation.

Unclear meanings can also create problems if you start exploring different treatment options. The word "allergy" is like one of those cats that eat at six different houses in the neighborhood: everyone feels as if they own it exclusively. A conventional allergist will understand one thing by "allergy," while a more unorthodox doctor may have a broader definition, and a herbalist or naturopath may use the word in a completely different way again.

This is an absolute jungle for the medically unqualified, and it can be an expensive jungle if you are looking around for an answer to your health problems. With the help of this book, you should be able to make sense of all this, and sort out the different and sometimes even contradictory advice on offer.

The word **allergy** was coined in 1906, when it was used to mean "altered reactivity"—any change in the way the body responds to the environment, whether immunity to a disease already encountered, or a sudden fit of sneezing from pollen. Immunity to disease was soon shunted off into a separate category altogether, leaving allergy with a narrower meaning: *any adverse reaction to substances that are normally harmless.* In this book, that meaning (definition 1) is covered by the word **sensitivity**.

One group of American doctors, who later became known as clinical ecologists, stuck with this definition. Their broad view of allergy is still found among some other doctors today, generally those whose approach to medicine is fairly unorthodox. It is a concept of allergy that is also shared by most practitioners of alternative or complementary therapies.

The rift between clinical ecologists and mainstream physicians occurred in the 1920s when the definition of allergy used by conventional doctors was narrowed further to mean *reactions to harmless items where the immune system is definitely involved*—definition 2. The term **immune sensitivity** is used in this book to convey that meaning.

In the 1960s, conventional allergists narrowed the definition of allergy again. It was an exciting time because the antibody known as immunoglobulin E or IgE (sometimes called the allergy antibody—see box on p. 12) had just been discovered. The new, tighter meaning of allergy was *reactions to harmless items where IgE is involved*—definition 3.

If asked to define allergy, most doctors would give the second of these definitions. (Although they might prefer not to think about the fact that this definition, applied logically, includes celiac disease—see p. 70.)

However, when they talk of "a tendency to allergy," "allergy treatment," "allergy shots," or "the allergy epidemic," doctors are generally using the third definition, and just mean IgE-mediated allergy.

This book deals with "allergy" in the very broadest sense of the word—all kinds of sensitivity. However— and this is purely for the purposes of clarity—where the word **allergy** is used in the text it always means **IgE-mediated allergy** (definition 3).

Other immune-mediated problems are called **non-IgE immune sensitivity** in this book.

Finally, any reaction where the immune system has no proven central role is called an **intolerance**. (As for other technical words, if you want to find the full definition, look in the index and turn to the page number shown in bold type.)

If you are reading widely on this topic, you may come across sensitivity used either according to definition 1 above, or as a synonym for intolerance. You may also encounter the word **hypersensitivity**. Doctors use this term to mean any immune system involvement (see p. 18). You may also see it used loosely in nonmedical literature to describe any adverse reactions or sensitivities.

Remember that medical politics and economics are a powerful force in all this debate over meanings.

Words are quite often redefined by medical interest groups (such as professional associations). Sometimes definitions change when there is a better understanding of diseases or conditions (see p. 24), and other times with the intention of staking out territory and claiming sole access to medical truth. To add to the long-standing battle over "allergy" there are now rival claims about the meaning of the word intolerance, with attempts to narrow the definition so that it only includes metabolic abnormalities (see box on p. 75).

When you talk with doctors, it will help enormously if, instead of saying you have a food allergy, for example, you just describe your symptoms. The important thing is to get along well and communicate clearly with doctors. Avoid using the word "allergy" unless this diagnosis has been medically established. Just describing how you react—the actual symptoms— is usually the best approach. If you need a general word for your condition, "sensitive" may be preferable to "allergic."

Allergies and inheritance
WHY IT RUNS IN FAMILIES

"My father had asthma as a child, and his sister had it too. In fact she died from it. My mother has never had any allergies, but one of her brothers had terrible hay fever all his life. Out of us four, only my brother Peter is completely allergy-free. I had bad eczema when I was small, as did my sister. So when our son developed eczema, and then asthma, and an allergy to house dust mites that made his nose run all the time, I wasn't entirely surprised." What Janey is describing is a good example of an **atopic family**—one where classical allergies, of one kind or another, affect several family members. The members of such a family are called **atopics**.

Atopics have an underlying tendency to allergy which, with luck, may never be expressed. But if they are unlucky, the tendency will lead to allergies, which can settle on the skin (atopic eczema), the nose (hay fever or perennial allergic rhinitis), the airways (asthma) or the mouth and digestive tract (food allergy). These diseases, which recur down the generations in atopic families like Janey's, are known as the **classical allergic diseases.**

The atopic tendency is coded into our DNA— in the genes that are passed from parent to child. There are also other genes that make asthma more likely to develop, and these can work in concert with the allergy-promoting genes to produce asthma in a child. And there are probably genes for dry skin, which contribute to atopic eczema.

Genes alone are not enough, however. Environment (in medical terms, *everything* external that affects an individual, including diseases, diet, cigarette smoke and other air pollutants, aller-

gens such as animal danders, dust mites or pollen, cockroaches, and even medical treatments) also plays a large part in promoting allergic reactions. In other words, genes and the external world interact to produce allergic disease. What happens in the months and years immediately after birth seems to be a crucial element.

This helps to explain why allergies are on the increase even though we are, genetically speaking, not so different from our grandparents or great-grandparents. It is also a considerable cause for optimism, since it means we may be able to reverse the trend in coming generations. All we have to do is adjust the environment, especially for newborns and young children.

Luckily, most of the problem factors are ones over which we have personal control, such as smoking by parents, diet, infant feeding, hygiene (*less* is better), antibiotic treatment, house design and furnishings (see pp. 11–12).

As unique as a fingerprint

Generally speaking, inherited traits such as height or skin color are governed, not by a single gene with a large effect, but by a great many genes each with a small effect. The many small effects add up to produce the final outcome.

Atopy is probably inherited in a similar way, which would explain why some people have a very strong tendency to allergies (they have lots of the wrong genes) while other people have only a mild tendency (they have just a few).

Current estimates hold that at least 20 different genes are involved in determining atopy and the number could be higher. This means that no two atopic individuals are going to be quite the same, because each will have a different combination of these genes. In the words of Dr. Vincent Beltrani, of New York's Columbia University, "it is not surprising that, as a result of all the possible genetic combinations and permutations, each atopic individual possesses a unique 'allergic fingerprint' and that not all atopic individuals have identical findings."

Multigene inheritance has another important effect, in terms of predicting who will develop allergies. The genetic risks from the two parents add up, so if both parents have allergies themselves or come from atopic families, the risks of the child developing allergies are much higher than if only one parent is atopic. The actual figures are uncertain because the results vary considerably from one study to another. If one parent is atopic, the risk can range from 20–58 percent, whereas if both parents are atopic, the risk ranges from 50–80 percent or even more.

Note that these are just *risks*—there are no certainties here because the actual mix of genes that a child receives is a selection—half of the mother's genes and half of the father's. There's no saying which half a child gets, because this is a random selection process, similar to the shuffling and dealing of playing cards. Luck plays a big part.

Naturally enough, both atopic parents and their doctors have asked whether there is any test that could assess the number of pro-allergy genes in a newborn and so predict the chances of allergy developing in particular children. That would allow more stringent anti-allergy measures (see pp. 238–47) to be taken for the children most at risk.

Various tests have been tried, and one does work, to a limited extent. It involves measuring the level of the allergy antibody, IgE, in a blood sample taken from the umbilical cord just after birth. Very high levels of IgE give some indication of the chances of allergies developing later, but the accuracy of the prediction is, unfortunately, not that good when the test is carried out in atopic families. The test doesn't reveal much more than is already known—that the baby has atopic parents.

The same test, when carried out on newborns who are *not* from atopic families, sometimes gives a much more useful and accurate result. In one study, 75 percent of babies with high levels of cord-blood IgE developed allergies a few years later, compared to only 6 percent of those with low levels. Unfortunately, the test does not always give such impressive results, and some disappointing studies have led doctors to conclude that it is not worthwhile as a standard test for all newborns.

This finding of high IgE in children from non-atopic families highlights an important point: genes that favor allergy are common. A lot of healthy people have them, but at levels that do not cause any symptoms—yet. This explains why, with the allergy epidemic, many new allergy sufferers are coming from families never affected by allergy before. As our lifestyle becomes more pro-allergy, a baby needs fewer of the pro-allergy genes to grow into an allergic individual.

Other forms of sensitivity

The multigene inheritance of classical allergy is very different from the inheritance of diseases such as primary lactase deficiency (see p. 79) where there is a single gene that is at fault. Generally speaking, all **metabolic abnormalities** (see box on p. 75) are inherited in this straightforward way, so they are an all-or-nothing affair: one child in the family gets the defective gene while another does not. No environmental triggers are needed to activate the defect.

In the case of food intolerance, if minor metabolic abnormalities play a part, as they may do for some sufferers, then there could be inheritance of the defect, but this will not necessarily lead to symptoms unless other intolerance-promoting factors (such as disturbed gut flora) are present.

Inheritance plays a part in several other forms of sensitivity. It is very important, for example, in celiac disease and dermatitis herpetiformis (see p. 70), which both stem from the same genetic feature. They are only expressed when wheat is eaten but the timing is important here—introducing wheat into a child's diet later, rather than during the first year of life, seems less likely to provoke the disease.

When celiac disease comes on in adult life, as it sometimes does, it suggests that some other environmental trigger was needed, in addition to wheat, to start the disease process.

A mast cell, magnified about 10,000 times. The black granules contain histamine.

How does allergy begin?

"At the beginning, I thought I just had a cold. I kept sneezing and coughing, and my nose was dripping. It got better on the weekend, and I thought—that's good, it's gone—but then on the Monday evening it started up again. The next thing I knew, I kept getting breathless. I'd been at the sawmill a month when it began. We were cutting planks of red cedar all day, and the dust was bad, it's true. But I didn't know that sawdust could cause you allergies. We were given dust masks, but they made you too hot. No one wore them. I found out later, from the doctor, that some men could work years at it before they got allergic to the dust, but with me it was just a month."

Like many people with work-related allergy, Dan can actually pinpoint the time he became sensitized—when he began making IgE antibodies against the red cedar dust allergen.

For allergies that are not caused by workplace allergens, this is rarely possible. The moment when symptoms begin may be obvious, but that is often long after sensitization (making IgE to the allergen) first occurred. Long-term studies of children show that they may start giving positive skin-prick tests to pollens (a sign that they are making IgE to those pollens) while they are toddlers, but not develop hay fever until 10 years later.

The basics of immunity

The **immune system** defends the body against infections and cancerous cells. One of its key jobs, before going on the offensive, is to recognize the difference between:
- self and non-self (e.g. the cells lining the lung, and bacteria trying to infect the lung)
- safe-non-self (e.g. a sandwich) and dangerous-non-self (e.g. *Salmonella* bacteria in the sandwich).

Through misregulation the immune system can cause:
- **allergies** (perceiving safe-non-self, such as pollen, as dangerous-non-self)
- **autoimmune diseases** (perceiving self as non-self).

The immune system consists of dozens of different kinds of cells (the **immune cells**) and a number of different **antibodies**—specialized "guided missiles" (see box on p. 15) that are produced by certain immune cells.

There is also a huge array of **messenger chemicals**, which send general instructions (e.g. "calm down!" "go for it!" or "exterminate!") from one type of cell to another.

Immune cells are self-contained units, many of them mobile and dispersed throughout the body. They travel around in the blood, and can move out of the blood vessels and into the surrounding tissues (skin, lung, nose, etc.)

These different components—immune cells, antibodies, and messenger chemicals—interact in very complex ways. When an **immune reaction** occurs—the immune system recognizes something, or mounts an attack on something—numerous different players are involved. All the reactions described in this book are very simplified versions of what actually happens.

Research shows that we are most vulnerable during the first two years of life as regards sensitization to allergens. Very often, sensitization occurs in the first few months of a child's life, and sometimes even before birth.

Why is a young infant so easily sensitized? The answer lies not with the baby, but with the pregnant mother-to-be, whose immune system has to overrule its natural inclination to attack anything that is non-self. Potentially, a woman's immune system could reject a fetus in just the same way that heart transplants are rejected. To prevent attacks on the fetus, the immune system is retuned during pregnancy, with one aspect of immunity—the part that's most keen to attack a foreign body—being damped down.

This aspect of immunity is co-ordinated by cells known as T-helper-1 cells, or Th1 cells for short. To protect the fetus, Th1 cells are asked to ease up during pregnancy. Meanwhile, since immune protection is still needed, their colleagues, called T-helper-2 cells or Th2 cells, become more active.

The classical allergic diseases

These four pages are concerned only with the classical allergic diseases, that is:

hay fever (an allergy to pollen)

perennial allergic rhinitis (a nasal allergy to a year-round allergen such as dust mites)

asthma where this includes an allergic reaction

atopic eczema (see p. 42)

urticaria (hives) where this is allergic in origin, and the accompanying **angioedema** (swelling that is due to fluid escaping from tiny blood vessels into the surrounding area)

anaphylaxis (a violent allergic reaction to food, insect stings, penicillin, latex, etc.)

food allergy (in most cases, an immediate and marked reaction to food, usually with symptoms in the lips and mouth, and/or widespread hives; in severe cases there may also be anaphylaxis)

Running the immune system

T-helper cells are, in a way, misnamed, because they do not help at all—they just give orders.

These are the supervisors of the immune reactions, telling other immune cells either to lie low or to get busy. Where Th1 and Th2 cells differ is in the types of immune cells they send into action. Among those who get their go-ahead from Th1 cells are immune cells that attack directly, without producing antibodies—these are the ones that reject transplants and could, if given free rein, reject a fetus or retard its growth.

The Th2 cells, on the other hand, have among their preferred troops the immune cells that produce IgE antibodies—the allergy-causing antibodies. So one effect of protecting the fetus from rejection is to push the immune system toward a greater tendency to allergy.

This shift of emphasis occurs in the mother's immune system, but it carries over into the immune system of the fetus because they are sharing the same blood supply, and the blood contains the messenger substances that fine-tune the immune system. Immediately after birth, the baby's immune system is still following the same pattern, continuing to upregulate Th2 cells and downregulate Th1 cells. This is a crucial factor in setting the stage for allergic sensitization.

Ideally, the world that the baby encounters just after birth should nudge the immune system in the opposite direction and get it operating in a non-allergic way. But the world in which we live is far from ideal in this regard.

For one thing, it is much too clean. As far as the immune system is concerned, "ideal" would mean encountering a bit of dirt, such as garden soil, in the early stages of life. The soil contains harmless bacteria that do not cause any symptoms, but do tweak the immune system toward Th1 cells and away from Th2 cells. Bacterial products that are found in household dust may do the same thing (see p. 21).

A long period of consuming nothing but breast milk would also suit the baby's immune system rather better than being fed on cow's milk formula or being suddenly weaned onto a number of highly allergenic foods, such as egg, wheat, soy (ubiquitous

What is an allergic reaction?

The basic cause of classical allergy is an immune reaction involving **mast cells** and **IgE antibodies**.

Mast cells are plentiful in the lining of the nose, the airways, and the digestive tract. They have counterparts in the blood, called **basophils**.

Seen under the microscope, both mast cells and basophils look very granular inside. The granules are tiny storage compartments, containing stockpiles of messenger chemicals, notably **histamine**.

Histamine causes several different reactions:

- contraction of muscle around the airways. This reduces the diameter of the airway, producing an asthma attack
- widening of blood vessels
- increased leakiness of the smallest blood vessels, allowing fluid and immune cells to escape into the surrounding area—for example, the skin or airway lining
- as a result of these two above effects, local swelling (called edema or angioedema) and irritation—in the skin this is experienced as urticaria, or hives, in the nose it causes blockage, itching, and sneezing
- if sufficient histamine is released into the blood, a drastic fall in blood pressure, due to widespread opening of blood vessels, and leakage of fluid into the tissues; this occurs in anaphylaxis (see p. 58).

Histamine is released when mast cells are activated, a process called **degranulation** because the cells discharge their storage granules.

Mast cells release other substances at the same time, some of which attract more immune cells to the area, causing more inflammation. They help to produce a "Late Phase Reaction" which occurs after the initial allergic reaction has died down, and lasts about 24 hours (see p. 13). Once activated, mast cells also start making messenger chemicals called **leukotrienes**, which are highly inflammatory.

What causes a mast cell to degranulate? The answer is found on the surface of the cells, where the allergy antibody, IgE, sits. One end of the IgE molecule is bound to the mast cell, and the other end can bind to the allergen concerned. In someone allergic to egg, for example, egg allergen will bind, with great specificity, to egg-specific IgE antibody.

For the receptors to pass a message to the mast cell there have to be two IgE antibodies specific for the same allergen on the mast cell—and the allergen has to bind to both these IgE molecules, so forming a link between them. This is the "go" signal for the mast cell to degranulate.

in processed foods), fish or peanuts, before it can handle them. Antibiotic treatment before age 2 also seems to be associated with increased risk of allergy. (Therefore if an antibiotic is suggested, you should discuss with your doctor if this is truly necessary—see p. 247.)

An ideal world for the immune system would also lack the by-products of cigarette smoking, whether in the blood of a pregnant woman or in the air that a baby breathes—both seem to promote the allergic tendency. In addition, the perfect world would lack central heating, wall-to-wall carpeting, draft-proofing, and thick upholstery. A house like this is heaven for dust mites but not for innocent young immune systems.

The problem with dust mites—apart from the fact that they breed like wildfire, and hole up in mattresses, armchairs and soft toys—is that they produce a highly allergenic protein in their droppings. This protein interferes with the membranes of cells, making them less stable. It irritates various immune cells, including mast cells (see box), and can even make mast cells degranulate, as if there were a true allergic reaction happening.

Once mast cells have done this, they release messenger substances that arouse the immune system and make a genuine allergic reaction— beginning with the production of IgE to the dust-mite allergen—much more likely. In other words, dust-mite allergen is an *agent provocateur*, an aggressive substance that actually provokes the immune system into reacting allergically.

Until recently it was widely assumed that allergens were just inoffensive, passive substances which the immune system happened to take objection to, in a distinctly unreasonable way. The new discoveries about dust-mite allergen raise the question: could other allergens be more aggressive than previously thought? Certainly the peanut allergen, or other substances found in peanuts, seems to destabilize cell membranes, which may explain why this powerful allergen so easily sensitizes young children.

The role of genes

Faced with this nonideal world, many children pull through without developing allergies, but others do not. This is where genes come in, making one child more susceptible to our allergy-promoting lifestyle and another child less so. Exactly how the genes make this difference is still not fully understood, but there are at least 20 genes involved (see p. 9), and it is clearly going to be a complex story. The overall effect of these genes is a greater tendency to make IgE, combined with mast cells and basophils (see box on p. 12) that are distinctly trigger-happy—much more eager to degranulate than in healthy individuals.

Given all the mayhem caused by mast cells and IgE, why does the body produce them at all? They cause a lot of damage to allergy sufferers and do little apparent good, at least for people in the Western world. The value of the mast-cell-IgE-reaction, for most of us, is historical—it wages war against large-bodied parasites such as tapeworms and schistosomes. (They are large by comparison with bacteria and viruses, and not easily tackled by other immune cells.) These unpleasant invaders have largely been eliminated in the developed world but are still rife in other countries. For millions of years such parasites were an inevitable part of human life, and this bit of our evolutionary past survives in our immune system.

The complexity of allergic reactions

"Each time the pollen season came around, I would start to get these pains, especially in my knees. I asked my doctor about it but she just looked at me rather oddly and said 'Take a painkiller.' I couldn't be sure it was linked to my hay fever, but the pains always came on just after the sneezing started. One year, it was worse than usual, and I felt very tired too. My face was all puffy and I could feel that something was seriously amiss. That, as I now know, was because my kidneys were being affected. It was years before the doctor would refer me to an allergist, and I actually got an explanation for all this. I think for a long time my doctor thought I was making it up, or just imagining the pain in my knees."

Karen suffers from a rare complication of hay fever involving an overload of pollen antigens and antibodies in the blood. Very large numbers of both are involved, and are bound to each other in dense tangled masses called immune complexes. Because these are carried around in the blood they are known as **circulating immune complexes**. They may be too large to be cleared quickly by the normal junk-munching systems that keep the blood clean.

Like a river choked with fallen leaves, that deposits some of the debris on its banks as it flows past, the blood inevitably leaves

behind some of the circulating immune complexes. They mostly become deposited in the tiny blood vessels called capillaries, particularly those in the skin, the kidney and the joints. Inflammation (see p. 140) here can cause a range of symptoms.

This problem is known to doctors either as **serum sickness** or **Type III hypersensitivity**. It is a well-known feature of several infections and of some autoimmune diseases.

Unfortunately, some family physicians are unaware of the potential for Type III hypersensitivity in allergies such as hay fever, as Karen discovered. As well as affecting hay fever sufferers, Type III hypersensitivity can also be a complication of reactions to penicillin and certain other reactions, such as insect-sting allergy.

When a reaction occurs to snake anti-venin—and it only occurs in an individual who has received snake anti-venin before—this too is Type III hypersensitivity. The snake anti-venin is cultured in horses, and the snake-bitten human who has received the snake anti-venin previously mounts a massive immune reaction *to the horse proteins* when snake anti-venin is injected for a second time. Large and numerous circulating immune complexes are formed, and although IgE is not involved, a very severe anaphylactoid reaction (see box on p. 59) follows.

Circulating immune complexes do not affect most allergy sufferers. But there are other immune responses that occur after the initial allergic response in *everyone* with allergies—they are termed the "**Late Phase Reaction**" to distinguish them from the immediate reaction.

The Late Phase Reaction starts 4–12 hours after the exposure to the allergen, and lasts about a day. It involves a number of different immune cells (including eosinophils—p. 19) and an even more varied array of messenger chemicals, making everything very complicated for medical researchers to investigate. When allergic symptoms become entrenched and difficult to treat, the Late Phase Reaction is usually implicated. Because the details are so complex, the Late Phase Reaction remains poorly understood at present.

Cross-reactions in allergy

For the rabbi's doctor, discussing the results of the allergy tests with his patient, it was an embarrassing moment. An allergy is not inborn, it is an acquired reaction—a response by the immune system to a substance it has already encountered at least once. So, in theory, nobody can be allergic to a food they have never eaten.

Naturally enough, the rabbi had never eaten shellfish—like pork, it is forbidden under Kosher law. But the nurse carrying out the skin-prick tests was unaware of this, and she had been told to test for all the common food allergens, so shrimp allergen was included. The test came up positive.

Fortunately, the rabbi had also been tested for inhaled allergens and had given a very strong positive reaction to dust mite. The likely explanation was clear: the rabbi had formed antibodies to a muscle protein of dust mite called tropomyosin, which is also found in shrimps and prawns. His antibodies against dust mite had cross-reacted with shrimp tropomyosin.

This does not mean that everyone who is allergic to dust mite will also react to shrimp. First they must have made antibodies to tropomyosin, rather than some other dust-mite antigen. Second, the antibodies must be recognizing a particular feature of dust-mite tropomyosin that closely resembles (chemically speaking) a particular feature of shrimp tropomyosin.

The important point about antibodies is that, on the one hand, they achieve results by being specific for their antigen (see box on p. 15), but on the other hand, they do make mistakes. In the case of allergies, this is sometimes an added problem for patients but is rarely life threatening. More seriously, there are other conditions, like celiac disease, where cross-reactions initiate attacks on the body's own components, causing severe symptoms.

Antibodies make mistakes because they recognize antigens by homing in on tiny chemical markers, not by looking at the antigen as a whole (see box on p. 15). Although this is a nuisance for allergy sufferers, it can be a bonus in fighting diseases. For example,

Antigens and allergens

An **antigen** is anything that elicits an **antibody** reaction. Each antibody is specific for a particular antigen.

When they tend to cause allergies (by provoking IgE antibodies rather than other kinds of antibody—see box on p. 13) these antigens are called **allergens**. Something such as ragweed pollen is both an antigen (because it elicits an antibody reaction) and an allergen (because it often elicits IgE antibodies in those who are allergy-prone).

when viruses (such as those that cause influenza) revamp their outer-coat proteins to evade the immune system, the chances are that some antibodies will still recognize them because a few of the original chemical markers persist.

Understanding cross-reactions

Many cross-reactions are between related species, and this makes sense in biological terms. The tropomyosin story is a good example—not only is tropomyosin found in dust mites and shrimps, but it also occurs in other crustacean shellfish, such as crabs and lobsters, in molluscan shellfish such as clams and oysters, and in insects. If one goes back over 300 million years, all these animals were just a twinkle in the eye of some primeval invertebrate, the common ancestor of them all.

Tropomyosin is one of those triumphs of the evolutionary process—a protein that reached near-perfection hundreds of millions of years ago, in the long-vanished ancestral species, and remains so good at its job that it has only been tinkered with by natural selection since then, never radically altered. In other words, because it works so well, it has been "conserved" by the various animal groups descended from the shared ancestor. Although there are some differences between the tropomyosins from different descendants, the similarities are considerable.

Relatedness counts here. Shrimps and prawns are pretty closely related, as anyone can see by looking at them. Their tropomyosins are extremely similar, as are many other allergens. You're unlikely to be allergic to prawn but not shrimp. The more distant the relationship, the more differences accumulate in the antigens, so a cross-reaction between dust-mite and shrimp is far less likely (the rabbi was unlucky).

Another conserved protein, parvalbumin, explains why people who are allergic to one type of fish are usually allergic to all kinds of fish (in spite of the fact that fish belong to several different families which are only distantly related). Those allergic to hen's eggs will probably be allergic to the eggs of all birds, because the primary allergens (ovalbumin) are so similar.

These conserved proteins produce cross-reactions across huge gulfs, in terms of zoological and botanical relationships. Far more easily understood are the cross-reactions between close cousins, such as dust mites and storage mites, wheat and rye, pine pollen and pine nuts, or ragweed and sunflower (both members of the daisy family).

Relatedness can be useful in explaining cross-reactions, but often fails when it comes to predicting them. Some related species do not show as many cross-reactions as one might expect. Peanuts are legumes (members of the bean-and-pea family, Leguminosae), and highly allergenic. One would expect some peanut-allergic individuals to be allergic to other members of the legume family, such as peas, beans, carob, and soy. In fact, although some patients give positive skin-prick tests to these peanut relatives, very few show actual symptoms when they eat these foods. Where symptoms do occur, they tend to be mild.

Paradoxically, those who are allergic to peanuts very often develop an allergy to tree nuts, and this usually spans several different kinds of tree nuts—yet botanically all these are very distant relatives. No tree nut is a legume and while walnuts and pecans belong to one plant family, almonds belong to another, hazelnuts to another, cashews to a fourth, and Brazils to a fifth different plant family. Here relatedness seems irrelevant, and it is shared lifestyle (surviving as a nut-producing plant) that is crucial.

A nut is just an oversized seed that has to survive being buried in the soil—either by the plant itself (in the case of peanuts) or by a nut-eating animal such as a squirrel. All nuts must resist rotting in the soil until the following spring, and therefore contain powerful bactericidal and fungicidal compounds. Some of these may have chemical similarities that cause cross-reactions.

These functional "lifestyle" allergens of nuts may be even more widely shared, with many seeds having something similar: recent research shows potentially cross-reacting allergens in wheat, rye, hazelnuts, sesame, and poppy. It is interesting that many people developing new allergies to sesame or poppy are already allergic to wheat and nuts.

A few cross-reactions seem to defy any explanation, such as that between dust mites and kiwi fruit—this appears to be just a case of chemical coincidence. Other cross-reactions that appear equally bizarre actually have a biological basis, notably that between latex (as used in medical gloves) and various fruits and vegetables, principally chestnut, banana, avocado, and kiwi fruit. This cross-reaction is due to a shared enzyme called a chitinase that protects plants against insect pests. Latex, of course, comes from the sap of the rubber tree: the tree needs such protection from insects and its sap is richly laced with chitinase.

How antibodies work— and why they make errors

Antibodies are catapult-shaped, with two **antigen binding sites** at the ends of the two arms. The other end of the antibody molecule—the handle of the catapult—is free to bind to cell receptors.

When an antibody binds to its antigen there is a "chemical handshake:" a very specific recognition event involving one of the antigen binding sites and a particular small site on the antigen molecule called the **epitope**. The two lock together. (Different antibodies, although specific for the same antigen molecule, may recognize different epitopes.)

The antibody is recognizing its antigen, but it is as if we recognized other people by homing in on one small part of them, choosing a different feature for each person, whatever is most distinctive about them—the quirky right eyebrow, the hook in the nose, or the mole on the cheek. The antibody does not "look at" the whole antigen molecule, but simply recognizes a characteristic cluster of chemical features at the epitope.

Cross-reactions occur because an antigen only has to resemble another molecule in one small area (the epitope) for a mistake to occur.

Breaking the mold
NEW DISCOVERIES ABOUT ALLERGY AND SENSITIVITY

"When I first arrived in Charlottesville in 1982, the senior allergist said 'I've got to warn you that here in Virginia we have patients who have very severe fungal infection of their feet, and they also have urticaria. If you treat their feet, their urticaria gets better.'" Professor Tom Platts-Mills of the University of Virginia in Charlottesville is recalling how his innovative studies of fungal infections and allergy began. That surprising observation about athlete's foot (a fungal infection) and urticaria (hives) was made by his predecessor, Professor John Guerrant.

"I followed his advice," Platts-Mills continues, "and found he was right. Then I started noticing asthmatics in our allergy clinic who also had fungal infections of their feet. They were mostly men with severe adult-onset asthma. We gave them skin-prick tests with the fungus *Trichophyton* and these were positive—showing they had an allergic reaction to it. So we tried treating them with antifungal drugs and the asthma got much better."

This discovery is not an isolated instance. Research over the last decade or so has revealed that allergic reactions to long-standing infections (**chronic infection** is the medical term) are far more common than anyone expected. Infections by fungi are frequent offenders.

An infection becomes chronic because, although the immune system tries to rout the infectious agent, it never succeeds. Making IgE may be part of that futile defensive effort. Once the immune system starts making IgE against the allergens produced by the infectious microbe, new symptoms may begin, or existing allergic symptoms may get much worse. The link between the infection and the allergy is far from obvious, however. Both the allergens and the IgE can be carried in the

Fungal infections

"Fungus" means everything from an edible mushroom or a huge bracket fungus to the specks of mold on stale bread or a shower curtain. Fungal infections are caused, not by mushroomlike fungi, but by inconspicuous moldlike forms, or by yeasts (which are single-celled fungi).

Once they are flourishing, some fungal infections may be seen as whitish or creamy-colored patches. But at an earlier stage, the fungi are so small that they cannot be seen without a microscope. They spread as invisibly as bacteria or viruses.

Some infectious fungi can exist in two different forms—a mycelial form (long thin strands, as in a mold) or a yeast form (single cells).

bloodstream, so the symptoms may be somewhere else in the body, far away from the site of infection.

If the symptoms of the infection itself are relatively mild, they may not receive medical attention. Infection-plus-allergy often explains severe long-term allergic problems for which no cause could previously be found. This is the kind of case that gets labeled as "intrinsic" or "endogenous". Most patients in this category have had years of simply being treated with steroids (often at high doses) to suppress the symptoms.

Sometimes the infection-plus-allergy is part of a larger picture, with other allergens or irritants also contributing to the symptoms, but with no stunning improvements when they are avoided because the allergic stimulus from the infection remains.

The links between allergy and fungal infections—all those that have been discovered so far—are described below. In such cases, antifungal drugs, taken by mouth, usually in capsule form, could be of value. They must be taken for an adequate length of time, normally several months.

Bear in mind that, with the possible exception of chronic sinusitis, an allergic reaction to fungal infection is a relatively uncommon cause of symptoms. It is important that, with the help of your doctor, you start with the more likely suspects such as airborne or contact allergens. These are described in detail, in Chapter 2.

Asthma

See pp. 36–41 for the common causes, and usual treatment, of asthma.

Trichophyton—the fungus that causes athlete's foot—can provoke allergic reactions that contribute to asthma. This fungus may also infect other parts of the body. *Trichophyton* diseases have names that begin with *tinea* (athlete's foot, for example, is *tinea pedis*). Other terms you may come across are intertrigo (an itchy rash that develops in skin folds) and onychomycosis (also called "ringworm of the nails" or *tinea unguinum*). The research on the link with asthma was published in the respected British medical journal, *The Lancet*. Very thorough treatment with antifungal drugs, taken in capsule form, is required.

Chronic urticaria

See pp. 54–7 for the many possible causes of chronic urticaria.

Trichophyton infections in any part of the body (see above) can provoke allergies, producing chronic urticaria. A great variety of other infections, including fungal, viral, and chronic bacterial infections, can be the root of the problem in chronic urticaria (see pp. 51–2). However, this may not be an allergic reaction. It could be a direct effect of the infection, provoking the immune system in such a way that it triggers mast cells (see box on p. 12) directly, without IgE.

Chronic sinusitis

See pp. 30–35 for the causes and treatment of chronic sinusitis.

Chronic sinusitis may be due to fungal infection with a subsequent allergy: **allergic fungal sinusitis**. Some doctors believe that a sensitivity reaction to fungal infection (not necessarily an allergic reaction) accounts for most chronic sinusitis, but this is disputed (see pp. 32–3).

Atopic eczema (atopic dermatitis)

See pp. 42–9 for the causes and treatment of atopic eczema.

The *Trichophyton* fungus can infect eczematous skin, though this is far less common than infection by *Staphylococcus aureus* (see p. 18). Among patients infected by it, there can be an allergic reaction to *Trichophyton* which makes the eczema worse.

There can also be an IgE reaction to a yeast, *Pityrosporum ovale*, in atopic eczema. This yeast is a commensal—a natural, and normally harmless, inhabitant of healthy skin. The inflammation of eczema makes the immune system far more irritable so that it reacts allergically to this yeast, an innocent bystander which it normally disregards.

Candida (see box on p. 83) can also provoke an allergic reaction in eczematous skin. While *Candida* is a commensal in the gut, it does not normally live on the skin. However, it may flourish in the disturbed skin of eczema patients.

Those with atopic eczema may also develop an allergic reaction to toxins from *Staphylococcus*

Fungi in the lungs

One form of infection-plus-allergy has been well recognized for many years—**allergic bronchopulmonary aspergillosis**, often shortened to **aspergillosis** or **ABPA**.

The problem starts with the fungus *Aspergillus fumigatus*, a ubiquitous mold that is abundant in damp straw, compost heaps, bird cages, and any decomposing material. Its spores are everywhere, and most immune systems quickly defeat them, but in some people, especially those with asthma, the spores begin to grow in the lungs. The fungus is found in the lung mucus, but does not actually invade the lungs. However, an allergic reation then occurs to the fungus.

This disease often goes together with asthma, or can be mistaken for asthma. There are several clues that point to aspergillosis:

- rubbery plugs of sputum, either golden-brown or green in color
- fever whenever the asthma is severe
- worsening symptoms despite treatment
- dependence on steroid tablets
- very high IgE levels in the blood

Allergic bronchopulmonary aspergillosis is treated with steroids to control the allergic reaction, and physiotherapy to clear the mucus from the lungs.

Antifungal drugs have not proved very effective in the past. There are some newer antifungal drugs that may well be more useful, such as itraconazole and terbinafine. These are not widely used for aspergillosis at present, except in patients who also have cystic fibrosis or an immune deficiency. Because there has been no large-scale trial of these drugs, they are not usually given to people who simply have aspergillosis. However, they are sometimes prescribed for people who are unable to take steroids, or are not responding to steroid treatment. Antifungal drugs may become more widely used in the next few years, so it is worth discussing the possibility of this treatment with your doctor.

aureus, a bacterium that often infects skin which is already inflamed by eczema and damaged by scratching. Antibiotics are needed to treat the infection (see p. 49).

A medical earthquake

The recent discoveries about infection-plus-allergy have not posed any serious challenge to conventional thinking about allergy, because a disease of just this kind—aspergillosis (see box)—was already well known. A far more fundamental shake-up of traditional ideas about allergy and sensitivity has been necessitated by new research into atopic eczema. It is little short of a medical earthquake in the basic concepts of allergy and sensitivity.

To understand the nature of this upheaval, you need to know about the time-honored system for classifying hypersensitivity reactions, which recognizes four distinct types:

- **Type I hypersensitivity**—the IgE-mediated allergies (see box on p. 12) such as hay fever.
- **Type II hypersensitivity**—irrelevant to allergy, these antibody reactions mainly occur after transplant surgery, if the transplanted organ is rejected.
- **Type III hypersensitivity**—caused by a massive overload of antibodies and antigen in the blood. It is a feature of certain infections and autoimmune diseases, and can also occur in allergic reactions, though this is rare (see p. 13).
- **Type IV hypersensitivity**—the odd man out, because antibodies are not involved, or are not of central importance. Immune cells that can launch a direct attack are the movers and shakers here. These attacking-cells are sensitized for a particular antigen, such as dust-mite or lanolin. Type IV hypersensitivity is a very slow reaction. Generally speaking, 48 hours passes, after an encounter with the offending substance, before the symptoms appear. The most common form of Type IV hypersensitivity is contact dermatitis (see p. 54).

Mystery has always surrounded atopic eczema. Although it crops up in the same atopic families that suffer from hay fever and asthma, and high levels of IgE in the bloodstream are typical of the disease, the actual role played by allergies in causing the symptoms is far from obvious.

The results of skin-prick tests—the standard test for an IgE-mediated reaction—are puzzling. Patients tend to give a lot of positive results, many of which don't mean much—the substances concerned do not provoke actual symptoms. On the other hand, skin-prick tests are often negative for substances that clearly do cause symptoms. Some children who regularly get eczema when they drink cow's milk, for example, give a negative skin-prick test to milk. This conundrum has puzzled allergists for several decades.

New discoveries about eczema do not entirely solve the puzzle, but they do go some way toward an answer, by revealing an immune response that cuts across the traditional categories. The most surprising fact is that even where skin-prick tests are positive and milk-specific IgE is involved in milk-induced eczema, this is not necessarily a standard IgE-mediated allergy.

While IgE antibodies may be involved, they are not necessarily teamed up with mast cells, their usual partners in crime (see box on p. 12). Instead, the IgE molecules are attached to special skin cells called Langerhans cells and dendritic cells. These have the role of picking up the antigen and showing or "presenting" it to attacking-cells in the skin (a task called **antigen presentation** which is the "go" signal that starts off all immune reactions).

The involvement of these attacking-cells, which are sensitized for a particular antigen, was a big surprise when first discovered. It makes this resemble a Type IV hypersensitivity reaction (see p. 18) rather than a Type I.

IgE is not essential here, it seems—some patients do not have IgE for the substance that triggers their atopic eczema—but when Langerhans cells and dendritic cells are associated with IgE they do become far more zealous. This excitement is communicated to the attacking-cells, which mount a more powerful attack.

It looks as if what really matters in atopic eczema is the presence of antigen-specific attacking-cells in the skin, plus the heightened activity of the Langerhans cells and dendritic cells. If the individual has IgE for the antigen, it can play a part, but it is not essential.

In other words, this reaction cuts across two different categories of immune response—Type I and Type IV. (However, the kind of antigens that provoke the reaction are typical of IgE-mediated allergy, rather than the kind of antigens that provoke contact dermatitis.) This has been exploited by researchers who are trying to assess whether patch testing (as used for contact dermatitis) with food antigens can be used to diagnose food-induced atopic eczema (see p. 69).

Why atopic eczema is a feature of atopic families is the crucial question that remains unanswered. One factor may be that high levels of IgE in the bloodstream (not IgE for a particular allergen, but total IgE) make the whole immune system more excitable and prone to overreact. The next few years will no doubt solve this part of the puzzle too.

Peacekeepers or aggressors?

"It is bad enough having a child on an ultrastrict diet—Tim can't have even a trace of cow's milk or else he becomes violently ill. What makes it worse is when people—teachers, for example— ask what's wrong. I take a deep breath and say 'eosinophilic esophagitis,' then watch their eyes roll in disbelief."

Tim's disease is caused by a particular type of immune cell called an **eosinophil**. In the right circumstances, eosinophils can be valuable—like IgE and mast cells, they are geared to destroying parasitic worms (see p. 13). Eosinophils produce some very toxic substances to kill these invaders, and it is the toxins that cause serious symptoms for Tim and others like him.

Any disease with "eosinophilic" in the name involves vast numbers of eosinophils converging on some unfortunate part of the body. In such diseases, the stimulus that attracts eosinophils often remains unknown, but once there, the toxins that they generate cause inflammation (see p. 140) of a particularly violent kind.

It is only in recent years that doctors have begun to distinguish between patients such as Tim and children with classical food allergy, and to understand the cause of Tim's symptoms. Several different forms of eosinophilic food sensitivity are now recognized (see p. 72). The exact relationship with IgE-mediated allergy remains a puzzle, because some sufferers make IgE to the culprit food but others do not.

That is not all—the eosinophil is finally coming out of the shadows and being recognized as an important agent in classical allergic diseases as well.

The fact that eosinophils appeared during the aftermath of an allergic reaction had long been known, but their role was misunderstood. What confused researchers was that eosinophils can break down histamine, the substance that kick-starts allergic symptoms (see box on p. 12). This ability gave eosinophils the appearance of peacekeeping troops, coming in at the close of battle to restore order. In fact, eosinophils are major aggressors— they do a whole lot of other things besides breaking down histamine, most of them pro-inflammatory. They can release toxins, just as they do in eosinophilic diseases (see above), and they attract other inflammatory cells into the area. In short, eosinophils play a big part in keeping allergic reactions going once the initial burst of activity is over. This "Late Phase Reaction" is enormously important (see p. 13).

Why are allergies on the increase?

"I can't think of *any* of our friends who don't have at least one member of the family with asthma, and often it's both children. If you go to a school sports event, you'll see the teachers going along the line of kids, saying, 'Have you taken your asthma medication?' It's so much a part of everyday life now," says Dee, a university lecturer from Melbourne, and an asthmatic. Allergies are increasing in all industrialized countries and Australia is one of the countries worst affected by the epidemic.

The word "epidemic" is now being freely used, even by the most conservative of medical scientists, to describe the increase in rates of allergy. All the classical allergic diseases seem to be on the increase, including:

- **atopic eczema**—in the U.S., up from 3 percent of children in the 1960s to 10 percent in the 1990s; in Canada, 20 percent of young children and 10 percent of older children may be affected.
- **hay fever**—affects more than 25 million Americans. Hay fever is now seen in 10–20 percent of Canadian children.
- **asthma**—in the U.S., cases have gone from 6.8 million in 1980 to some 15 million today. Among 5—14-year-olds, 7.4 percent have asthma. From 5 percent in Canadian children 20 years ago, rates are now close to 20 percent in children in Hamilton, Ontario, and 12 percent in Saskatoon.
- **peanut allergy** seems also to be increasing, but there are no hard figures.

Are other immune diseases increasing?

These two pages deal solely with the classical allergic diseases (see box on p. 11). Many doctors have the impression that eosinophilic disorders (see p. 72) are also becoming more common, and some think that there are more cases of adult-onset celiac disease than previously.

To the question "why?" there is no simple answer—the causes are many and various. But one thing is abundantly clear: this is a disease of modern, Westernized society. Travel to rural Africa or Asia, among people living a simple subsistence lifestyle, and you will find little or no sign of allergic diseases. There are no words in their languages for asthma or hay fever, because these are virtually unknown.

As soon as these people become more affluent, and change their lifestyle, allergic diseases appear, and the number of cases steadily rises over the years. Sometimes this coincides with a move to the towns, but it can also occur when people stay right where they are—as in Taiwan, where allergies rose dramatically with increasing affluence and a more Westernized way of life.

In the case of asthma, everyone is keen to blame air pollution, particularly traffic pollution. But a look at the research shows the link to be largely a myth. Certainly, polluted air can trigger off attacks in someone who already has asthma—but the effect is not huge, and this is not the same as causing asthma to develop in the first place. And while growing up in polluted air can increase the chances of children developing asthma, it makes only a small difference, one that simply cannot account for the massive asthma epidemic. The hollowness of the pollution argument is spectacularly evident when you consider rural New Zealand, where asthma rates are among the highest in the world, yet there are no factories, and sheep heavily outnumber cars.

Allergy to dust mites has also received a lot of publicity, and it does play an important part. Our warm, draft-free and thickly carpeted homes allow these tiny creatures to breed with abandon (see p. 114) and many people with perennial rhinitis, asthma, or atopic eczema have an allergy to dust mites. Recent research shows that dust mites play a far larger role than anyone previously suspected: the dust-mite allergen actually provokes immune cells (see p. 12), and once an allergy to dust mite has begun, other allergies become more likely.

But blaming dust mites as the supreme cause of the allergy/asthma epidemic (as some do) is as mistaken as blaming pollution. The proof in this case comes from the highlands of New Mexico where dust mites cannot survive because the air is much too dry. Allergies, including asthma, are just as common there as elsewhere in the Western world.

Spoiling the immune system

Thanks to discoveries made during the past decade, we are now beginning to understand what has made the younger generations—those born since the early 1960s—so much more susceptible to allergies. The new data reveal that the way you bring up a child's immune system matters as much as the way you bring up the child itself. You can "spoil" an immune system all too easily, by protecting it from life's natural challenges and obstacles.

As a small child, I ate a spoonful of soil. My mother was horrified but research now shows that she should not have been. Exposure to certain bacteria in the soil, known as mycobacteria, is probably just the kind of education that a young immune system needs. These bacteria cause no ill-health, no symptoms at all, but they are thought to have an effect on the immune system, pushing it away from allergic reactions (see p. 11).

Children playing outdoors have probably always eaten soil, either intentionally or by accident—licking a grubby finger. Country people used to say, philosophically, "You eat a bushel of dirt before you die," and they were probably right. Indeed, you may well *need* to eat a bit of dirt before you can live happily in an allergen-packed world. A preliminary study from England has found that immunizing asthmatics using an extract from soil bacteria improves their asthma control significantly.

A study from Britain's University of Bristol shows that children who wash their hands more than five times and have two baths a day are almost twice as likely to get asthma as children who wash their hands less than three times a day and have a bath every other day. The grubbier children are probably being protected from asthma by acquiring minor infections, with few or no symptoms. These infections could include both soil bacteria and germs that are spread from one child to another.

Other research reveals that children with older brothers and sisters are less likely to suffer from certain allergic diseases than only children or firstborn children. This seems to be due to the spread of infectious diseases, because mixing with lots of other children in daycare produces more infections but also gives protection against allergy. Studies from the former East Germany, where many children went to daycare at an early age, demonstrate that if children from small families went to daycare aged 6–11 months they were substantially less allergy-prone than if they went later. The allergy risk was highest for only children who did not go to daycare until they were over 2 years.

Researchers in Colorado have recently tackled this subject from a different angle completely, analyzing house dust for the levels of bacterial endotoxins—substances that are produced by many bacteria and which have a powerful effect on the immune system. If the house dust contained high levels of endotoxins, babies brought up in that house were less likely to give positive skin-prick tests to common allergens. The babies from very clean houses, with low levels of endotoxin in the dust, were the ones with allergic reactions. (Fortunately, it is possible to have a dusty house with very few dust mites—see p. 115.)

The **hygiene hypothesis**, as it is known, could also explain the strange history of hay fever. For the first century of its existence, hay fever was a disease of the urban upper classes, only gradually working its way down to the poor and to rural communities: this fits in well with the gradual spread of more hygienic ways of life. In most parts of the developed world today, it shows no class distinctions, but recent investigations have found a lower rate of hay fever among children raised on a farm with animals compared to children living in the same villages without farm animals.

In addition to greater hygiene, the following aspects of modern living appear to promote an allergic tendency in children:
- smoking by the mother during pregnancy and after;
- exposure to a virus called Respiratory Synctial Virus (RSV) during infancy, which provokes an IgE-reaction (see p. 37);
- breathing nitrogen dioxide from gas stoves, and formaldehyde from various household sources (see p. 129); the poor ventilation of many modern houses, and the far greater time spent indoors aggravates the problem by increasing exposure to these irritants, and to allergens such as dust mites and animal danders;
- bottle-feeding and/or abrupt and early weaning onto a variety of foods;
- taking antibiotics in infancy (see p. 247).

This knowledge allows parents to reduce the risk of allergies developing in their own children, as described on pp. 238–49.

Age and allergy
DOES EVERYONE GROW OUT OF IT?

If you have a child with allergies, sooner or later some friend or relative will tell you not to worry because your child "will probably grow out of it." Your doctor may well say the same thing. But what does this mean? Do all children shake off their allergic symptoms as they get older? If the symptoms go, is the underlying disease completely cured? And why treat allergies if they disappear of their own accord? The truth is that the relationship between allergy and age is incredibly complex. The best anyone can offer is a broad overview of how allergies change with age, with few explanations of the underlying mechanisms, and absolutely no predictions of what the future holds for any particular allergy sufferer.

It is certainly true that the classical allergic diseases, such as atopic eczema, hay fever, and childhood asthma (see box on p. 11), frequently seem to disappear as children grow up. Babies tend to shrug off certain food allergies (such as allergies to cow's milk and egg) by the time they are toddlers, and a fair number of asthmatic children lose their symptoms before they are 10 years old. Others do so in their teens or their early twenties.

Unfortunately, the disappearance of symptoms does not mean that the underlying disease has necessarily disappeared, particularly in the case of asthma. Quite a few young adults find themselves wheezy and breathless again in their late twenties or thirties, especially if they take up smoking. One study of children who wheezed before the age of seven found that:

• 25 percent lost their asthma for a time—anything between 2 years and 25 years—only to get it back again by their early thirties. Some recovered and relapsed more than once.

• Over 70 percent shook off asthma and were still symptom-free by their early thirties when the study ended.

• Only 2 percent remained asthmatic throughout and still had asthma in their thirties.

Realistically, anyone who has ever been asthmatic should regard themselves as "at risk" indefinitely and never be careless with their health. If you had asthma as a child, don't smoke, keep away from smoky bars and clubs, eat a good diet with plenty of fruit and vegetables (see p. 206), and avoid things you know you are allergic to, such as animals or dust mites.

Workplaces with high exposure to allergens, such as sawmills, bakeries, or laboratories using animals (see pp. 133–4) are not recommended for those with a history of allergy. Anyone who has ever had eczema should also take care with cosmetics and soaps, choosing the gentlest brands. They should also protect their hands (see p. 135) and avoid hairdressing or bricklaying as an occupation, or anything else where skin irritation is likely.

Moving on

Growing out of classical allergies seems to be a consequence of the child's immune system changing and maturing as it grows. This same process, unfortunately, can also substitute one allergic disease for another.

"When Alex developed eczema as a baby I hoped that she'd grow out of it in time. Well she did, gradually, and by the time she was five it seemed to have cleared up, but then she started having a snuffly nose that never really went away. A year or so later, she began wheezing whenever she got a cold, and this has now developed into asthma." The pattern described by Alex's mother will be familiar to many parents, who watch their children slowly work their way through all the allergies in the medical textbooks. Doctors call it the "**atopic march**" or "**allergic march**."

Fortunately, even this type of allergic pattern can have a positive outcome eventually. Many such children improve in time, and develop into healthy adults.

In the meantime, there are several itchy, wheezy, or sneezy years to get through, and since childhood is a time to be enjoyed, not endured, treatments that alleviate the symptoms of allergies are generally welcomed. Being energetic, healthy, "normal," and able to join in with sports and other activities is particularly important for a child's social development and self-confidence.

Treating the symptoms also prevents any long-term and irreversible damage, such as the thickening and loss of elasticity that occurs in the airways of children with untreated asthma.

At the same time as treating the symptoms, it makes sense to maximize the chance of the allergies or asthma diminishing. Parents can tip the odds in the right direction by providing an environment that reduces the chance of new allergies developing. A detailed action program is described on pp. 248–9.

Allergies that begin in adult life

What about those people who develop classical allergic diseases for the first time as adults—or even in old age? Will they too "grow out of it" with the passing years?

Only a minority of people develop such allergies for the first time as adults, although the numbers seem to be increasing. The older you are when your allergies begin, the less likely you are to ever throw them off. On the positive side, they are unlikely to get a great deal worse than they are at the outset, especially if you take care of yourself and keep the air at home as unpolluted and allergen-free as possible (see pp. 114–31).

In the case of asthma that develops in adulthood, there may not be an allergic reaction involved. Whereas allergies play a part in asthma for 80–90 percent of children, the figure is thought to be lower for adults. Nevertheless, it is worth investigating the possible role of allergens, because avoiding them is one of the most effective treatments.

The outlook for food intolerance

Food intolerance causes a wide variety of symptoms, from infant colic to migraine. A full list is given on p. 76. Although far less is understood about food intolerance than about true allergies, there is much more certainty about the future for affected individuals. With rare exceptions, people find that the problem clears up as long as they totally avoid their problem food for a year or two. After this period of strict avoidance, they can eat the food again in moderation but should never forget that the problem can return. Eating the culprit food very regularly will turn the clock back and all the original symptoms will return. Anecdotal evidence shows that this change for the worse may be irreversible for people with severe reactions such as rheumatoid arthritis.

Safety first

Anyone who suffers the life-threatening allergic reaction known as anaphylactic shock (see p. 58) is probably going to have this for the rest of their days. Some children become tolerant of food allergens in time (allergies to milk, eggs, or soy may well disappear, whereas fish or peanut allergies usually persist) but before concluding that there is no longer any risk, extremely careful testing should take place. Skin tests or RASTs (see pp. 91-2) can show if there is still a potential for allergy to the food. There should be resuscitation equipment on hand as severe reactions sometimes occur with skin tests. Never give the child any of the food to eat, until it has first been tested in other, less risky ways. For example, if your doctor has experience with food allergy, and feels it is safe, you can smear a little on the face to see if there is any reaction. If there is none within 24 hours, put a tiny amount on the outer lip and watch again.

If both these tests produce absolutely no reaction, then a very small amount of the food can be eaten as a test: this should be done under medical supervision with resuscitation equipment available. The amount can be slowly increased with successive tests, until it seems certain that no reaction will occur even with a normal portion.

the diseases

In medical terms, this chapter covers a lot of ground. First there are the **classical allergic diseases** (see box on p. 11) such as hay fever, and true food allergy, caused by the allergy antibody, IgE (see box on p. 12). Then there is **non-IgE immune sensitivity**, a category that includes a number of quite different diseases, caused in a great variety of ways. They also vary in severity—there are serious lifelong problems such as celiac disease and minor short-lived ones such as contact dermatitis from garden plants.

Finally (pp. 74–85) the chapter looks at diseases where the immune system seems not to be involved, or plays only a minor role: the **intolerance** reactions to food and synthetic chemicals. These are diverse and, in most cases, rather mysterious in origin. They would not be described as "allergies" by most doctors, though they often are by practitioners of alternative therapies (see p. 6).

These categories are not nearly as neat and tidy as they might sound. Some problems refuse to fit anywhere, atopic eczema caused by food, for example. A percentage of children with this problem have IgE to the food concerned, while others do not—so where does it belong?

If you were expecting an answer to this question, you will be disappointed. Nor, quite often, are there certain and honest answers to questions such as "Does my baby really have asthma?" or "Can you be sure it's irritable bowel syndrome?" There are no answers to such questions because most diseases do not exist in neat compartments, and the words we use to describe them really denote rather abstract concepts.

This does not mean that the terms used to describe diseases are invalid—doctors and medical researchers invent them to try and make sense of a complex, confusing, and sometimes foggy reality. They also argue over them, split them, unite them, and redefine them. There is a constant desire to get the medical picture of that foggy reality more precise and accurate.

Over time, thanks to huge amounts of research effort, things gradually get clearer. You'll no longer hear a doctor talk about rheumatism for example, because it was long since realized that this category is useless—it includes a number of diverse diseases. And while doctors might say "food poisoning" or "heart attack" or "skin cancer" to a patient, they use much narrower and more precise terms when talking among themselves, and when ordering tests or prescribing treatment. Each of these categories has been split into several well-defined subcategories.

Ideally, this process of splitting continues until each disease category has a set of well-defined symptoms (this set is known as a **syndrome**), plus a few simple and definitive diagnostic tests. This will probably depend on the cause of the disease (the **mechanism** in medical jargon) being clearly understood. Once the mechanism is clear, then a disease category is a truly satisfactory tool for diagnosis and treatment.

Of the disease categories in this book, only a few, such as celiac disease and hay fever, have reached that happy state. The majority are still debatable.

Some disease terms describe a set of symptoms with no clear underlying cause, for example, "irritable bowel syndrome." Others describe a well-defined response by the body, that can be caused in many different ways—an end point that can be reached by various routes. This is true of "asthma" or "urticaria."

A third type describes a much less well-defined cluster of symptoms. Idiopathic food intolerance, chemical intolerance and yeast overgrowth all fall into this category. A few doctors don't even see some of these clusters as real diseases because the symptoms involved are so vague and so widely encountered. Some of the arguments used to dismiss idiopathic food intolerance are dissected on pp. 74–7. A key point made against these diseases is that the symptoms they produce are nonspecific—common symptoms such as headache, fatigue, and diarrhea, which can arise in a great variety of ways. Ever since Pasteur and the germ theory, medicine has been based on the idea of each disease having *specific* symptoms and *specific* causes, and it has roared ahead on the basis of this

assumption. This is the prevailing paradigm of modern medicine, and like all paradigms it blinds people to facts that don't fit. Evidence is accumulating that there *are* diseases that have multiple, nonspecific, and variable symptoms. Chronic Fatigue Syndrome (CFS—see box on p. 85) is one of these, and its recent transformation from a doubtful diagnosis to a disease recognized by conventional medicine suggests that the paradigm might be starting to crack.

To sum up, the business of identifying and naming diseases is a complex and uncertain process, in which the concept of most diseases is only ever that—a *concept*, subject to change and refinement. This does not make it worthless—quite the opposite. These concepts are the best we can do at the present time, and accurate diagnosis is the key to getting the best treatment available now.

With regard to diagnosis and treatment, this book covers a very wide spectrum of medical opinion, from the entirely orthodox to the frankly wacky. It aims to give an objective view of these different opinions and approaches, using the evidence currently available, in the hope that this will help readers to improve their health while wasting as little as possible of their time or money. In using this information, you should always try to work closely with your doctor (see pp. 94–5), respecting the depth and breadth of knowledge that conventional medicine has to offer.

Hay fever

Foxtail grasses release their pollen—a potential source of hay-fever symptoms.

"I gradually recognized that it was not an ordinary cold and that the symptoms were much worse on the golf course or even during a nice day rowing on Loch Lomond." Dr. John Morrison Smith, then a medical student, began suffering from hay fever in the late 1930s. "At first I did not know what I had, and neither did any other doctor I encountered in the next two or three years . . ."

All the classical allergic diseases (see box on p. 11) seem to be increasing, but none has exploded quite so dramatically as hay fever. The physicians of ancient Greece described asthma and food allergy, and the Romans recorded allergy to horses, but there were no reports of hay fever. The only account—and it is a doubtful one—comes from Persia in A.D. 925. Two hundred years ago, hay fever was unknown—and careful research by medical historians has shown that this was not a case of it simply being ignored, or misinterpreted as a cold.

The first case was reported in 1819, but even in the 1930s it was so rare that a succession of Scottish doctors and medical students were baffled by Dr. Morrison Smith's symptoms. Today everyone knows what hay fever is, since huge numbers of people sneeze and sniffle their way through the pollen season. There are no certain explanations for this meteoric rise, but greater hygiene (see p. 21) may be an important factor.

Symptoms of hay fever

The common symptoms of hay fever are well known:
- itchiness of the nose, mouth, throat, and eyes—often the first sign
- a streaming and/or blocked nose
- frequent sneezing
- red, watery eyes (very rarely, hay fever affects the eyes only, with no symptoms in the nose)

Less commonly, there may be:
- dryness of the throat if the nasal blockage results in constant breathing through the mouth
- no sense of smell due to a blocked nose (but nasal polyps can also cause this—see p. 30)
- a feverish sweaty feeling (but the body temperature is usually normal)
- swelling and inflammation of the eyelids, sometimes leading to blistering and ulceration: *there is a risk of blindness if this is not treated promptly*
- recurrent sinusitis (see p. 30)
- earache, a stuffy feeling in the ears, or "glue ear" (see p. 29)
- itching in the ears

Some sufferers also experience:
- Oral Allergy Syndrome (an itchy tingling mouth) from certain fruits, nuts, and vegetables (see box on p. 63)
- a skin rash from pollen falling on the skin (direct contact with the leaves of the offending plants, or with droplets of moisture from them—as when mowing a lawn or using a trimmer—may also produce a rash)

Even more rarely (and controversially) there can be:
- stomach upsets or even colitis (inflammation of the bowel), possibly due to pollen swallowed with food or in the saliva
- irritation in the vagina
- migraine
- kidney inflammation (nephritis), leading to puffiness of the face and hands, and possibly other symptoms
- joint pains

The last two are probably caused by pollen allergens bound to their antibodies and carried in the blood (see p. 13).

Diagnosis

The standard diagnostic tool here is the prick-puncture test (see p. 91). In diagnosing hay fever there are three separate questions:

1 Is it actually hay fever?

2 Which pollen or pollens are responsible?

3 Are there allergens other than pollen also involved?

Don't be surprised if none of these questions are asked. In most countries, if you have hay-feverlike symptoms during the pollen season, the doctor will conclude that you have hay fever—and that will be the end of that.

If hay fever seems plausible to you, and you respond to drug treatment, or manage well on pollen avoidance (see p. 126), then there is probably no reason to go further. Should you want a more thorough investigation, you will need to be persistent. These are good reasons for requesting a full diagnosis:

• Your symptoms are worse in the pollen season, but they never really go away, suggesting that you may also be allergic to year-round allergens, such as dust mite or molds. It is worth knowing which ones, so that you can avoid them. If you live in an area such as California or Florida that is always warm, it may be that your culprit pollen is in the air year-round—even so, knowing which pollen it is can help with avoidance. Around the Mediterranean, the pollen from cypresses can keep hay fever going through the winter (or cause symptoms in winter only).

• Your symptoms are sometimes worse when they should be better. If you feel worse indoors with the windows closed, this could indicate that a seasonal indoor allergen is the culprit—mold spores or cockroach perhaps (cockroach is often a summer allergy in regions with cold winters—see p. 118).

• Your symptoms begin before the pollen season begins, or go on long afterward. Or the severity of your symptoms does not match the daily pollen count for your suspect pollen. In North America, the molds Alternaria and Cladosporium release their spores all summer, especially during the grass season (June–July) and ragweed season (August–September). Allergy to these molds can easily be mistaken for pollen allergy. You would need skin-prick tests for both these molds and for grasses.

• You are much worse near home than elsewhere. It could just be a garden plant or tree. As one California resident observed, "The worst offender was an olive tree on our front lawn. It's been removed."

• You want to plan holidays free from the culprit pollen. Moving house—especially if you have the option of moving to a region with different vegetation—can also be a spur to finding out exactly what your allergens are.

• Testing with individual pollens, rather than with a mixture of pollens from different species of plant is best—it tells you precisely which plant you need to avoid. In the case of grasses, however, testing with a pollen mix is fine.

Treatment

Too many people allow hay fever to spoil the summer months because they are anxious about taking drugs, or feel that it is nobler to suffer. This book is not in any way complacent about the dangers from drugs (see Chapter 5), but when it comes to hay fever there really is very little cause for concern. The risks with drugs used for hay fever are absolutely minimal, and it is such a waste to miss out on the best time of year.

Most hay fever responds very well to treatment with antihistamines (see p. 138). If they make you sleepy, persist for a while, because this side effect often wears off—or ask for one of the new non-sedating forms. The sleepiness is annoying, but it is only a minor side effect, and not an indication of the drug causing any serious harm.

Cromoglycate drops (for the eyes or nose) do not work for everyone, but if they work for you, go for them. These are absolutely the safest of the anti-allergy drugs. Steroid sprays or drops for the nose (see p. 144) are also recommended. The dose of steroid involved is usually very small, and there is little risk of serious side effects. If you suffer stinging, burning, or dryness, it might be due to preservatives in the drops, not the drug itself (see p. 33). Steroid drops for the eyes should be used cautiously and only under medical supervision (see p. 144). Don't use over-the-counter decongestant drops for more than three days (see p. 29).

Allergy shots usually work very well for hay fever and are well worth the effort. They tend to reduce other symptoms besides the classical nose and eye symptoms—hives, for example, if this is due to pollen. Some hay fever sufferers feel they do well with homeopathy (see p. 216) or acupuncture (see p. 214), although these therapies are controversial for hay fever treatment.

Pollen asthma

Some people with hay fever also have pollen asthma. Their asthma is worse in the pollen season but it usually persists all-year round (either because there are other allergens or irritants involved, or just because the inflammation of the airways is self-perpetuating) whereas hay fever itself clears up. Treating the hay fever fully with antihistamines helps considerably with the asthma symptoms.

A blocked or runny nose
THAT LASTS ALL YEAR

"Everyone has heard of hay fever, but it's news to most people that you can have this sort of problem all year round," complains Elizabeth. "Before we got the treatment sorted out, Benny was 'the kid with the constant cold,' and I did notice other mothers looking less than enchanted at the prospect of his coming over to play."

Benny suffers from allergic reactions to dust mites and cats that cause hay-fever-style symptoms (see p. 26) all year round. This condition doesn't even have a common name—the medical one is **perennial allergic rhinitis**—yet it is one of the most common allergic diseases.

Any **airborne allergen** that is found in the air all year round can cause perennial allergic rhinitis:

- Dust mite and cockroaches are the main suspects in most parts of the world. Particles from other insects, such as midges and mosquitoes outdoors, and Asian lady bugs, houseflies, bloodworms (used for fish food) or carpet beetles indoors, can also cause nasal allergies.
- Mold spores can be the problem: they are found both indoors and out.
- In some regions, certain types of pollen are airborne year round (see p. 27).
- All pets other than fish produce airborne allergenic particles (even snakes).
- Allergens encountered at work (see p. 133) can also produce symptoms in the nose. *This is a warning sign you should not ignore*—it often means that occupational asthma is on its way (see p. 132).

Occasionally, the offending substance is being eaten not inhaled. This is less common, so you should investigate inhaled allergens first, before trying an elimination diet (see p. 29).

Skin-prick tests (see p. 91) will help to identify any airborne allergens that are responsible, but where food is the culprit, skin-prick tests are often negative (see p. 69).

Aspirin-sensitive triad and NARES

Diagnosis of perennial allergic rhinitis is complicated by the fact that there are two other conditions—called **aspirin-sensitive triad** and **NARES**—that produce similar symptoms and involve the immune system but are not, strictly speaking, allergies.

Aspirin-sensitive triad is so-called because it involves three distinct symptoms:

- perennial rhinitis
- polyps in the nose—little fleshy growths that can kill your sense of smell and, secondarily, your taste
- asthma

People with aspirin-sensitive triad tend to collect all three symptoms gradually, in no fixed order, over a period of years or even decades. Many are sensitive to aspirin and related drugs, and almost everyone with these symptoms develops this sensitivity eventually.

Aspirin sensitivity can come on very suddenly and produces a reaction akin to anaphylaxis (see p. 101). This can be fatal, so it is best to avoid all aspirin-like drugs, *even though you have not reacted to aspirin in the past*. Aspirin-like drugs, also called nonsteroidal anti-inflammatory drugs (NSAIDs), are found in painkillers, arthritis drugs and cold remedies—check with a pharmacist before you buy (see p. 151).

The initial letters of Non-Allergic Rhinitis with Eosinophilia have been stretched a bit to get NARES. (This is a medical joke—the Latin word *nares* means nostrils.) The problem is caused by eosinophils (see p. 19), which flock into the nose and cause severe inflammation. Some people with NARES go on to develop aspirin-sensitive triad.

Collateral damage

Having the nose swamped with mucus can lead to secondary problems in the ears, sinuses, and airways.

If the tube that leads from the ear to the nose (the Eustachian tube) becomes blocked, then fluid cannot drain away from the middle ear. This is called secretory otitis media, or **glue ear**—it dulls the hearing and causes an unpleasant "popping" sensation. The ears may also feel blocked and itchy, but if children have had this problem since they were tiny they may not complain because they assume that's just the way ears are supposed to feel. Deafness or a delay in starting to talk are often the first signs.

Sinusitis is another possible complication, because fluid from the sinuses should also drain into the nasal cavity. With the ouflow blocked, mucus builds up in the sinuses and can become infected by bacteria (see p. 30).

Postnasal drip can also occur with perennial allergic rhinitis. The overabundant mucus runs down the back of the nose, into the throat, and then the airways. This leads to a persistent cough, with sputum production. It may occasionally be mistaken for asthma.

When the rhinitis is treated effectively, all these problems should sort themselves out, although additional treatment is usually necessary in the case of persistent sinusitis (see p. 33).

Treatment

Where an allergen such as dust mite or mold spores has been identified as the source of problem, eradicating it from your house (see Chapter 4) will make a huge difference, and may avoid the need for drugs. If the allergen is unavoidable, immunotherapy (see pp. 164–9) or some alternative form of desensitization (see pp. 210–13) could be very helpful.

Where drugs are needed, nose drops are best. They get the drugs right to the target, so doses are minimal, which means very few side effects. The drugs used are:

- cromoglycate, to prevent the allergic reaction before it starts (see p. 148)
- antihistamines, to block the allergic reaction before it produces inflammation (see p. 138)
- steroids, to calm down inflammation (see p. 144)

Steroid nose drops are also useful for NARES and aspirin-sensitive triad. If you are taking steroid drops continuously, your doctor should check the membranes inside your nose every six months. Make sure you put the drops in correctly, especially if you have polyps (see p. 144).

If you suffer stinging, burning, or dryness, it might be due to preservatives in the drops, not the drug itself (see box on p. 33), so talk to your doctor about a different formulation.

Don't use over-the-counter decongestant drops: they do nothing to treat the allergy or inflammation, and are little more than a "chemical crowbar" to open up the nose. Your nose gets used to them in a few days, and when you stop using them you get "rebound congestion"—absolute and total blockage. It does wear off eventually, but is unpleasant meanwhile. If you are suffering this problem at this very moment, *don't* put more decongestant drops in—your nose needs to go "cold turkey" to recover.

If none of the anti-allergy drugs works, but decongestant drops do, then you probably have a nonallergic disease called **vasomotor rhinitis**. The symptoms are very similar to allergic rhinitis, but without the sneezing and itching. (This is also called skier's nose or jogger's nose because cold air and/or exercise may cause the profuse watery nasal discharge. Other triggers include hot or spicy foods, and weather changes). See your doctor again, because there is an effective treatment using anticholinergic drugs such as ipratropium bromide (see box on p. 156). Acupuncture (see below) can also be tried.

An elimination diet (see p. 194) will diagnose any food reactions. It works wonders for some people with severe and unexplained perennial rhinitis, including people with such a flood of mucus that they can scarcely work or live normally. You should certainly give this diagnostic diet a try if there are clues that suggest food is the culprit (see p. 69) or if no airborne allergen can be identified.

Acupuncture is worth trying, to reduce the blockage in the nose and stem the flow of mucus, because the autonomic nervous system (see box on p. 235) plays some part in the symptoms of allergic rhinitis (and is the sole cause of the symptoms for those with vasomotor rhinitis).

Very occasionally, psychological or emotional reactions play a part in perennial allergic rhinitis, with symptoms getting significantly worse during stressful events. One possible manifestation of this is **postcoital rhinitis**, where sex brings on rhinitis (and sometimes asthma as well). However, postcoital rhinitis may be another manifestation of vasomotor rhinitis. (Check also that you are not just allergic to the dust mites in your bed.)

A nose by any other name . . .

Rhinitis means inflammation (-itis) of the nose (rhin-). The same Greek word gives us rhinoceros—"nose-horn."

Sinusitis

Sinus cavities are something that most people just don't know they have. It's only when they start to hurt that you find out where they are. "There is this terrible throbbing pain above and around my eyes, and in my cheeks. It's the most unpleasant feeling, but it's hard to describe to anyone who hasn't felt it," says Gina, who suffers from chronic sinusitis (long-term inflammation of the sinus cavities). There are no figures, but chronic sinusitis seems to be increasingly common.

A sinus cavity has no function, it is just empty space without which our skulls would be much heavier. In other words, these airy spaces seem to have evolved simply to help us feel more "light-headed." If you have sinusitis, unfortunately, you feel just the opposite. "I had sinusitis for years," says Dr. Wellington S. Tichenor, a New York allergist who now specializes in treating chronic sinusitis. "I kept working but felt like I wanted to die."

Sinus cavities are lined with a membrane which is essentially similar to that lining the nose. It contains immune cells and can produce mucus when necessary. Most of the time it doesn't need to produce much, because relatively few microbes or foreign particles get into the sinus cavities.

Any mucus that is produced should escape from the sinus cavities through narrow drainage channels, called ostia, leading to the nose. Unfortunately, the ostia are very narrow—the diameter of a pinhead—and U-shaped, making them prone to blockage. And that is not the only problem. These drainage channels are situated at the top rather than the bottom of the main sinus cavities—this arrangement was fine for our ancestors who walked on all fours, and therefore did not have to fight gravity when clearing their sinuses. Sadly for us, natural selection has not got around to reorganizing things yet. It would be a completely hopeless arrangement if not for the tiny hairs known as cilia, which lie like a carpet across the membranes lining the sinus cavities. The cilia beat rhythmically, 18 times a second, to waft the mucus upward to the top of the sinus cavity.

This is a far-from-perfect system, and it is hardly surprising that it sometimes goes wrong. Chronic sinusitis can begin in at least three different ways:

• the sinus membranes become inflamed due to an allergic reaction—see p. 28 for likely airborne allergens.

• the drainage channels from the sinus cavities become blocked due to events in the nose (infection or allergy) or due to the growth of **polyps** (noncancerous jellylike lumps that can block the drainage channels). When mucus cannot drain away, it stagnates in the sinus cavities, encouraging infection by bacteria or fungi. These infections cause inflammation.

• a bout of acute sinusitis (see box), due to bacterial infection, never really goes away and the persistent infection causes long-term inflammation. Note that this is unlikely: it is rare for acute sinusitis not to clear up.

Whether the problem begins through allergy or blockage or infection, once it has begun a vicious circle can be set up all too easily. Mucus output increases when there is inflammation, blocking the drainage channels even more, so the sinus cavities become clogged up and increasingly uncomfortable. More mucus pooling in the sinus cavities perpetuates any existing infections and fosters new ones.

All this infection results in more severe inflammation, causing the membranes that line the sinus cavities to swell up. Inflammation also makes polyp growth more likely. The cilia may be lost or severely depleted, and the mucus gets thicker. All this means yet more blockage. To cap it all, there can be allergic reactions to some of the microbes involved (see right), fueling the inflammation further.

The body's own attempts to clear the sinuses are defeated, and the problem is also very resistant to medical treatment. This may make depressing reading, if you have chronic sinusitis, but don't despair. Understanding the complexities of the problem is a large part of the battle. Chronic sinusitis is not invincible, if you have a good doctor to help you—that means a doctor who also understands these complexities.

The symptoms of sinusitis are:
- Pain and a sense of swelling or unpleasant fullness around the cheeks, or over and between the eyes. This is rare in children.
- Earache or headache; pain around the teeth
- Reduction in the senses of smell and taste
- Sore throat
- Coughing, particularly at night
- Postnasal drip (mucus from the back of the nose running into the throat and airways)
- Bad-smelling breath
- Feverishness
- For some people, severe fatigue, poor concentration and even (but very rarely) psychiatric symptoms
- Irritability, especially in children

Note that any of these symptoms can be caused in other ways, and even if you have several of them, you may not necessarily have sinusitis. On the other hand, sinusitis can go unrecognized—to some people it may seem like nothing more than a lingering cold.

Acute or chronic?

In medical terms, "acute" means short-lived, while "chronic" means long-lasting.

Acute sinusitis—a short, sharp dose of it, lasting less than 3 to 4 weeks—usually follows on from a cold. Colds are caused by viruses, but a bacterial infection can follow, and it is the bacteria that move into the sinus cavities and cause trouble. Some people are far more susceptible than others and have an attack of sinusitis after every cold.

Chronic sinusitis means symptoms lasting more than 3 months, according to some authorities, but the time point is a little arbitrary. This article deals with chronic sinusitis.

If your sinusitis has been going on for between 4 weeks and 3 months you will obviously be asking, "Is this acute or chronic?" At this point, no one can say, but you would certainly be wise to seek some expert medical treatment now, on the basis that it could be the start of chronic sinusitis. Tackling chronic sinusitis before the problem becomes entrenched and complex is a good plan.

Allergy and chronic sinusitis

Chronic sinusitis is not necessarily an allergic disease, but it can be connected with allergies (or other forms of immune sensitivity) in various ways:
- Allergic reactions can occur in the sinuses, usually in conjunction with allergic reactions in the nose.
- Even if the allergic reaction does not affect the sinuses directly, allergic reactions in the nose can block the drainage channels from the sinuses, causing an accumulation of mucus there. This may lead to sinus infections.
- Once sinusitis has begun, infectious fungi (molds) in the sinuses may provoke allergic reactions, or other forms of immune sensitivity. This allergy to "the enemy within" fuels more inflammation and more mucus production. Right now, **allergic fungal sinusitis** (as it is known) is a source of heated debate—see p. 32. Allergic reactions to some of the bacteria that are present may also occur.
- Chronic sinusitis—however caused—can contribute to asthma. Research on children with both sinusitis and asthma found that 80 percent no longer needed asthma drugs once their sinusitis had been treated, and 85 percent no longer wheezed. The link may be due to postnasal drip, increased mouth-breathing, or to a nerve connection between the sinuses and the airways (the sinobronchial reflex) that can stimulate airway inflammation. Alternatively, the sinusitis may simply fire up the immune system with messenger chemicals in the bloodstream, resulting in more powerful responses throughout the body.
- Chronic sinusitis can also be a rare cause of long-standing hives, and treating the sinusitis can result in a prompt and remarkable clearance of the skin symptoms.
- Some people who have chronic sinusitis are sensitive to aspirin (see box on p. 28)—a sensitivity that is also linked with chronic urticaria, and with asthma, nasal polyps, and rhinitis (the aspirin-sensitive triad). Avoiding aspirin and all other aspirin-like drugs (see p. 151) may substantially improve the sinusitis.

Diagnosis

Because so many different factors can play a part in chronic sinusitis, diagnosis should, ideally, consider the problem from several different angles:

- The sinuses are viewed using X-rays and CT or CAT scans (computed axial tomographic scans—they use X-rays but give a much more precise picture). These reveal how badly swollen the sinus membranes are, which sinus cavities are blocked, and how much mucus has collected in the sinuses.
- Endoscopy (see p. 92) may be used to look inside the sinus cavities. Polyps are best located by this method.
- Where allergies seem to be part of the picture, the doctor may employ prick-puncture tests (see p. 91) to identify allergies to airborne allergens (from dust mites, molds, pets, pollen, cockroaches, etc.).
- Laboratory tests on samples taken from your sinus cavities will be used to show which bacteria and/or fungi have set up home there. There may also be a hunt for the immune cells known as eosinophils (see p. 19) or the typical debris that they generate. The presence of large numbers of eosinophils indicates involvement of the immune system, for example, classical allergies, NARES, aspirin-sensitive triad, or allergic fungal sinusitis (see below).
- Skin testing with the fungi (molds) that have been found growing in the sinus cavities may also be tried, if allergic fungal sinusitis is suspected.
- In severe cases, there may be tests of immune function, to see whether this is depressed in any way.
- Children may be tested for an inherited disorder that affects the cilia, or for cystic fibrosis—mild forms may have escaped detection, and can produce both chronic sinusitis and wheezing.

The enemy within

The biggest controversy in sinusitis research at the moment concerns **allergic fungal sinusitis**. The orthodox view of this condition is that:

- it affects a small minority of chronic sinusitis patients—fewer than 10 percent
- there is a true IgE-mediated allergic reaction to the fungus (mold) growing in the sinus cavities. This allergic reaction is detectable with a prick-puncture test (see p. 91). Immune cells known as eosinophils (see p. 19) are also key players in the inflammatory reaction to the fungi, but it is an IgE-response to the fungi that draws the eosinophils into the sinuses.
- there is clear evidence of fungal infection in the membranes of the sinus cavities

A rare complication

In rare cases, the fungi involved in allergic fungal sinusitis can be invasive, spreading from the sinuses to the surrounding bone. This problem needs prompt and thorough treatment with antifungal drugs.

- there may also be "fungus balls"—a solid mass of fungus inside the sinus cavity. Or there may be "allergic mucin," a dark sticky mucus containing fragments of the fungus.

In 1996, researchers at the Mayo Clinic in Rochester, Minnesota, caused a ruckus by claiming to have identified a different form of allergic fungal sinusitis that is overlooked by standard diagnostic techniques, and which affects 96 percent of patients with chronic sinusitis.

This is a staggering figure—96 percent means, in effect, that they are claiming to have found the fundamental cause of virtually all chronic sinusitis. "Up to now, the cause of chronic sinusitis has not been known. Our studies indicate that, in fact, fungus is the likely cause of nearly all of these problems," states Dr. David Sherris, one of the researchers.

According to the Mayo Clinic team:

- the fungi (molds) are growing in the mucus of the sinus cavities, not generally in the membrane itself. They are not detected by normal diagnostic methods, which tend to ignore the mucus. A special method of collecting the mucus is required to detect the fungi.
- the immune reaction to the fungi is not usually an IgE-mediated reaction, so prick-puncture tests are often negative.
- finding evidence of unusual numbers of eosinophils is adequate for diagnosis of allergic fungal sinusitis because the eosinophils are the prime movers in this sensitivity reaction to the fungi, as in several other diseases (see p. 19).

"We can now begin to treat the cause of the problem instead of the symptoms," says Dr. Eugene Kern, head of the research team. There is a lot of skepticism about these claims among other sinusitis specialists, and so far no new treatment for chronic sinusitis has emerged. The Mayo Clinic researchers say that they are in the process of developing a drug treatment, but that it will take several more years before it is generally available. Existing antifungal drugs (taken in capsule form) could not work on this particular form of allergic fungal sinusitis (if it exists) because the drug does not get into the mucus. Any new treatment would probably involve inserting an antifungal drug directly into the sinus cavities, which is far from easy.

All we can do for now is wait and see what emerges from the

ongoing research. The current treatment for allergic fungal sinusitis involves all the usual methods (see right) with special emphasis on steroids to calm the inflammation, plus antifungal drugs where fungal infection is detectable in the membrane. Allergy shots can be useful to reduce the immune reaction to the fungus.

Clearing molds from your home may be beneficial (see p. 34). Indeed, simply reducing the humidity in the house (see p. 119) may help, as dampness is linked with allergic fungal sinusitis—it is more common in humid regions of North America.

Treatment

Sinusitis can be very hard to treat, particularly if it has been going on for a long time. You need a really committed attitude if treatment is to be successful.

These treatments must all be given at the same time:
- Antibiotics for two to three weeks minimum (it takes this long because the antibiotic has such trouble getting into the sinus cavities—a shorter course may not clear the infection completely, leading to relapse). It must be the right antibiotic—commonly used ones such as penicillin, tetracycline, and erythromycin are unlikely to work because the bacteria are usually resistant to them.
- Steroid drops in the nose to combat the inflammation. It is important to put these in correctly, so that they have maximum effect (see p. 144), especially if you have polyps.
- Antifungal drugs (taken by mouth) if allergic fungal sinusitis has been diagnosed. Sometimes these have a dramatic beneficial effect on chronic sinusitis that has previously resisted treatment.

The following treatments are intended to reduce congestion and drain mucus from the sinuses. They are regarded by some doctors as options that simply help to relieve discomfort, and are therefore used only when required. Other doctors see these treatments as an essential part of a full-scale treatment of chronic sinusitis, to be used simultaneously with antibiotics and steroids. In their opinion, the work of the drugs is helped by also clearing mucus and unblocking the drainage channels.
- Irrigating the nose and sinus cavities daily with sterile salt water (saline). Your doctor will show you how to do this.
- Tablets that reduce the congestion in the nose.
- Nose drops that reduce congestion, but for three days only (see p. 29).
- Steam inhalations to loosen the mucus. There are special steam vaporizers on sale (ask at a pharmacy), but you can just inhale steam from a bowl of boiling water, with a towel over your head to keep the steam in. Adding eucalyptus oil

to the water may help. For a quick-and-easy version, warm up a damp facecloth in the microwave and place it over your nose. Some doctors recommend having a steam vaporizer beside the bed at night, when nasal blockage is most likely to occur, but if you have allergies to dust mites or molds, this is not a good idea in the long term, as a damp bedroom will favor both (and could encourage allergic fungal sinusitis). You may also be given other drugs, such as steroid tablets. The new antileukotriene drugs (see p. 149) are also being tried, with some success. A few sinusitis specialists also use a drug called guaifenesin which thins the mucus.

Problems with nose drops
Nasal drops and washes contain preservatives and other nondrug ingredients. Some of these may act as irritants—or the pH (acidity or alkalinity) of the preparation might cause problems. If you experience burning or irritation after inserting drops or irrigating the sinuses, ask your doctor or pharmacist about trying a different preparation.

Antibiotic resistance

Bacteria are becoming resistant to the effects of antibiotics: it is probably the biggest headache facing modern medicine.

This is emerging as a particular problem in chronic sinusitis because many patients have been dosed very regularly with antibiotics. Although most of the bacteria have been killed each time, the fact that the sinus cavity is so clogged up with mucus, and so badly accessed by the bloodstream anyway, means there is always some nook or cranny where a few bacteria survive because they have not been exposed to the full lethal dose of the antibiotic. As you might expect, these survivors tend to be the "tough ones"—those bacteria that are not just well hidden but also the least sensitive to the antibiotic.

Repeat this process many times, with frequent courses of antibiotics (separated by intervals during which the hard-to-kill bacteria multiply in numbers) and what happens? Eventually you breed a race of bacteria that are completely resistant to one or more of the antibiotics taken.

If you ever get to this point with your sinusitis, treatment is going to be extremely difficult. That's why it is so important to treat infections really thoroughly, and get rid of them completely. Expert medical help is essential for this treatment campaign.

Too many people with chronic sinusitis are careless about taking their antibiotics regularly, or feel ambivalent about them and stop the course before it's complete, or don't see the doctor again when the tablets are used up. This is courting disaster.

Don't start antibiotic treatment for chronic sinusitis until you are sure you can see it through to the end. If you have doubts about taking antibiotics, try all the other treatments and self-help measures first. They may be sufficient, especially if you find you have an allergy underlying the chronic sinusitis and can tackle this successfully.

Should there be no improvement, you could then go on to the antibiotic program.

Antihistamines may be prescribed to treat any allergic reactions, but some specialists feel that they can also aggravate the problems. In their experience, antihistamines dry out the mucus so that it sticks to the walls of the sinus cavities, rather than being ushered out by the cilia. Drying out the mucus may make you feel better initially, by reducing the pressure inside the sinus cavities, but it makes matters worse in the long run. (This effect may not be present with newer nonsedating antihistamines, which have less drying potential.)

Anticholinergic drugs (see p. 156) are sometimes prescribed for chronic sinusitis, but they too can dry up the mucus and should be used cautiously.

After three weeks, if the sinusitis has not improved substantially, a different antibiotic is given. If there are any bacteria resistant to the first antibiotic infesting your sinus cavities, the new antibiotic is intended to kill them off.

Should you still have sinusitis after another three weeks, you will be given yet another antibiotic. Changing the antibiotic, and taking prolonged courses, is the best way of exterminating the bacteria completely, which prevents the development of antibiotic-resistant bacteria (see box).

It is crucial that you always see the doctor promptly at the end of each course, so that there is no gap between the courses—do not give the bacteria any opportunity to build up their numbers again. The last antibiotic treatment should continue for at least a week after symptoms clear up.

Dealing with allergic reactions is also important:
• If you cannot get allergy tests, try to work out for yourself if an allergen is playing a part. Ask yourself if there were any changes in your life before the sinusitis began, such as getting a new pet, moving house, increased exposure to molds or dust mites, or starting a new job with exposure to allergens. When thinking about this, remember that allergies to newly encountered allergens do not develop immediately—it may take months, or even years. Try avoiding the allergen concerned and seeing if you improve.
• Should you discover that an allergen is at the root of the problem, but have difficulty reducing your exposure to the offending item, try to obtain allergy shots (see p. 164).
• If you suspect allergic fungal sinusitis (see p. 32), it is well worth eliminating any mold growth in your home (see p. 120). One research study showed that the molds growing in a patient's sinus cavities were often the same as those growing in the patient's house. It is possible that, by inhaling the mold spores from molds in their houses, sinusitis sufferers are continually reinfecting their sinuses.

Various other self-help measures can be valuable during this medical treatment.

- Reduce your exposure to cigarette smoke (including other people's) to an absolute minimum. Cigarette smoke acts as an irritant to the nose and sinuses, but, more importantly, it paralyzes the cilia, preventing them from shifting mucus out of the sinus cavities.
- Avoid breathing other irritants, especially ozone (see p. 130). Think about the chemicals you use both at work and at home—could any of these be irritants that are aggravating your sinusitis?
- Don't drink too much alcohol—it dries out the sinus membranes and makes matters worse.
- Drink plenty of water, to keep your mucus from becoming too dry and therefore hard to shift.
- Try to breathe through your nose as much as possible. The amount of oxygen in your sinus cavities drops drastically if you breathe through your mouth, and the low oxygen level probably fosters the growth of certain bacteria. Devices, such as nose clips, that help keep the nose open at night may be worth trying.
- Some people find that garlic, eaten or sniffed, and spicy foods such as chili and hot curry help.
- If you suspect that your sinusitis might be related to food sensitivity (see p. 68), consider trying an elimination diet to identify the culprit food.
- Observe your reactions immediately after eating—some foods, such as yeast and red wine, can cause an immediate swelling of the nasal membranes in certain people. So can sulfite food additives. Avoid such items if you are affected.
- Treating gastroesophageal reflux (acid regurgitation from the stomach after meals) can improve sinusitis.
- Some patients experience good effects from acupuncture although there are no observable changes on CAT scans. Other alternative therapies, such as homeopathy or Chinese herbal medicines, have not been investigated scientifically, but some patients report good results.

Prolonged courses of antibiotics destroy many of the beneficial bacteria in the intestine, and may cause long-term bowel problems. It makes sense to take a probiotic (see p. 205).

Surgery for sinusitis

Chronic sinusitis sufferers may be offered surgery to remove polyps, or to correct anatomical problems such as a deviated septum (the central division of the nose).

These operations can be very useful, but if you have asthma, try all other options first, because surgery to the nose can sometimes make asthma much worse.

Surgery on the sinus cavities themselves is also a possibility, when sinusitis does not respond to medical treatment. The least invasive surgical procedure is functional endoscopic sinus surgery. The operation enlarges the natural drainage channels, so that mucus drains away more easily. This rarely cures chronic sinusitis completely, but it usually makes it much easier to manage. Once the drainage channels are larger, antibiotics can be put directly into the sinus cavities, for example, avoiding the need for antibiotic tablets.

It makes sense to try and maximize environmental measures and medical therapy before considering surgery. Some patients for whom surgery seemed the only answer found they did not need an operation once their allergies were treated.

If you decide on having an operation, make sure your surgeon has a proven track record with *this type* of surgery. Don't be afraid to ask searching questions about how many operations of this kind the surgeon has done, how many he or she carries out per year, and the complication rates (how often things go wrong). It's a delicate job, and you want a real expert.

Asthma

Tom sorts mail on a night shift. "After work, I come out of the sorting office—it's about five or six in the morning, and really cold—and when I suddenly hit the cold air, I feel as if I just can't breathe. My chest clamps up like anything, so much that it hurts. Then, when I get in the car and put the heater on, it's fine again."

What Tom is describing is **bronchospasm**, the key event in asthma—a sudden, but reversible, tightening of the bands of muscle that surround the airways. The narrowed airways stop air from leaving the lungs at the normal speed, which means the lungs are still half-full when it's time for the next in-breath. Taking more air into half-full lungs produces pain and tightness in the chest, as the lungs become overinflated. (This can be alarming, because it can seem like pain from the heart, but it is just the rib joints and chest muscles hurting as they become stretched.)

Insufficient oxygen reaches the bloodstream because there is so much stale air in the lungs, so the asthmatic also feels breathless. Meanwhile, the air being forced through the narrowed airways makes a whistling sound called **wheezing**.

Those are the common symptoms of asthma, but there are others:

- Coughing, rather than wheezing, is the main symptom for some people (see box on p. 40).
- Sometimes there is vomiting during an asthma attack, especially in children, because the overexpanded lungs put a great deal of pressure on the stomach.
- A few asthmatics suffer narrowing in the trachea (the upper part of the windpipe) rather than in the airways lower down, and therefore feel as if they are being strangled.

Bronchospasm is just the endpoint of the disease process in asthma, a process that begins with **inflammation of the airways**. Although the airway muscles relax when an asthma attack is over, and you therefore feel much better, the underlying inflammation of the airways remains.

Airway inflammation may be caused, or partially caused, by allergy. Among asthmatic children, allergies exist in 80–90 percent of cases. However, the presence of allergies does not necessarily imply that they are an important cause of the asthma.

Inflammation makes the lining of the airways swell up, which itself narrows the airways a little. The inflamed airway lining often makes more **mucus** than usual, in an effort to protect itself (this is basically a healthy response—mucus mops up irritating dust particles so that they can be ejected by coughing—but it's excessive in asthma). This mucus can clog up the airways even more. Finally, the inflamed airways send nerve impulses directly to the airway muscles, telling them to contract.

Mucus alert

Asthmatic mucus is white or clear, and sometimes frothy. Greenish or yellowish mucus suggests an infection and should be reported to your doctor.

In severe cases of asthma, a lump of mucus can completely block an airway, leading part of the lung to collapse.

What causes asthma?

This question can be answered at three different levels:

1 What makes someone predisposed to asthma?
2 What starts asthma off—in other words, what starts the inflammation process in the airways?
3 What triggers asthma attacks?

What makes someone predisposed to asthma?

The predisposition to asthma is partly inherited (see p. 8) and partly a matter of lifestyle: a poor diet makes asthma more likely (see p. 206), as does an over-sterile environment (see p. 21).

What starts asthma off?

The predisposition to asthma sets the stage, but it does not, in itself, set off the inflammation of the airways. That may be started by an allergic reaction to something in the air—such as dust mite or pet allergens.

Alternatively, the initiating factor could be a viral infection, especially a kind known as Respiratory Syncytial Virus, or RSV—there are epidemics of RSV every two or three years. Those predisposed to asthma may make an abnormal kind of immune response to chest infections caused by viruses, a response that shifts the balance of the immune system toward Th2 cells—see p. 11—and allergy-type reactions.

A heavy dose of certain irritants, such as chlorine, or the substances used in spray-painting cars, can also initiate asthma; this mainly occurs in a workplace setting, causing **occupational asthma** (see p. 132).

What triggers asthma attacks?

Once the inflammation of the airways has begun, the airways are "twitchy"—oversensitive—and the airway muscles contract at the smallest provocation. Irritants in the air, such as tobacco smoke, can then trigger an attack, as can a great variety of other things—from cold air or the scent of hyacinths, to thunderstorms, laughter, or anxiety—see p. 39 for a full list. Exposure to the allergens that started the inflammation will also trigger an asthma attack, as will a virus (viral) infection such as a cold or flu.

For many asthmatics, the breathing pattern is disturbed by the asthma attacks and may remain abnormal between attacks. Hyperventilation or "over-breathing" can begin quite easily for asthmatics and then adds to the overall problems. It may be difficult to tell if you hyperventilate or not, because your habitual pattern of breathing will seem normal to you, but there may be telltale symptoms such as dizziness, tingling of the hands and feet, numbness, and muscle cramps. For a full list of symptoms, see p. 227.

Mind power

The muscle of the airways is the kind of muscle over which we have no conscious control, like that of the heart. It is known as **involuntary muscle**, whereas mucles in the arms and legs, which contract or relax when we tell them to, are called **voluntary muscles**. Studies with biofeedback have shown that asthmatics may, with training, gain some degree of control over these involuntary muscles. Experienced yoga practitioners are able to influence various involuntary muscles, including those in the airways.

There are also various ways in which the mind, or a person's social and emotional situation, can make asthma worse (see p. 234), but the damaging idea that it is an entirely "psychological" disease is now discounted.

Allergens and irritants

Understanding the difference between allergens and irritants is important for asthmatics. Allergens are specific—either pollen is an allergen for you or it isn't, depending on how your immune system reacts to it. They are also a basic cause of asthma—they start it off.

Irritants, on the other hand, are nonspecific: they affect every asthmatic if sufficiently concentrated, causing bronchospasm by aggravating the airway lining. And, at the levels usually encountered, they only cause trouble because the inflammation of the airways has already occurred. Irritants include cigarette smoke, other smoke, and some industrial fumes, ozone (see p. 130), sulfur dioxide (given off by some foods and drinks—see box on p. 207), fly spray, air freshener, or other aerosols.

Diagnosis

There are four separate aspects to diagnosis:

1 Is this really asthma or something else entirely?

2 Is it combined with other diseases and how are they affecting the asthma?

3 What is the basic cause of the inflammation in the airways and can this be avoided?

4 What sort of factors trigger the asthma attacks?

You may not get this full diagnostic program, but you can probably help in finding answers to some of the questions.

Is this really asthma or something else entirely?

There are no tests that can diagnose asthma with complete certainty, but the average case of adult asthma is pretty easy to spot, and the same is true for children over five. It is also true, however, that some patients now described as asthmatic would have been given a different diagnosis (for example, wheezy bronchitis) 30 years ago. To some extent, this is because asthma was under-diagnosed in the past: doctors were hesitant about giving a diagnosis of asthma, because of the supposed overtones of psychosomatic disease. Sweeping away that stigma has been of immense value, but certain patients (especially young children) may now get diagnosed as asthmatic without sufficient evidence. However, there are also many instances of asthma being missed.

These are two tests that should be carried out before a diagnosis of asthma is given. (However, they cannot be reliably performed on children under 5 years.)

1 Peak flow is the top speed of the outgoing air from your lungs, usually measured with a simple portable machine called a peak flow meter. Because of the narrowed airways, asthmatics have a lower peak flow than normal.

2 Spirometry, a more sophisticated test of pulmonary function, is commonly used to measure the lung capacity and extent of airway narrowing.

Asthma may be difficult to diagnose in certain situations:

• In babies, who often wheeze, especially when they have colds or chest infections. This generally clears up later and does not automatically develop into asthma. There is great controversy about whether wheezy babies should be labelled "asthmatic" or not, and how bad the wheezing should be before they are given asthma drugs. Views on this vary from one doctor to another. For older children who wheeze only when they get chest infections, most doctors feel it is valuable to use asthma drugs—such treatment does not "turn wheezing into asthma" as is sometimes claimed. (There are several things you can do to minimize the chance of early wheezing turning into asthma later—see pp. 244–9).

• When the main symptom is coughing (see box on p. 40).

• When asthma occurs only at night. In some asthmatics, even intensive testing reveals no abnormality in the airways during the day. The only way to diagnose the condition is to use a peak flow meter at home, morning and evening.

• When there is a sudden one-off asthma attack in response to a powerful allergen load. This sometimes happens to hay fever sufferers at the height of the pollen season (especially during thunderstorms). Some doctors will want to start asthma drugs immediately, but it may be better to get the hay fever well controlled with antihistamines and see what happens. Often there are no further asthma attacks.

Then there are conditions that can be mistaken for asthma:

• In children, an inhaled object—such as a button—becoming stuck in the airways. In babies it can also be inhalation of milk; if so, the "asthma" comes on mainly after feeding.

• Post-nasal drip (see p. 29).

• Heiner's Syndrome—(see p. 72).

• Bronchiolitis: a viral infection (generally caused by RSV—see p. 37) that affects the small airways (the bronchioles) of babies and toddlers. Unlike asthma, it usually produces fever.

• Gastroesophageal reflux (GER), or the rising of food from the stomach into the esophagus. (This is commonly called heartburn, after its most typical symptom, but you can suffer from GER *without* having heartburn.) GER can aggravate existing asthma, and it can also be an asthma mimic. Babies, children, and adults can all suffer from this problem. There will usually be clues such as symptoms that come on at night after a late supper, or whenever lying down.

• Hyperventilation (see p. 227) in nonasthmatics can be misdiagnosed as asthma if it causes breathlessness.

• Aspergillosis (see box on p. 18).

• Problems with the vocal cords. Habitually contracting the vocal cords on the in-breath makes a loud wheezing sound and can cause breathlessness. This problem can mimic asthma, but it also affects those who really are asthmatic. The cause is usually psychological.

• Low-level carbon monoxide poisoning, generally from gas fires, which can cause breathlessness and fatigue.

• Bronchiectasis: stretching and damage to the airways caused by diseases caught in childhood, such as pneumonia or whooping cough. This causes lifelong breathlessness.

• Emphysema (see p. 39).

Is it combined with other diseases, and how are they affecting the asthma?

Any allergic problems in the nose will contribute to asthmatic symptoms in the lungs, because there are nerve connections between the two. Long-term sinusitis can also make matters worse. Optimum treatment for the nasal and sinus symptoms (see pp. 28–35) will help considerably with the asthma.

One unlikely source of asthmatic symptoms has only recently been recognized: allergies can develop to the fungi causing athlete's foot, or other diseases (see pp. 16–17).

GER can contribute substantially to asthma, as described on p. 38. Your doctor can advise on treatment.

For older people, especially veteran smokers, asthma may be part of a larger picture of inflammation and damage to the air sacs of the lung (emphysema) and/or to the airways (bronchitis). This mosaic of problems is known as chronic obstructive pulmonary disease (COPD) or chronic obstructive repiratory disease (CORD). It may be difficult to tell if there is asthma present, or how much it is contributing to the overall problem.

Since many patients with COPD are helped by asthma drugs, and trying out the drugs does no harm, doctors often prescribe them just to see what happens.

What is the basic cause of airway inflammation?

Skin tests are usually needed here, to check for allergic reactions. However, simple detective work may pinpoint allergens without the need for tests. The likely suspects are all airborne allergens—see p. 28. Remember that the reaction does not generally start as soon as exposure to the allergen begins: there is a time lag. So a new dog or cat, or an allergen encountered at work, may cause no trouble for the first year or two.

Some irritants can also be a basic cause of asthma, but only if encountered in high doses, which usually occurs in the workplace (see box on p. 132).

In all cases, removing the allergen or irritant from the airways should be a top priority. The sooner you can end the exposure, the more likely you are to shake off the asthma, rather than have it for ever. Once the inflammation of the airways is firmly established, it just fuels itself—so act quickly.

In a minority of cases, **food sensitivity** is the initiating cause of asthma. The reaction to food is delayed, so the link will not be obvious. Skin-prick tests for the culprit food are usually negative, so an elimination diet (see p. 194) is needed to diagnose this problem and identify the food concerned. Those most likely to benefit are brittle asthmatics (those most severely affected). There are various other clues that food could be a factor (see p. 69).

When asthma begins in adulthood, there may be no clear initiating cause—it is just a question of long-term damage and irritation to the airways. But there can be allergens playing a part, so it is worth investigating this possibility.

What sort of factors trigger the asthma attacks?

Most asthmatics will recognize one or more of these as triggers:

- exercise (because breathing hard dries out the airways)
- the allergens responsible for the asthma, e.g. cat allergen
- colds, flu, and chest infections
- cold or dry air
- strong smells including perfume and fragrant flowers
- irritants in the air (such as cigarette smoke and other indoor pollutants, traffic fumes, industrial pollutants); indoor pollution is often the worst, especially if you have a gas stove without adequate ventilation, so there is a lot you can do to improve the air you breathe (see pp. 128–30)
- sulfur dioxide given off by preservatives used in some food and drink (see box on p. 207)
- weather conditions, particularly thunderstorms
- laughing, sighing, yawning, coughing, or any other altered breathing pattern
- stress or anxiety
- strong emotions such as fear, anger, or excitement
- situations or people that evoke unpleasant memories—including traumatic childhood memories; sometimes psychotherapy is needed to sort such problems out (see p. 233).

Recording your symptoms day by day should help to identify the triggers that are most powerful for you. Generally speaking, such triggers should be avoided, but this is not the case for exercise, which does much more good than harm, in the long run—without exercise, your asthma will get far worse (see p. 41).

Take care with aspirin

Aspirin sensitivity can develop unexpectedly in asthmatics, especially those with allergic rhinitis and/or nasal polyps (see p. 28). It can produce a severe, even fatal, asthma attack. Remember to avoid all aspirin-like drugs (see p. 151).

Just a cough?

For some, coughing is the main symptom of asthma. Known as **cough-variant asthma**, this is not always diagnosed correctly, especially in children. For children with recurrent coughing (two or more episodes per year of coughing without a cold) it may be a long time before the doctor considers asthma. But other doctors may diagnose a coughing child as "asthmatic" all too readily, without doing enough tests. The important point is that asthma involves episodes of bronchospasm—contraction of the airway muscles. Without this it is not asthma. Bronchospasm can be detected by medical tests such as peak-flow readings. Wheezing is one possible sympom of bronchospasm, but coughing is another.

If there is only coughing as a symptom, and never any wheezing, this is probably not asthma. Among children with this pattern of symptoms, allergies are unlikely to be involved. The cause of such coughing may be:
- In children, the effects of parental smoking.
- In those with perennial allergic rhinitis or chronic sinusitis (see pp. 28–9 and 31), mucus from the nose running into the lungs. This is called **postnasal drip** and produces a persistent cough.
- In the middle-aged, **eosinophilic bronchitis**. This is caused by an influx of eosinophils (see p. 19) into the airway lining, causing inflammation. Allergies do not seem to play a part (it is no more common in atopics than anyone else), and the airway muscles do not contract abnormally. Treatment is with inhaled steroids.
- In atopics (those prone to allergies), a condition sometimes called **atopic cough**. It involves eosinophils congregating in the trachea (windpipe) and bronchi, but not in the lower airways. There is inflammation but no airway narrowing. Very little is known about this disease at present; it may or may not involve allergies. Again, inhaled steroids are effective.
- For a few people, habitual coughing. This is usually an expression of some underlying emotional difficulty and responds to psychological treatments. The cough often has a honking or barking sound.

Any of these can be misdiagnosed as asthma. For patients with eosinophilic bronchitis or atopic cough, this is no tragedy as they will probably get the right treatment (inhaled steroids) anyway.

Treatment

The first and most important aspect of asthma is environmental control—to try and minimize contact with allergens and irritants. If you are asthmatic and you smoke, you must stop, because this will only make matters worse by stoking up the inflammation. Any other smokers in the family should accept that from now on this is an outdoor activity.

One of the aims of good asthma treatment is to calm the airways down, so that they are less sensitive and "twitchy." This means tackling the inflammation. You can do this with **preventer drugs** such as steroids or cromoglycate- (cromolyn) type drugs (see p. 157), or with the new antileukotriene drugs (see p. 159), or you can simply remove the basic source of the trouble, if it is a domestic allergen such as a cat, dog, or dust mite.

Treating associated diseases, such as sinusitis, hay fever, perennial allergic rhinitis, gastro-esophageal reflux (see p. 38), and even athlete's foot (see p. 16), can also help in reducing the airway inflammation. Eating a better diet may make a further contribution to calming the airways down (see p. 206).

The second strand of treatment is to deal with bronchospasm (contraction of the airway muscles) when it occurs. This is done with **reliever drugs** such as Ventolin (see p. 152). Note that these only relieve the symptoms of an asthma attack and do not address the underlying problem of inflammation. Excessive use of reliever inhalers (more than once a day) indicates loss of asthma control, which, in severe cases, can lead to a fatal or near-fatal asthma attack (see p. 153).

At one time, reliever drugs were the mainstay of asthma treatment, and were perceived as entirely safe, while preventer drugs such as steroids were only given to those with severe asthma. All this has changed, and most asthmatics, other than those with very infrequent attacks, are now given a preventer. If your drug regime has not been reviewed for some time, make an appointment with your doctor and check that you are getting the best of the modern treatments.

Drug treatment of asthma is not something you can just hand over to the doctor—it requires a lot of personal decision-making. If you usually get worse when you have a cold, for example, you need to increase your dose of preventer as soon as a cold appears, to stop the inflammation before it starts. You also need to know when an asthma attack is serious enough to warrant calling an ambulance. A **management plan**, worked out with your doctor, is a useful aid in such decisions (see p. 95). Using a peak flow meter night and morning to monitor your asthma will also be valuable (see p. 95).

The third strand of asthma treatment is to deal with associated problems:

- panicky reactions during asthma attacks— which make matters infinitely worse—can be dealt with by meditation, yoga, relaxation techniques, or martial arts training (see p. 222).
- hyperventilation, which plays a much larger role in asthma than previously suspected, can be tackled by a variety of methods (see p. 228).
- losing weight, if you are very heavy, will help ease the burden on your breathing.

Exercise and asthma

Exercise-induced asthma is best tackled, paradoxically, by getting exercise. As your fitness improves, you don't pant so hard when exercising, so your airways dry out much less. Countless asthmatics will tell you that once you overcome the first hurdle—of wheezing the minute you start to exercise—things get a great deal easier. You will need reliever drugs, and possibly extra preventer, to help you over this hurdle, but it's worth it.

Warming up with a few sharp sprints, separated by a rest period, will also help. (If you get an asthma attack while exercising, however, you should always stop—carrying on regardless can be fatal. Always have your reliever inhaler with you when you exercise and use it if you get an attack.) Swimming is an excellent starting point for unfit asthmatics, because the moist air prevents the airways from drying out. Once you are fitter, regular strenuous exercise makes the breathing muscles stronger, which is of great benefit—this can also be achieved with operatic exercises, and with mechanical lung exercisers (see p. 231).

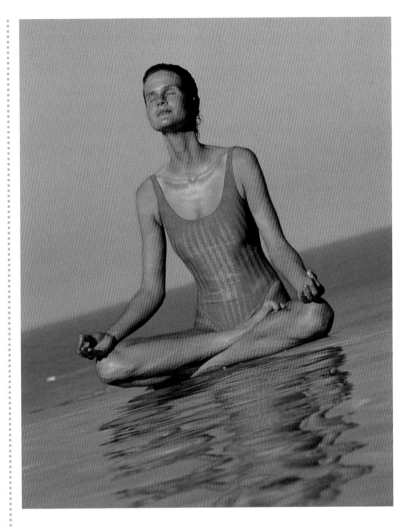

Don't underestimate asthma

Asthma can be fatal. Close to 6,000 Americans and more than 700 Canadians die from asthma every year. If you often wake up in the night with asthma, you cannot keep up with most other people your age, or are frequently breathless when climbing stairs or walking uphill, then your asthma is not under control. The same is true if you need your reliever inhaler more than once a day, or frequently need steroid tablets. Review your treatment with your doctor because you probably need more preventive treatment (see p. 157).

Recognizing an asthma attack and knowing when to call for help, or go to the hospital, is also crucial (see p. 100). Fatal asthma attacks often come on very quickly—half those who die do so within two hours, a quarter die within 30 minutes. Those who die are generally people who have neglected their preventer medication, or have been exposed to very high levels of allergens.

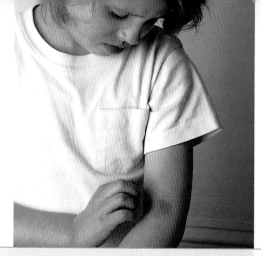

Atopic eczema

A Greek word meaning "to boil over" or "to erupt" is the source of the medical term "eczema." It refers, of course, to the way in which the skin erupts into a rash, but it could equally well describe the eruption of controversy around this disease. No other allergic disease is quite such a cauldron of dissent—indeed, even the question of whether it *is* an allergic disease remains unresolved. These controversies directly affect the treatment of atopic eczema, so it is useful to understand them if you or your child have eczema.

The disagreement begins with the question of what causes atopic eczema.

Let's start with the one point that everyone agrees on: dry skin plays a fundamental role. Those with atopic eczema have dry skin, not just in the eczematous areas, but in other parts as well, sometimes all over the body. The skin cells are less efficient than normal skin cells at retaining water.

Everyone would also agree that there is **inflammation** of the skin—a reaction that is produced by the immune system. But when it comes to the question of what *starts off* the inflammation there are huge differences of opinion among specialists treating atopic eczema—these specialists include dermatologists, allergists, and pediatricians.

Given that people with atopic eczema are atopic—that is, allergy-prone—and that most of them have huge amounts of the allergy antibody, IgE, going round in their blood, it might seem plausible that an allergic reaction to some external item kicks off the inflammation. And when skin-prick tests to common allergens such as dust mite are tried, there are usually a large number of positive results.

But many of these turn out to be false positives—when tested more directly, the allergen concerned does not actually play a part in causing the skin symptoms. This has led some specialists working with eczema, mainly dermatologists, to believe that allergic reactions play little part in either initiating or perpetuating atopic eczema.

In their view, the basic cause of atopic eczema is dry skin and a generally over-wrought immune system, not specific allergic reactions. To these doctors, positive skin-prick tests are *all* false positives in atopic eczema—that is, irrelevant to the disease process.

A positive skin-test result, they believe, simply indicates that the skin of atopic eczema sufferers is in a highly sensitive state, not that the allergen concerned plays any causative role.

What the words mean

Eczema is not a disease in itself. The word refers to a certain type of reddish rash—a rash that can be caused in a variety of ways. The type of eczema that affects people of an allergic disposition (atopics) is called either **atopic eczema** or **atopic dermatitis**.

The word **dermatitis** just means inflammation of the skin. Most doctors consider it to be synonymous with **eczema**, but some give it a slightly broader meaning.

Allergists tend to take a different view—but even here a wide range of opinions exists. Just to complicate matters, new research by allergists suggests that what is happening in atopic eczema is not necessarily allergy, but **immune sensitivity** (see p. 6). While some with atopic eczema may have a true allergic reaction, others may have a different type of immune reaction (see pp. 18–19), or even a mixture of the two.

Research using direct challenge tests (see p. 90) has identified some of the things that could provoke such sensitivity reactions:

- cow's milk or other food—a prime suspect in babies and young children (see p. 68). Note that the response to food is usually delayed, occurring some hours after the offending item is consumed.
- dust mites, pollen, or molds
- cats, dogs, rabbits, and other furry pets

The eczema symptoms can be provoked either by airborne allergens falling on the skin, or by direct contact (mite allergens in the bed, skin contact with pets, lying on grass for those with grass-pollen allergy). The rash tends to occur on skin not covered by clothes. But it can sometimes be localized to the most sensitive areas of skin, for example in those who react to dust mites but have eczema on the eyelids only.

Additionally, experiments show that even when allergen is *only inhaled* it can sometimes provoke eczema symptoms. The allergen reaches the skin in the bloodstream. This means that the skin reaction could occur anywhere on the body, not just on exposed skin.

The next step

Whatever causes atopic eczema, it provokes the most horrendous itching, as every eczema sufferer knows. The itch cries out to be scratched, and scratching is the major cause of the visible rash. *If left untouched, the skin does not erupt into eczema*, although it may well turn red, and there are still distinct changes in the skin that can be seen with a microscope.

Once eczema has erupted, the skin is no longer an intact protective layer that neatly separates "in-here" from "out-there." The skin becomes more permeable and loses its own natural moisture far more readily, so the dryness gets worse. At the same time allergens and irritants penetrate far more easily, causing yet more inflammation.

Something else compounds the damage: once atopic eczema is established, the immune system starts making IgE antibodies to the body's own proteins, especially those found in skin cells. This helps explain why atopic eczema can become so severe and so entrenched.

The wandering rash

For a baby with atopic eczema, the face, and especially the cheeks, are commonly affected, but there may be a rash all over the legs, the backs of the arms, and the back. As the months go by, the rash settles on the lower legs, and spreads to the fold of the elbow, and then the fold at the back of the knees—by about three years of age, the main problem for most children.is this **flexure eczema.**

In adults, eczema is often found in quite restricted areas, such as the hands, scalp, lips, eyelids, or chest. It may be located around the nipples—a sensitive spot where rubbing by clothing is enough to initiate a rash.

Atopic eczema is always in a process of change, and different parts of the body may display different stages of the rash:

- The rash is red and usually dry at first, and there may be not a great deal to see. In this early stage the visible signs may be minimal, while the itchiness can be colossal. Sometimes there is oozing of clear fluid.
- Occasionally the first phase is more marked, with dense patches of small red bumps or tiny blisters. On the hands, these may merge to form much larger blisters.
- Infections tend to change the appearance of the rash (see p. 44).
- With time the skin becomes thicker and paler with fine scales. It may form leathery patches (called **lichenification**), especially if there is habitual scratching or rubbing. This is known as **chronic eczema**.
- When the eczema clears, there may be an area of skin that is lighter in color, or darker, than the surrounding skin.

Infections—another vicious circle

When eczema erupts and the skin barrier is breached, infections frequently become a problem. A regular source of trouble is the bacterium *Staphylococcus aureus*, the cause of the infection called impetigo. This microbe invades eczematous skin very readily, causing a prolific ooze with golden-yellow crusting.

Staphylococcus aureus produces a toxin known as a "superantigen," which revs up the immune system to even more furious effort. This effort does not, unfortunately, oust the bacteria, but it does make the skin inflammation even worse. To add to their woes, many who are afflicted with atopic eczema start making IgE antibodies against *Staphylococcus aureus* toxins.

Infection with fungi is an occasional problem in atopic eczema (see p. 49), and there may be sensitivity reactions to these fungi.

The herpes virus, responsible for cold sores, can also invade eczematous skin, though this is much rarer. It worsens the eczema and produces flocks of small red bumps, each with a tiny dimple or blister at the center—*this needs urgent treatment*.

Irritants and stress

People with atopic eczema are far more susceptible to everyday irritants such as soap, traces of detergent left behind in clothes, wool and rough synthetic fabrics. Chlorinated water, either in swimming pools or from the tap, can also aggravate the skin, and even "hard" water (found in areas with chalk or limestone bedrock) may be a factor.

Some air pollutants may play a part in atopic eczema. Researchers in Germany found that children living close to busy highways, or in homes with a gas stove and no extraction hood (see pp. 128–9), were more likely to develop eczema. Formaldehyde fumes, often found in houses (see p. 129), are sometimes a factor when eczema affects the face and hands.

Various other things can irritate the skin and make atopic eczema flare up:
- cold weather
- dry air
- sweating heavily; clothes or shoes that trap sweat may also cause problems
- dust-mites, which can act as an irritant, even if not an allergen
- tobacco smoke
- solvents and other chemicals encountered at work
- irritant fabrics such as wool; also some carpeting
- contact with cosmetics and perfumes
- skin contact with fruit (especially citrus), vegetables, sauces, ketchup, juices, and some other foods. The spray generated by peeling potatoes can produce eczema on the face.

Anything that increases blood flow through the skin makes the itching worse:
- heat, especially a hot bath or being too hot in bed
- anger or embarassment
- hot drinks of any kind
- coffee, tea, and alcohol because of the druglike substances they contain
- vinegar and spicy foods
- chocolate, soy sauce, yeast extract, orange juice, tomatoes, and other foods that are rich in amines (see p. 200)

Various changes in the body can make the eczema worse:
- teething, in babies
- colds and other viral infections
- in women, certain phases of the menstrual cycle

Many eczema sufferers are aware that their skin gets worse when they are upset, stressed, or anxious (just before examinations, for example). Like other allergic diseases, atopic eczema is not *primarily* psychological but, once it has begun, psychological factors can play quite a big part.

Contact sensitivity

People with atopic eczema can develop contact dermatitis (see p. 54)—to nickel, for example, or perfume. There is always this risk with regularly applying creams to your skin, especially anything containing fragrance or lanolin. Antihistamine and antibiotic creams also carry this risk.

Even the ingredients in the creams prescribed for eczema—such as moisturizers and steroids—can sometimes provoke contact dermatitis. Creams are more likely to contain sensitizing ingredients than ointments. Very occasionally, the sensitivity is to a preservative or emulsifier that is widely used in different ointments and creams, which means that switching brands yields no improvement. Steroid suspended in petrolatum (petroleum jelly) is the least likely to cause reactions.

The rash produced by contact dermatitis looks no different from atopic eczema, so this sensitivity will be far from obvious. It will just seem as though the atopic eczema is not getting better.

Talk to your doctor if you think there may be a problem of this kind. He or she can check by using the suspect cream on one side of the body and a different-but-equivalent product on the other side. Patch tests (see p. 92) may also help to identify contact sensitivity.

The good news . . .

. . . for children and teenagers, is that if you have eczema as a child, your chances of developing acne during your teens are greatly reduced.

Diagnosis

There are five separate aspects to diagnosis:

1 Is this really atopic eczema? There are no clear-cut tests for atopic eczema. Instead the diagnosis is based on a "points system"—how many of the typical features of atopic eczema are present? The doctor adds them up, and if there are enough, then it's atopic eczema. Sometimes all the typical features are there and this is obviously the right diagnosis, but in other cases there may be room for doubt. The doctor should rule out the possibility of contact dermatitis (see p. 54), especially if you have eczema only, or mainly, on the hands.

2 What avoidable irritants are making the skin worse?

3 Is the eczematous skin infected? The signs of infection are usually clear, but not always, especially with fungal infections. Steroid creams can sometimes mask the overt signs of infections: if atopic eczema is not responding to treatment, this possibility should be investigated.

4 Are there any allergic reactions to those infections? Or to the normally harmless microbes that live naturally on the skin (see p. 17)? Interpretation of allergy tests to these is difficult because people with atopic eczema make a lot of IgE. Adults with persistent atopic eczema that is getting worse rather than better are the most likely candidates for such tests.

5 Are there allergic reactions (or other sensitivity reactions) to food, or to allergens such as house-dust mite?

This fifth aspect of diagnosis is where controversy is rife. Many dermatologists feel that atopic eczema is treated quite adequately with moisturizers and steroid creams. The search for allergic/sensitivity reactions—in other words, for basic causes—seems unnecessary for most patients, or more trouble than it is worth. Indeed, some believe that looking for such sensitivity reactions is actually mistaken because they are not basic causes (see p. 42).

Other specialists disagree, and feel that allergic/sensitivity reactions are a basic causative factor in atopic eczema. They concede that there are many false positives, but in their opinion, there are enough true positives in the skin-prick test results to make it worth sorting them out from the false positives. Except for patients with very mild eczema, such doctors prefer to identify and eliminate the root causes, if possible.

Patch tests are now used by some of these doctors (see p. 69)—yet another contentious issue! The time-honored use for patch tests is in contact dermatitis, and there is a lot of resistance to using them for atopic eczema. Traditionally, the immune reactions involved in atopic eczema and contact dermatitis are seen as entirely different—the former involving IgE and being a quick reaction (identified by skin-prick tests), the latter involving immune cells and being much slower (identified by patch tests). New research into atopic eczema shows this view to be overly simple (see pp. 18–19) and provides a rational basis for using patch tests.

If, as a patient or a parent, you are keen to search for fundamental causes, remember that this should *never* displace treatments to quell infection or restore the protective structure of the skin. When these treatments are neglected the whole problem can get far worse, because of the vicious circles that sustain atopic eczema.

Sweaty sock dermatitis

More correctly known as "juvenile plantar dermatitis" this rash on the feet affects an awful lot of atopic children. It is frequently misdiagnosed as athlete's foot, and treated with antifungal drugs. The important clue can be found by looking between the toes: if there's no rash there, then it is not athlete's foot.

Treatment

Treatment for atopic eczema has five possible angles:

1 calming the inflammation
2 avoidance of scratching and rubbing
3 caring for the skin and restoring its normal structure
4 treating infections
5 avoiding allergens

One or more of these aspects may be neglected, depending on what kind of specialist you are seeing. Some allergists may not put enough emphasis on skin care, for example.

Calming the inflammation

Steroid creams are the mainstay of atopic eczema treatment because they calm the inflammation in the skin. The creams do carry a risk of side effects, but are safe when used correctly (see p. 147). An over-fearful attitude to steroids creams can mean that the eczema never gets under control, and this can mean using more steroids in the long run. When treating an outbreak of atopic eczema with steroid cream, it is vital to continue applying the cream until the "hidden healing" has occurred (see p. 146)—don't stop as soon as the skin *looks* better.

Tar-based ointments have a much milder anti-inflammatory effect and can be helpful for areas of thickened skin. They were once widely used for atopic eczema, but are used less now, in part because they stain fabrics and smell unpleasant. Sometimes they irritate the skin, too, and there are concerns about safety: they contain carcinogens, and significant amounts are absorbed into the bloodstream. However no evidence has been found that these cause cancer, despite intensive searching.

Antihistamines (in tablet or capsule form) are sometimes used and while they may not help the eczema much, some evidence suggests that they could reduce the risk of asthma developing later (see p. 249). Some doctors believe that sedative antihistamines used at night can help reduce the tendency to itch and scratch, which worsen eczema.

Powerful drugs such as cyclosporine are sometimes used in severe cases of atopic eczema, to damp down the immune response. They must be taken by mouth and can affect other parts of the body, not just the skin. Very careful monitoring is needed. A new immune-modulating drug called tacrolimus, which works when applied directly to the skin in a cream, may soon become available.

Sunlight is often beneficial, because it suppresses the inflammatory processes in the skin. However, not everyone improves with sun exposure—some get worse. Careful experimentation is the only way to find out: build up the length of sun exposure very gradually, starting with less than an hour a day.

Medical treatment with UV (ultraviolet) light can produce the same effect as sunshine and suppress inflammation. This treatment may be prescribed, but you should not try it for yourself with a sunlamp. In PUVA treatment, a plant-derived substance called psoralen is given by mouth, or applied to the skin, to enhance the response to UV light.

Kicking the scratching habit

Scratching is a substantial part of the problem in long-standing atopic eczema. Experiments with healthy people and mechanical "scratching machines" show that perfectly normal skin will erupt into eczema if it is scratched intensively.

There is no steroid cream powerful enough to counteract the effects of scratching. But if scratching stops, then the skin can—with the help of medication—heal up.

Note that "scratching," in this case, includes rubbing the itch (directly or through clothes; using a hand, wrist, chin, leg, foot, or *any* other part of the body), touching or picking at the skin, rubbing against sheets, furniture, or another person, or using a towel, facecloth, or hairbrush to rub the skin. All these activities can be habitual and *quite unconscious,* if atopic eczema has been present for more than a few months—you just don't realize you're doing it most of the time.

For many with atopic eczema, another problem creeps in—scratching without itching. This may be just habit, a response to boredom, stress, or anxiety. Scratching alone can set off itching, and a scratch-itch-scratch cycle ensues.

The first step in combatting scratching (for an adult or older child) is simply to notice how often scratching occurs. Doctors at the Chelsea and Westminster Hospital in London issue their patients with little hand-held counting devices (tally-counters), and ask them to press the button on the device every time they scratch or rub. Over a period of days, patients discover—usually to their own amazement—just how often they do scratch. The point of the exercise is simply to become conscious of the scratching impulse, and to notice the situations that typically provoke scratching. You could use a small pocket-sized notebook and pencil to achieve the same end.

Once this awareness has been gained, then you are in a position to break the scratching habit. The methods involved—called "habit reversal"—were first developed by a Swedish dermatologist, Peter Norén. It takes about 2 to 4 weeks for most people, but the change is long-lasting. Most eczema sufferers find that they recoup their time investment rapidly, once they are free from the chore of dealing with chronic eczema.

When you notice that you are about to start scratching, and before the urge to scratch overwhelms you, take control and do something deliberate with your hands—for example, clench your fists, while breathing deeply and slowly. Think cool nonitchy thoughts. The urge to scratch may pass. If it doesn't, then you can allay the itch by pinching the itchy area gently, or pressing your fingernail into it, or *lightly* applying a little moisturizer.

In the bath or shower, don't use facecloths, and never rub or scrub the skin. Dry off by gently patting with a soft towel.

The aim is to get scratching episodes down to fewer than 10 per day. In achieving this goal, relaxation exercises, stress-management techniques, hypnotherapy, or autogenic training (see p. 222) can also be very helpful, especially if you sometimes scratch in tense situations.

With small children, the parents have to do the noticing. Most are unaware just how much their child scratches or rubs the eczema—babies often rub against the side of the cot.

Once the awareness is there, a child over four can usually be taught the habit-reversal technique described above. With a younger child, the parents must distract the child when scratching is imminent, by talking or playing. If the child is scratching while asleep, parents should pick the child up and, very gently, hold the child's hands away from the body. Situations and activities that commonly provoke scratching should be avoided, or planned for. Give the child something to hold while dressing and undressing, for example—keep the hands busy. But *never* say, "Don't scratch"—it usually has the opposite effect in the long run.

For the first four days and nights, while you are trying to break the scratching habit, the child should never be alone, even for a minute—someone who is able to distract the child from scratching should always be there, and awake. Fortunately, children lose the habit far more quickly than adults.

Keep a child's fingernails very short and smooth them with an emery board too, so that if any scratching does occur the effects are minimized. (Soft-cotton mittens, to be worn at night, are often recommended, but the cotton itself can be used to rub the skin—observe your child carefully! The same is true of allover cotton suits.)

For this antiscratching program to be effective in healing the skin, there must be a *determined effort with drug treatment at the same time*. You should be using a steroid cream of *sufficient strength*, twice a day, and plenty of moisturizing treatment.

By taking this "Combined Approach," as Dr. Christopher Bridgett and his colleages at the Chelsea and Westminster Hospital call it, you should be able to clear the eczema completely, even if you have had it for years and have tried innumerable different treatments. Once this has been achieved, you can maintain an eczema-free state by watching carefully for any outbreaks of itching, redness, or roughness, and treating them immediately with a short course of steroid cream (see p. 146).

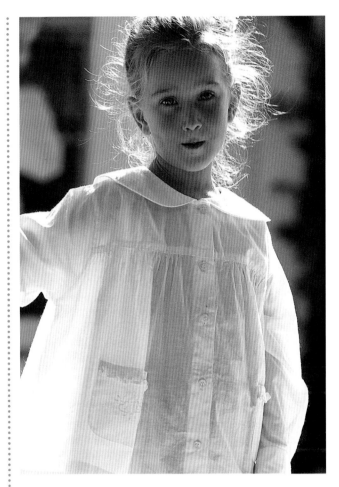

Will it clear up?

Small children with mild eczema generally grow out of it by the age of two. Those who have eczema after this age tend to show a big improvement at puberty. Sometimes, however, the eczema can disappear at puberty, only to reappear later: so continue to be careful with your skin.

Atopic eczema is frequently the first sign of a tendency to allergies and asthma (see p. 22). Given this early warning sign, parents should take steps to avoid allergies developing, or at least reduce their severity (see pp. 244–9).

People with both asthma and atopic eczema frequently notice that when one improves the other seems to get worse. There is no explanation for this as yet.

Moisturizers—how to use them

Moisturizers do two things: they trap the water already in the skin, and they lubricate the skin, making it less brittle.

A moisturizer is designed to leave an oily layer on the surface of the skin that stops the skin's natural moisture from escaping. The most effective preparations, from this point of view, are petroleum jelly, ointments, such as Vaseline, which form an uninterrupted waterproof layer: these are sometimes called **occlusives**. They contain no water, unlike creams. Although a cream forms a less formidable barrier to the escape of moisture from the skin, it does provide some moisture itself, which can soak into the skin.

The most important thing is to have something that you like using, so that you apply it regularly. There are lots of moisturizers available, so ask the doctor for different ones to try.

Applying moisturizer well is crucial:

- Apply moisturizer before your skin gets dry, as a preventive treatment.
- There's no need to rub in your moisturizer (this can be a form of scratching). Just apply it very lightly.
- A thin layer is all that's needed. A thick layer keeps in heat, which aggravates the skin.
- Always apply within three minutes of a bath or shower.
- In addition, apply every 3 to 4 hours during the day. Carrying moisturizer around with you is helpful—the little plastic containers in which camera film is sold are useful for this.
- Ask the doctor to prescribe moisturizer in large quantities, to make sure you have enough. But beware of infecting big containers with *Staphylococcus* bacteria and then reinfecting your skin. Pump-action dispensers are safer.

Moisturizer can also be smeared onto bandages that are then wound around the affected areas at night to reduce the itch—or you can use ready-made "wet-wraps" (ask your doctor about these). As long as the bandages/wraps are immovable, they will reduce nocturnal rubbing and scratching.

Avoid lotions, and any non-prescribed creams, as most contain fragrance or other ingredients that can irritate the skin. Choose bath oils with care—some contain alcohol, which is an irritant.

Skin care

First, avoid all the irritants that you think may affect your skin. Give clothes an extra rinse cycle in the washing machine, to remove all detergent. Wash all new clothes before wearing them, to remove chemicals such as formaldehyde. Wear soft cotton or silk next to the skin.

Where eczema affects the hands, special care is needed (see p. 135).

Water can be both good and bad for eczema. When you soak in a bath, water is absorbed by the skin cells, which helps correct the dryness of the skin. But when you get out of the bath, and the skin dries, the outermost layer shrinks and develops microscopic cracks, making it even less waterproof than it was before. The way around this problem is to apply a moisturizer immediately after a bath or shower—gently pat the skin until partially dry, and apply the moisturizer immediately so that it can trap the water in the skin.

For anyone with a severe flare of eczema, current recommendations are:

- soak in lukewarm water for 20 minutes, twice a day
- pat dry
- quickly apply steroid cream to the eczematous areas, then moisturizer over the top, and to all other dry-skin areas.
- make sure the moisturizer goes on *within 3 minutes of emerging from the water*.

This works well for some people, but not all. For a few eczema sufferers, the effect of taking natural oils out of the skin (which soaking does, to some extent) may outweigh the benefits of putting water in. Or they could be sensitive to something in the tap water—the chlorine, perhaps, or pollutants. It may not be obvious that this routine treatment is not helping. As Dr. Michael Tettenborn, a British pediatrician with long experience of atopic eczema, observes: "By the time they're referred to me, children are usually on the standard regimen of two soaks a day. One of the first things I do, as an experiment, is tell the parents to just bathe them once a week and use a moisturizer and tissues to keep them clean the rest of the time. Some children do a lot better after that."

Tackling infections

Where infection of eczematous skin occurs, antibiotics, antifungal drugs, or antiviral drugs (depending on the type of infection) are essential. Learn to recognize the early signs of an infection developing, and seek medical help promptly.

This is particularly important in the case of herpes (cold sore) infections: a severe infection of eczematous skin with herpes can even be life-threatening. Avoid contact with anyone suffering from cold sores.

If you would prefer not to take antibiotic tablets, you could talk to the doctor about the possibility of using an antibacterial ointment containing the drug mupirocin, available in the U.S., but not in Canada. This is a relatively new treatment.

Undetected fungal infections can be a cause of severe atopic eczema that does not respond to treatment. A recent study at the University of Virginia, showed that for some adults with disabling eczema, a prolonged course of itraconazole (the drug that kills the widest range of fungi) can work wonders. Antibiotics may well be needed at the same time.

Infection of the hands with the fungus that causes athlete's foot can sometimes be the main factor in persistent hand eczema. Occasionally it is *only* the feet that are infected with this fungus, and the hands just "come out in sympathy." Treating the feet cures the hands. Contact dermatitis of the feet can produce the same strange "echo" of eczema symptoms on the hands.

Some doctors believe that overgrowth of yeasts in the gut, combined with an allergic reaction to them, occasionally plays a part in atopic eczema. Children whose skin is very red, and who are not responding to standard treatment for eczema, are likely candidates. This is a controversial area, as explained on p.83.

Allergen identification and avoidance

Where pollen is the culprit, there is usually a marked eruption of eczema during the pollen season, so the link is obvious. By contrast, 75 percent of eczema sufferers who are sensitive to dust mites don't notice the connection because the exposure to mite allergen is constant.

If you want to investigate the possible role of everyday allergens, and cannot get skin tests, then simply avoid the allergen and observe the effects. Given that a child with atopic eczema is at high risk for developing other allergic symptoms later, it makes perfect sense to avoid these allergens anyway, especially dust mite. Follow the avoidance programs described in Chapter 4.

The vexed question of investigating food sensitivity is considered on p. 68.

Assuming allergens have been identified, is there any alternative to avoidance? Unfortunately, conventional immunotherapy does not work well for atopic eczema: in fact it can make the skin worse. Doctors practicing enzyme potentiated desensitization (see p. 211) claim good results with atopic eczema. However, this is still considered an experimental treatment.

Additional treatments

Giving up coffee, or stopping smoking, sometimes clears atopic eczema symptoms completely.

There are a few reports of probiotics (bacterial replacers) helping with atopic eczema. They are worth a try (see p. 205), especially if you have taken frequent courses of antibiotics. Some adults with hand eczema lose their symptoms when taking a supplement of Vitamin E.

Evening primrose oil helps some eczema sufferers (see p. 221). Chinese herbal treatments, taken as a tea, may also work for atopic eczema, but be extremely wary of Chinese "herbal creams" for eczema (see pp. 220–21).

An unsuspected problem

Nickel, and other metals, if at high levels in the diet (see p. 55), can cause symptoms resembling atopic eczema in people who are sensitized. The fold of the inner elbow, the sides of the neck, and the skin around the genitals and anus are commonly affected. Recurrent episodes of hand eczema, especially if it is a blistering rash, may also be a sign of metal sensitivity.

Hives and swelling

The stinging nettle is a fearsome plant which, if it touches the skin, produces a mass of itchy bumps. This rash looks and feels so similar to **hives,** that the botanical name for the nettle, *Urtica*, has provided the medical term for the rash, **urticaria**.

This resemblance between hives and the rash caused by nettle stings is no coincidence: the liquid that the nettle plant injects into the skin with its spiky hairs contains **histamine**, which is also the main messenger chemical produced during allergic reactions.

When histamine causes fluid to seep out into the surrounding area of deeper tissue, a diffuse swelling known medically as **angioedema** results (*angio*-means blood vessels, *edema* means swelling caused by excessive fluid). Histamine has many effects on the body (see box on p. 12), among them making the smallest blood vessels more leaky. The histamine also causes intense irritation, leading to itching and sometimes burning. Hives typically have a central, white, raised, superficial area, called a **wheal**, caused by fluid leakage, surrounded by an angry red area, called a flare or erythema—thus the description of urticaria as a "wheal and flare" reaction. (A positive prick-puncture test—see p. 91— produces a small hive.) Hives can be single or multiple, small or giant, and can blend together into large patches. Small hives are often round, whereas large ones are often very irregular.

Hives and angioedema can occur together or separately. Hives is a symptom that can be caused in countless different ways. The symptoms are produced by a release of histamine from mast cells (see box on p. 12) deep in the skin, but the triggers that activate the mast cells are many and various.

These triggers can sometimes be very difficult to identify in the case of **chronic urticaria** and angioedema ("chronic" means that the symptoms have been present for some time). Prolonged and careful investigation may be needed (see pp. 51–3).

In **acute urticaria** and angioedema—a severe but short-lived reaction—the trigger is usually obvious. It is often an insect sting, a food, or a drug such as penicillin, and the symptoms are due to an IgE-mediated allergy (see box on p. 12).

Sex and hives

A few women suffer acute urticaria after sexual intercourse, due to an allergy to semen. In some cases it appears all over the body, not just around the vagina, and asthma or anaphylaxis can develop (see p. 58). This problem is "not readily recognized by the medical community," to quote doctors at the University of Cincinnati, who have studied it intensively. This is an IgE-mediated allergy, but is usually an allergy to proteins supplied by the partner's prostate gland, rather than to sperm themselves. Quite often (and this is a puzzle) it occurs on first intercourse. Skin-prick tests with the partner's semen should confirm the diagnosis.

Using condoms usually solves the problem. (If the symptoms persist in these circumstances, the possibility of latex allergy should be considered.) Allergy shots using the partner's semen are also very effective. For women who have not had immunotherapy and want to conceive, artificial insemination with washed sperm, free of the offending allergens, can be used. The drug sodium cromoglycate (see p. 148) can be used within the vagina before intercourse, but only for localized reactions. Use of this drug may allow conception.

Drugs such as penicillin, taken by the man can get into the semen in trace amounts and cause urticaria, or even anaphylaxis, in women already sensitized to the drug. It is also believed possible that food allergens eaten by the man, and transmitted by the semen in minute amounts, could affect women with severe IgE-mediated food allergy. However, there is no concrete evidence of this.

There can also be IgE-mediated allergic reactions in the vagina to spermicides or to very low levels of *Candida*, but these tend to cause more persistent symptoms of itching, or burning and irritation, rather than acute urticaria. This is often wrongly diagnosed and treated as if it was caused by a recurrent *Candida* infection.

Because acute urticaria comes on immediately after the encounter with the food or other allergen, there is generally no difficulty in identifying the culprit—if a child takes a mouthful of egg and within minutes his lips and face are swollen and puffy, you know he's allergic to eggs.

Acute urticaria and angioedema are key symptoms of food allergy (see p. 62) and often form part of the catastrophic allergic reaction known as anaphylaxis (see p. 58). Hives due to foods or insect stings often last only a few hours. Hives due to drugs may last days or weeks until the drug is totally eliminated from the body. Viral infections, especially in children, are a common cause of hives lasting days or weeks. The reason for this is unknown.

Chronic urticaria

First the good news: if you have had chronic urticaria for less than six months, it may well clear up of its own accord—it does so in about 50 percent of cases.

Anyone who has been suffering for more than six months has a much smaller chance of spontaneous recovery (only 6 percent), so treatment is advisable. Those who see a conventional allergist about their problems may then be told the bad news: "a cause can be determined in only 5–20 percent of chronic urticaria cases," to quote one authority; or "90 percent of the time your physician will not be able to find the cause of your hives," in the words of another.

Luckily, it isn't true. Some research teams studying chronic urticaria intensively have got the proportion of patients with unexplained symptoms down to 23 percent. Indeed, a recent paper from doctors at the University of Munich in Germany states: "there are probably few truly 'idiopathic' cases of urticaria"—in other words, few cases in which no cause can be found for the disease.

The common identifiable causes of chronic urticaria include:
• in the "**physical urticarias**", simple physical triggers such as cold, heat, superficial pressure, deep pressure (as from sitting on a chair, though the symptoms may not come on until some hours later), vibration, exercise, contact with water, and exposure to light, sunlight, or UV light. Sensitivity to pressure may result in **dermatographism** or **dermographism**—skin that can be "written on" because it produces a wheal in response to a fingernail being lightly dragged across it.
• in **cholinergic urticaria**, activity by the branch of the nervous system called the parasympathetic (see box on p. 235), that is thought to directly trigger mast cells. This type of urticaria has a typical rash with very small lumps surrounded by areas of redness. It is triggered by warmth (after exercise or a hot shower, for example), or by emotional stress, and is found mainly in teenagers and young adults, who seem to grow out of it in time
• a type of autoimmune disease in which the body produces antibodies against IgE, or against the receptors for IgE; these rogue antibodies can activate mast cells directly
• autoimmune thyroid disease, especially in women
• a rare disease called mastocytosis, in which the number of mast cells in the skin is abnormally high
• immunoglobulin deficiencies, especially of IgA
• a cancer (*the most unlikely of all these causes*)

Some other causes for chronic urticaria, which can be investigated after the common causes have been ruled out, are:
• A chronic infection elsewhere in the body, often unrecognized. Possible culprits include long-term sinusitis or throat infections; tonsillitis; infected teeth;

Could it be the "ulcer bug"?

Some research suggests that *Helicobacter pylori* in the stomach—recently identified as a cause of stomach ulcers—may also be a source of chronic urticaria. The data is conflicting on this point, but if other investigations have got nowhere, and you have an active *Helicobacter* infection (shown by antibodies in the blood, a breath test for urea, and a stomach biopsy), then it is worth trying an eradication program. This is a tough treatment—you take three antibiotics together for 1 to 2 weeks, followed by another stomach biopsy, then a second round of antibiotic treatment if the bacteria are still found. Don't accept a less rigorous treatment program than this.

middle-ear infections; intestinal parasites; inflammation of the gallbladder, kidneys, ovaries, or uterus; athlete's foot or related fungal infections (intertrigo, onychomycosis, tinea); prostatitis; Epstein-Barr virus; and cytomegalovirus. If there is diarrhea and inflamed joints as well, *Yersinia* infection is a possibility. These infections seem to have a direct effect on the immune system, which causes mast cells to release histamine.

• a reaction to a food additive or to alcohol; these may act by triggering mast cells directly, as in false food allergy (see box on p. 67)

• a reaction to nickel in food among those with skin sensitivity to nickel (see p. 55)

• drug sensitivity—often to aspirin or aspirin-like drugs (see p. 151); but it could also be antibiotics, sulfonamides, morphine, or other narcotics. A recent case of chronic urticaria in a child was found to be due to an aspirin-like drug in her teething gel.

• chemical intolerance (see p. 84)

• unusual sensitivity to histamine found naturally in wine and aged cheeses such as Camembert; histamine produced by bacteria in the gut can also cause problems, and this may be linked to gut flora imbalance

• a reaction to the preservatives, (for example parabens) used in creams and ointments. Where urticaria occurs in direct response to something on the skin, it is called **contact urticaria**.

• sensitivity to food or pollen (relatively rare causes)

• contact with latex, pets, or other items (these too are uncommon causes)

• premenstrual changes in hormones

• problems with **"Candida"**—this is highly controversial; some sufferers probably do have yeast overgrowth in the gut, but it may not be *Candida* yeast (pp. 82–3)

• very rarely, chronic urticaria is an early symptom of adult-onset celiac disease (see pp. 70–71)

Is it an allergy?

Acute urticaria is usually a symptom of IgE-mediated allergy (see box on p. 12), but **chronic urticaria** is a different matter. Although atopic people are rather more likely to develop chronic urticaria than nonatopics, there is no firm link with true allergy. When a food or drug is responsible for the chronic urticaria, often no IgE antibodies to the offending item are found.

Allergists check for physical urticarias with an ice cube, heat, a UV lamp, water, and other relevant stimuli. And they will eliminate the possibility of an inherited defect or a more serious underlying disease by taking blood tests and skin biopsies.

Should a physical cause for your symptoms, such as cold or exercise, be found by the basic tests, you will probably be advised simply to avoid these triggers. This is good advice, especially for cold-induced urticaria, which can get worse and develop into cold-induced anaphylaxis (see p. 59). However, some people with a physical urticaria have multiple causes for their symptoms, including intolerance to a commonly eaten food. Dealing with other causes—by identifying and avoiding the culprit food, for example—may mean that cold, exercise, or whatever is no longer a trigger. So an elimination diet (see pp. 194–7) is worth a try. For example, one patient with cold urticaria found that, by avoiding milk she no longer had problems with the cold and could even take up skiing.

The downside of this aspect of chronic urticaria is seen when *both* causes are intermittent. The fact that two (or even more) factors have to be present at the same time to produce symptoms can make identification of those causes very difficult.

Investigating chronic urticaria

If you have chronic urticaria you will almost certainly need the help of a specialist. However, there are some simple investigations that you could do for yourself at home.

You will probably have a good idea of the cause already if you have one of the physical urticarias (see above), and you could devise commonsense tests—with an ice cube, for example—to confirm your suspicions.

Look at the list of other possible causes on pp. 51–2, and investigate those that do not require specialized medical tests. Do your symptoms come on during the summer—could it be pollen, or just heat or sunlight? Is there anything you are in contact with regularly (such as ointments, creams, latex products, or pets) that could explain your symptom pattern? These are *not* the most common causes of chronic urticaria, but they are ones you could track down for yourself.

Food allergy can kill...

An elimination diet may be useful for investigating possible causes of chronic urticaria, **but not for acute urticaria**. Those who have prompt reactions to food, symptoms in the lips and mouth, or positive skin-prick tests, should *never* undertake food testing at home without their doctor's agreement and careful preliminary testing (see box on p. 23). If you ever have suffered anaphylaxis, an asthma attack, or any swelling of the throat from a food, do not test it except under medical supervision with resuscitation equipment available.

Unfortunately, chronic urticaria comes and goes all the time, and it can be affected by the temperature, emotional stress, and a range of other factors. There could be more than one trigger, with both needed to start the symptoms. You will have to make an accurate daily record of your symptoms, and keep an open mind, to have any hope of puzzling this problem out.

Another self-help measure is to investigate the effects of dietary changes. Get your doctor's agreement before you start.

- First try an additive-free diet for 6 weeks. You must also cut out alcohol, spices, and all aspirin-like drugs—see p. 151 for details.
- A low-histamine diet (see p. 200) may be helpful: some people with chronic urticaria are thought to be unable to detoxify histamine in food. A low-amine diet (see p. 200) is also worth trying.
- If there is no response to this, or only a partial response, go on to a low-carbohydrate diet, while continuing with histamine avoidance—the idea is to minimize the production of histamine by bacteria in the gut. The diet reduces the food supply of these bacteria by reducing starchy foods (such as bread, cookies, cakes, potatoes, pasta, pizza, pastry, rice) and fruit and vegetables, especially those with relatively indigestible residues that go through into the intestine, such as spinach. This is not a particularly healthful diet, and is not recommended long-term. Should it help with your urticaria, take a probi-

otic to repopulate the gut with beneficial bacteria (see p. 205), and then experiment with gradually reintroducing various foods.
- You could also carry out an elimination diet to look for food intolerance (see pp. 194–7), but this is a rigorous diet, and food intolerance is a relatively unusual cause of chronic urticaria, so you may want to explore other possibilities first.
- The role of yeast overgrowth in the gut (see pp. 82–3) causing chronic urticaria is controversial. It may be worth investigating if all else fails.

Drug treatment

Investigating the causes of chronic urticaria could take some time, and it is important to control symptoms in the meantime. The best treatment is a non-sedating antihistamine, as used for hay fever (see p. 139). Some doctors add another type of drug, called an H-2 receptor antagonist, normally used for those with stomach ulcers. It blocks a different kind of receptor for histamine, and because the two drugs together block *both* kinds of histamine receptor (H-1 and H-2), the combination may achieve better control of chronic urticaria.

If you are sensitive to colorings, other additives, or to any foods, you should obtain special additive-free, food-free formulations of these drugs.

Antihistamines can become ineffective if taken continually for years. Switching to another kind of antihistamine may help. Steroid tablets (see p. 141) may be used for particularly troublesome cases.

The new antileukotriene drugs (see p. 149), appear to be potentially very useful for chronic urticaria.

Treating solar urticaria

In the case of severe solar urticaria—a reaction to sunlight—total avoidance is clearly very difficult and sunblock creams don't help. Even thin clothing may let through enough sunlight to cause a reaction. Often, however, there is a spectrum of light that inhibits the reaction, if given promptly after exposure. Careful testing will reveal the wavelength of light that has this curative effect. Alternatively, there are light treatments, similar to those used for atopic eczema (see p. 46), that can desensitize the skin. You will need a very good dermatologist to explore such treatment options with you.

High doses of antihistamines can also help, by reducing the itchiness of the rash, but your skin will probably still turn very red in the sun. Fortunately, solar urticaria seems to become less severe with the passing years. In particular, the hands and face, which are constantly exposed to light, become less sensitive.

Contact dermatitis

"I got this terrible itchy rash on my face, worst of all on my eyelids," Barbara recalls. "My dermatologist did a load of tests on my back, then said it was a reaction to nail polish. That seemed crazy, because my fingers were fine. But he said that it was where I had been touching my face, and that the skin around the nails was OK because it's a whole lot less sensitive."

Direct contact of the skin with the **sensitizer**—in Barbara's case an ingredient of nail polish—is the usual source of trouble in contact dermatitis. But things can get complicated, as Barbara discovered. Pets or clothing can also pick up the sensitizer, and then transfer it to your skin. Creams can rub off from your partner onto you, usually in bed at night, and cause you contact dermatitis while leaving your partner unaffected. Men urinating after touching a sensitizer such as poison ivy may get a rash on the penis only. (Poison ivy is dealt with on p. 56—these two pages deal with all other forms of contact dermatitis.)

The sensitizer in contact dermatitis may be either:
- an irritant, often something encountered at work, which will produce contact dermatitis in anyone, given enough exposure. This is known as **irritant contact dermatitis.**
- an antigen, which can provoke the immune system into a **delayed hypersensitivity** or Type IV hypersensitivity reaction (see p. 18). These **antigen sensitizers** affect some people but not others. The reation usually occurs about 48 hours after exposure, but the time lag ranges from 12 hours (if the reaction is recurrent) to a week (if it is newly acquired). The response provoked by this second type of sensitizer is sometimes known as "allergic contact dermatitis," but given the tight definition of allergy being used in this book (see pp. 6–7), that term is not appropriate. There is no IgE involved, and the problem is no more common in atopics than in anyone else.

    Quite often a person's contact dermatitis is caused by both irritants *and* antigens.

Cross-reactions

The immune cells that produce contact dermatitis recognize their antigen by means of receptors on the cell surface. These receptors work in much the same way as antibodies, so they can produce cross-reactions (see p. 14).

Many different antigen sensitizers exist, including:
- Nickel, cobalt, and chromium. Much more rarely, silver and gold. Nickel leaches out of jewelry, the metal studs of jeans, and other items in contact with the skin. Chromium sensitivity is typically caused by exposure to cement.
- Fragrances and other ingredients (for example, lanolin and preservatives) in perfume, cosmetics, and toiletries.
- Sunscreens, and medicinal drugs applied to the skin in creams, including antihistamines, some antibiotics, benzocaine, and steroids. Likewise preservatives and other additives used in these creams.
- Garden plants and weeds, particularly those of the daisy family, such as chrysanthemums, marigolds, ragweed, and feverfew. These plants are so common that the source of the rash often goes unrecognized. Primroses and primulas, Algerian ivy, hydrangeas, and tulip bulbs are also frequent culprits. With some plants the sensitizer is in the sap; with others it is in the leaves, or the hairs on the stems. Several lawn weeds produce a rash only when the skin is also exposed to sunlight.

• Plant extracts used in herbal medicines, and in many "natural" or "herbal" type cosmetics and toiletries. Some of these cross-react with garden plants such as feverfew; others cross-react with fragrances, while some are just powerful sensitizers in their own right (tea tree oil and propolis, for example).

• Glue, resins.

• Latex, used in rubber gloves, balloons, condoms, rubber bands, eyelash curlers, makeup sponges, and elastic. The substances that provoke a contact dermatitis reaction to latex are additives called rubber accelerators, whereas immediate IgE-mediated reactions (see box on p. 12) are due to the natural proteins in latex.

• Textile dyes, leached out of clothing and bed sheets by perspiration.

Getting into the system

Sometimes a sensitizer becomes airborne and is inhaled, then carried around the body in the blood. There is a reaction affecting the skin of the whole body, but especially those areas previously affected by direct contact. Medical workers sensitized to drugs, and then exposed to them in the air at work are vulnerable in this way. This reaction is known as **systemic contact dermatitis**, because the sensitizer gets into the whole system.

If the sensitizer, or something very similar to it chemically, is found in food, or is taken as a medicine, this too can cause a systemic reaction. Some physicians now believe that absorbing nickel from food may produce systemic reactions in a few patients. Patients with this problem vary greatly in terms of symptoms. At least five different symptom patterns are seen:

1 long-standing hives (chronic urticaria) sometimes with swelling (angioedema)

2 a widespread rash that resembles atopic eczema. The distribution of the rash may be all over the body, or it may favor the folds of the elbows, the eyelids, sides of the neck, and skin around the genitals and anus.

3 an all-over itchy rash that defies diagnosis

4 recurrent episodes of hand (and occasionally foot) eczema, often a severe blistering rash.

5 eczema around the anus and genital area only.

Most of those affected are young women, the group most likely to have contact sensitivity to nickel. More surprisingly, according to one study, over 40 percent of patients have *never* noticed any rash due to contact with nickel. However, they do generally show sensitivity to nickel when patch-tested. These women improve considerably on a low-nickel diet.

People who are sensitized to chromium or cobalt may also respond to these metals when they absorb them from food. A recurrent blistering hand rash is especially likely. Some of the most severe cases of this are seen in patients with a sensitivity to both nickel and cobalt.

If you have a longstanding and unexplained rash that fits one of the descriptions above, and if you have tried all the standard treatments without success, then a low-nickel diet (see p. 199) may be worth investigating. Talk to your doctor first. A low-chromium or low-cobalt diet is more difficult (see p. 200).

Diagnosis

The **patch test** (see p. 92) is the only test for contact dermatitis. Once the offending substance has been identified, you should be given:

• the name of the antigen, plus any synonyms

• typical places where it might be found, or substances in which it may be an ingredient

Prevention

To prevent the development of nickel sensitivity, avoid earrings containing nickel—which means any made of relatively cheap metal. Choose high-carat gold or stainless steel. For those who can't imagine life without jeans, the metal studs can be covered (on the back, where they contact the skin) with a piece of adhesive tape.

When shaving, men should use an electric shaver, not a razor. One study showed that razors triple the risk of developing fragrance sensitivity to aftershave.

Treatment

Once sensitivity has begun, it is probably going to be with you forever, so avoiding the sensitizer is necessary. You may be able to protect your skin with clothing or gloves, but make sure the material used really will keep out the sensitizer concerned—ask your doctor (preferably a dermatologist) for advice. Barrier cream very rarely works.

Special attention is needed for your hands if they are affected (see p. 135). If the skin is already inflamed, avoid using creams and ointments containing known contact sensitizers such as antihistamines, neomycin and some other antibiotics used in creams, benzocaine, and tea tree oil.

By using these medications you could perpetuate the rash or make it worse.

You may need steroid creams from your doctor to get the dermatitis under control. Occasionally steroid tablets are given for a short time.

Poison ivy and poison oak

Poison ivy, poison oak, and poison sumac are a major cause of contact dermatitis in North America. All belong to the same plant genus, called *Toxicodendron* (previously *Rhus*). The offending substance in these plants, an oil called **urushiol**, is an antigen that can provoke a delayed hypersensitivity reaction (see p. 18).

Urushiol is one of the most powerful sensitizers known, and 85 percent of people will eventually develop contact dermatitis to it, given sufficient exposure. Sensitivity can develop in as little as 7–10 days from first exposure (which is symptomless, and may go unnoticed), but many people have low-level exposure for several years before becoming sensitized.

Other plants in the family Anacardiaceae, to which *Toxicodendron* belongs, have similar oils—sufficiently similar to provoke a cross-reaction. The Japanese lacquer tree is one such, and lacquered items from China and Japan can cause a rash to those with poison-ivy sensitivity. During President Richard Nixon's visit to China in 1972, several members of the presidential party developed embarrassing rashes on their thighs and buttocks, as a result of contact with recently relacquered toilet seats. The Chinese themselves are not affected by the lacquer, since they do not have poison ivy to sensitize them.

Cashews and mangoes also belong to this family, and a consignment of cashew nuts contaminated with fragments of the shells (only the shells contain the offending oil) has, on one occasion, caused an outbreak of illness among those sensitized to poison ivy. This is an example of **systemic contact dermatitis**—the sensitizer getting into the system and causing widespread symptoms. Mango rind can do the same thing, so always eat them peeled. Ginkgo is unrelated, but its fruits also seem to provoke a cross-reaction, so do not eat these.

Diagnosis

The skin reacts to poison ivy within 12–48 hours usually, but the rash can take several days to erupt. Initially, the skin becomes red, then bumps or blisters break out. The rash may show up in certain areas as a line, where a leaf has brushed across the skin.

Swelling may occur, and the rash is generally very itchy. The blisters eventually start to weep, and a yellowish crust forms. When this fall off, the skin underneath is very sore.

Poison ivy rash can become infected by bacteria, especially if the blisters are scratched, and the infection may cause fever.

Assuming there is no infection, the worst is over after 5 days, and the rash disappears without treatment over the following 2–3 weeks. Widespread exposure in a highly sensitive person can produce a more generalized illness, and very occasionally the kidneys are affected.

Most people with sensitivity to poison ivy know what the problem is and do not need further diagnosis. Patch tests can be used if there is uncertainty, but are best avoided since they can be misleading (false positives—see p. 91—are possible). What is more worrying is that the test itself can actually sensitize someone who is not already sensitized to poison ivy.

Prevention

First and foremost, learn to recognize poison ivy, poison oak, and poison sumac, and take care to avoid them. The old saying, "Leaflets three, let them be," is worth remembering. Poison ivy and poison oak both have slightly glossy leaves grouped in threes—their most typical feature. Both are very widespread, growing in woods, yards, and fields, up to an elevation of 4,000 feet. Poison ivy, found right across North America but especially in eastern and central areas, grows as a small shrub, a climber, or a low creeping plant. Poison oak, found in the West, grows taller, and the leaves are more lobed, something (but not much) like an oak leaf. Study the drawings on p. 57—or ask someone who knows to point the plants out. You can also find photographs of these plants on the Internet.

Poison sumac, also called poison dogwood, is a small tree up to about 6 feet in height, which favors swampy areas far from civilisation. The leaves have 7–13 leaflets, arranged around a central stem, as in a true sumac. Unlike the true sumac, the leaflets have no serrated edge, and the fruit is a cluster of green berries hanging downward, not in an upright red "candle."

Even in winter, they can cause a rash, therefore it's important to learn to spot the berries, which are the main identifying features in the colder months.

Covering all exposed skin with clothing will help if you are in an area that is heavily infested with these plants. A new barrier lotion, available in the U.S. without a prescription, contains the active ingredient Bentoquatam, which helps protect against poison ivy, poison oak, and poison sumac rash. This product is not available in Canada.

Double trouble

If poison sumac is burned and the smoke inhaled, sensitized people will suffer severe irritation of the nose, throat, and lungs. The smoke can also coat the skin with urushiol and provoke a dermatitis reaction.

Wash all clothes and shoes that may have been in contact with poison ivy to remove the urushiol—make sure they do not brush against anything or anyone before being washed. The same goes for pets, garden tools, backpacks, and other equipment. The oil remains potent for up to a year.

There is no form of immunotherapy available for poison-ivy dermatitis. Native peoples used to feed their children small amounts of the leaf, but the effects were doubtful, and the side effects (when it went wrong) were serious; so don't try it! Attempts to produce a scientific version of this treatment have largely failed.

Treatment

Washing the skin within 5–15 minutes of contact with the plants can prevent the rash completely—use mild soap if possible; but prolonged immersion in a running stream will work when you are out hiking. The oil is unstable in the presence of moisture. Alcohol can also remove the oil if there is no water available. Remember to clean under the fingernails.

Until you have washed, avoid touching any other part of the body with the part that has contacted poison ivy. The oil, and thus the rash, is easily spread. (However, It is a myth that the fluid in the blisters can spread the rash.)

Once the rash has developed, there is not a lot you can do to stop it, but you can ease the symptoms by soaking in a cool bath with baking soda added, or by applying compresses of cold water or Burow's solution (ask your pharmacist). Antihistamine tablets (available without prescription) and calamine lotion may also ease the itch, but some physicians are skeptical about their usefulness.

Avoid using antihistamine creams or benzocaine creams which can themselves produce contact sensitivity (see p. 54).

Non-prescription steroid cream (hydrocortisone cream) can be useful, especially if applied in the very early stages of the rash, before any swelling or blistering occurs.

Cover the blisters once they break, to prevent infections. Don't use soap or alcohol on the skin at all once the rash has begun, as these will irritate. So may lotions, but a general moisturizer (fragrance- and lanolin-free) can be useful in the later stages, when the skin often feels very dry.

It is worth going to see a doctor only if you have previously had a very severe reaction to poison ivy, if the rash covers more than 20 percent of the body, or if it is on the genitalia or near the mouth or eyes. You may benefit from a stronger steroid cream, available only with a doctor's prescription. This must be used at an early stage to be of value.

Steroid tablets or injections are often used for severe cases. Such courses can safely be taken up to four times a year.

However, it is much better to avoid poison ivy if you can, rather than relying on steroid tablets, which have potentially serious side effects if taken for prolonged periods. A physician's help is also needed if the rash is infected—a bright red color and oozing pus are the key signs.

Poison ivy can grow as a low shrub, 21–30in/53–76cm tall, or as a vine. The leaves are glossy green in summer, turning yellow or red in the fall.

The fruits of poison ivy are greenish white berries.

petiolule

The shape of the leaflets is very variable. To distinguish poison ivy and poison oak from other plants with three-lobed leaves, look for the long stem on the central leaflet (called a petiolule).

Poison oak has more lobed leaves than poison ivy, but they are very irregular in shape, unlike a true oak.

Poison oak can grow as a vine or a shrub.

In winter, look out for the leafless stems of poison ivy and poison oak, as they can still produce a rash.

Anaphylaxis
ALLERGIC COLLAPSE

The Egyptian Pharaoh Menes was the first recorded victim of anaphylaxis, over 4,000 years ago. Hieroglyphic inscriptions in his tomb reveal that he was stung by a wasp and died soon afterward.

The term anaphylaxis was coined in 1902, by a French doctor, Charles Richet, who derived it from two Greek words. There is disagreement about how to translate it—"repeated reaction" or "excessive reaction" are two possibilities.

"Excessive" is an appropriate description, as anyone who has suffered severe anaphylaxis will confirm. The symptoms of anaphylaxis include:

- itching all over
- hives (see p. 50) anywhere on the body
- widespread swelling under the skin caused by fluid escaping from the blood vessels into the tissues (angioedema)
- sometimes hoarseness due to swelling of the larynx
- difficulty in breathing, swallowing, or speaking
- coughing, wheezing
- occasionally, sneezing and a blocked nose, and/or symptoms in the eye
- a flushed face and a general feeling of warmth
- rapid pulse, palpitations
- anxiety, disorientation, and (most characteristically) a sense of doom
- cramping pains in the stomach, vomiting
- incontinence or diarrhea
- dizziness, faintness, and collapse due to a sudden fall in blood pressure.

It may take less than an hour to progress from the first itchiness to the final—often fatal—symptoms. *Prompt action is vital*—read p. 98 *now* so you know what to do if the worst happens. Sometimes things go much more slowly, and anaphylaxis takes an hour or more to start, but it can still be a very serious reaction.

Another name for the later stages of this devastating reaction, including collapse, is **anaphylactic shock**—or it may be described as a **severe systemic reaction**. "Systemic" means that it involves the whole body (owing to allergens traveling in the bloodstream) rather than just affecting that part of the body where the allergen made contact. A **cutaneous systemic reaction** is one that simply affects the skin, producing the first three symptoms only. (Note that some doctors use anaphylaxis in a narrower sense, to mean only anaphylactic shock.)

Anaphylaxis can kill in a variety of ways:

- the drastic fall in blood pressure can do it
- the swelling in the throat
- a fatal asthma attack

Recent research has shown that most of those who die are asthmatics. Heart failure during anaphylaxis, or due to treatment, is also a possibility, especially in older people.

For those who have near-fatal attacks, there is a risk of kidney failure or brain damage.

Recognizing anaphylaxis

In the early stages of the reaction it may be difficult, even for a doctor, to be sure it really is anaphylaxis. Fainting or a panic attack can look very similar. But those who are simply fainting are pale and have a slow pulse, whereas those suffering anaphylaxis are usually pink in the face and have a fast pulse. If someone is just fainting, their blood pressure normalizes and they start to recover when they lie down, but this is not true for anaphylaxis.

There are many different causes of anaphylaxis:

- Food allergy (see pp. 62–67).
- Insect-sting allergy or snake-venom allergy (see pp. 60–61). Even leech bites can provoke anaphylaxis.
- Latex allergy, a problem that mostly affects hospital workers, others who wear latex gloves for work, and children who have had a lot of surgical operations (for example, those with spina bifida). Once sensitized, there may be a reaction to balloons, elastic bands, condoms, and rubber gloves.
- Drug allergy, most commonly to penicillin.
- Vaccines, although this is rare (see box on p. 249).
- The extracts used for allergy shots (see p. 164).
- Prick-puncture tests, though this is rare; anaphylaxis is more common with intradermal tests.
- Allergy to substances used in other medical procedures, such as radiocontrast media used prior to X-rays.
- Exercise—usually strenuous exercise, but some unfortunate people are affected by simply walking or raking leaves. As well as the usual symptoms of anaphylaxis, there may also be headache, extreme perspiration, and choking. Some people are only affected if there are other triggers as well (see below).
- Cold—this is a rare and extreme form of cold urticaria (see p. 51). Swimming in cold water is the usual trigger, and the anaphylaxis may lead to drowning—great caution about outdoor swimming is needed in those who have severe cold urticaria since this could progress to cold anaphylaxis.
- Semen—anaphylactic shock can occur, but the reaction is usually milder than this, and it is rare for semen allergy to be life-threatening. There are effective treatments (see p. 50).
- Beta blocker drugs, used for heart problems, can transform a mild allergic reaction into severe anaphylaxis, by preventing the body from protecting itself (see p. 150).

Even when all these potential causes have been investigated by an allergist, there remain cases of **idiopathic anaphylaxis**, where no trigger can be found. Such mystifying patients are far from rare, and the cause is not psychological in the majority of cases. Fortunately, this unexplained condition is very rarely fatal.

With exercise-induced anaphylaxis, identifying the cause may be tricky. Some people only react to exercise if they have eaten beforehand, or eaten a particular food—shellfish, alcohol, tomatoes, cheese, celery, strawberries, wheat, and peaches are the most common offenders, but it could be any food, and you may need an elimination diet (see p. 194) to pinpoint the culprit(s). Certain individuals require the additional trigger of aspirin-like drugs (see p. 151) or extreme weather conditions (heat, cold, or high humidity) to react to exercise. You need to keep a detailed record of what occurred just before each attack.

Treatment

You should see an allergist, to confirm that you really have suffered anaphylaxis and to identify the cause if possible.

To protect yourself in future, carry an autoinjector containing epinephrine (see p. 150) and wear a MedicAlert bracelet or pendant, just in case you arrive in hospital alone and unconscious one day. This is particularly important if you are allergic to latex (surgical teams need to know that their gloves could kill you), penicillin, other drugs, or radiocontrast media.

Great caution about triggering factors is necessary, especially where anaphylactic shock has occurred. Make sure to tell all the medical staff you deal with—including dentists—if you have an allergy to drugs. Allergy shots (see pp. 164–9) may be helpful for triggers that are hard to avoid, especially insect stings, but it must be done carefully.

Avoiding all exercise is obviously a bad idea, and by being careful about what they do, most people with exercise-induced anaphylaxis can remain fit. Indoor exercise may be a good choice if weather extremes affect you. Drugs such as antihistamines (see p. 138) and cromoglycate (see p. 148), taken before you start, can be very helpful. Both are safe enough for daily use and it is better to take this preventive medication than to resort to epinephrine injections at regular intervals. It is important to stop exercising as soon as any symptoms start, even if they are minor.

Make sure those you play sports with know about your problem, so they can call an ambulance in an emergency. Solitary jogging is a bad idea if you have ever had severe anaphylaxis. Those with exercise-induced asthma as well should take additional precautions (see p. 41).

Fortunately, exercise-induced anaphylaxis often clears up spontaneously after a time. The same is true of cold anaphylaxis, and some food allergies in children (see box on p. 23), but not the other kinds of anaphylaxis.

Anaphylactoid reactions

When there is a massive release of histamine from mast cells, but IgE is not involved, an **anaphylactoid reaction** ensues. This looks exactly like anaphylaxis, and can be just as deadly.

For example, the antivenin given for snakebites, if antivenin has been given before, will provoke such a reaction: the circulating immune complexes (see p. 13) are present in such numbers that they spark off a system called **complement**, which in turn triggers the mast cells. False food allergy and histamine poisoning (see box on p. 67) can also provoke anaphylactoid reactions.

Insect-sting allergy

"I'd been stung by bees before, but that time it was different. I started to itch like mad, all down my body, I felt sick and it was hard to breathe or talk. I went dizzy, and the next thing I knew, I woke up in hospital." Hilary was lucky to survive this experience—anaphylaxis (see p. 58) to a bee sting. It kills more than a hundred North Americans every year. The tragedy is that these deaths could, in most cases, be prevented.

Insect-sting allergy is caused by the body making IgE antibodies (see box on p. 12) against the insect's venom. Because the venom enters the bloodstream, there are symptoms in distant parts of the body—a **systemic reaction**. In its mildest form, this may just cause itching, hives, and swelling all over the body. A more severe systemic reaction can be fatal.

Very rarely, there are further reactions after the initial crisis has passed. Some people who have had a severe systemic reaction, or multiple stings, develop an inflammation of the blood vessels, the kidneys, or the nerves. This is due to circulating immune complexes—see p. 13.

Assessing the risk

Venom allergy is alarming, and you need to have a realistic idea of how great a risk is involved:

• The ordinary reactions to insect stings—itching, pain, redness, and some swelling around the sting—are not due to allergy but to toxins in the venom.

• Anyone can develop an allergy to insect stings—you don't have to be atopic (prone to allergies). But atopics are more likely to have severe anaphylaxis if they become allergic to venom. Routine skin-prick testing of atopics is, however, not considered worthwhile because false positives are so common. Taking the general population, 10–30 percent of adults give a positive skin test to at least one venom, but only 1–5 percent of adults have a systemic reaction.

• Some people have more pronounced local reactions than is normal, with extensive swelling around the site of the sting,

peaking after 2 to 3 days. This may or may not be an allergic reaction (one involving IgE). About 10 percent of people affected in this way will eventually have a full allergic reaction.

• Suffering a lot of stings at once will produce a body-wide toxic reaction, from the sheer volume of venom injected. This is not the same as an allergic reaction, but the effects can be similar and emergency treatment may be needed. (Very occasionally, multiple stings seem to cure a preexisting allergic reaction to venom, but it's just as likely to be the death of you, so don't try it.)

• A **cutaneous systemic reaction** is one that affects the skin in parts of the body far distant from the sting site, causing itching, hives (urticaria), and swelling (angioedema). It indicates a genuine IgE-mediated allergic reaction. An adult who has had such a reaction may well progress to a severe systemic reaction, and would benefit from immunotherapy. This is not true for a child under 16: the risk of a severe systemic reaction next time is only 10 percent.

• A **severe systemic reaction** causes allover skin symptoms, as above, plus anaphylactic symptoms such as swelling of the throat, wheezing and breathlessness, faintness, stomach pain, vomiting, diarrhea, and collapse. Someone who has survived one such reaction will not necessarily react in the same way again—the risk of a similar or worse reaction is, surprisingly, only 30–60 percent. But it's wise to be cautious.

• Children under 10 have much less chance of a fatal reaction than teenagers or adults. Older people with heart conditions or bronchitis are most at risk of dying.

Diagnosis

If you have had a bad reaction to a sting, there are two effective forms of treatment—epinephrine and allergy shots—which could save your life if stung again. See the doctor as soon as you can and take the insect with you, if you have it, or the sting. If not, try to identify the insect using a field guide.

Unfortunately, many people never see their insect assailant. In these circumstances, make a record of where you were at the time, as this may give vital clues. If a child is the victim, get as much detail as possible about what happened, when, and where. Did they feel a sting go in? On which part of the body? Try to locate the site, as this may assist with diagnosis.

Prick-puncture tests and intradermal tests (see p. 91) are the next step. The usual procedure is to test with all the venoms from stinging insects found locally. You may react to more than one, because the rate of false positives—a positive test but no allergic reaction—is high.

There are also rare individuals who are genuinely allergic but give a negative skin test. A blood test known as a RAST (see p. 92) may be positive but—very rarely—this too gives a doubtful result, with barely detectable levels of antivenin antibodies.

Treatment

Prompt first aid can save the life of those with venom allergy (see p. 99). Most deaths occur within the first hour. (A severe reaction can also begin some hours after the sting, but never more than 24 hours afterward.)

Anyone who has had a systemic reaction to an insect sting should be referred to an allergist. In the meantime, your GP should prescribe an auto-injector loaded with epinephrine, in case you are stung again. Make sure you have proper training in using it (see p. 150).

Avoidance of the insect is essential (see pp. 112–13). Wear a MedicAlert or similar bracelet or pendant (see box on p. 95), in case you are stung while alone and fall unconscious.

Immunotherapy is invaluable for this allergic condition. It reduces the risk of another systemic reaction to a mere 3 percent, and for the unlucky few who do succumb again, the reaction is much less severe. Try to get this treatment if you can (see pp. 164–8). Beekeepers do particularly well on immunotherapy and most are able to go on keeping bees thanks to this treatment.

Mosquitoes and midges

The received wisdom on biting insects such as mosquitoes and midges is that, while inhaled particles from them can cause allergic symptoms in the nose and lungs (see p. 28), their bite injects little or no allergen—so allergic reactions to their bites are extremely rare.

New research is beginning to question this view. Doctors at the University of Manitoba have identified what they call "Skeeter syndrome": a very large swelling around the area of the bite, plus fever. The problem is usually misdiagnosed as an infection deep in the skin (cellulitis), despite the fact that the swelling comes on within hours—much too soon to be an infected bite.

Conventional skin-prick tests for mosquito bites will probably be negative because the commercial test extract is made from the whole bodies of mosquitoes, and this contains very little of the allergen from the salivary glands. (The dedicated Canadian researchers made a test extract by carefully dissecting the salivary glands from no less than 370 mosquitoes!)

"Skeeter syndrome" is seen most often among young children and those with lowered immunity.

In addition, there is one report of an asthmatic who suffered asthma attacks in response to mosquito bites. Immunotherapy gave her protection.

Those with dermatographism (see p. 51) often show an unusually large local reaction to mosquito and other insect bites, but this is simply due to the general sensitivity of their skin.

Snake-venom allergy

Not all snake bites are instantly fatal. Some snakes, such as the rattlesnake, deliver a bite that many people survive. But others do not—an anomaly that may be explained by allergic reactions. Research shows that those who are bitten once run the risk of developing IgE antibodies against snake venom. (If already sensitive to bee venom, there may be a greater risk.) This can result in anaphylactic shock if they are bitten again, on top of the symptoms caused by the toxins in the venom. The risk of death then shoots up dramatically.

Some general practitioners or family physicians may not be aware of this possibility and not offer appropriate treatment for the allergic reaction. The distinctive symptoms of anaphylaxis—symptoms that are not seen with ordinary snake-bite reactions—include itching, hives, general swelling (angioedema), wheezing, and breathlessness. (Reactions to the antivenin given for snake bites are dealt with on p. 13.)

Food allergy

Could you be killed by a kiss? For those with very severe food allergy—the "exquisitely sensitive" as doctors call them—a microscopic amount of the food is enough to provoke a severe reaction. A smear of the food left in a badly washed cooking pot can do it, or a trace left on a grill or work surface. And the killer kiss has *nearly* occurred on at least two occasions. A young man with fish allergy kissed his girlfriend shortly after she had eaten fried mackerel and had to be given emergency treatment for the consequences. In another incident, a young boy was kissed affectionately by his aunt, who had just consumed some peanuts. She had forgotten about his peanut allergy and was horrified to see, within a few moments, his lips and face swelling with the allergic reaction.

Both these reactions were extreme examples of **IgE-mediated food allergy**, one of the **classical allergic diseases** (see box on p. 11). This kind of response usually occurs immediately after eating the food and first affects the lips, tongue, and mouth, and often the throat. Much less commonly, it can occur some hours later and affect the stomach and intestines—see p. 64. In babies with food allergy, a delayed reaction that manifests as stomach pain, vomiting, and diarrhea is actually more common—see p. 65.

In its mildest form, IgE-mediated food allergy produces a tingling or itching of the mouth, sometimes with slight swelling of the lips, mouth, and face. More severe reactions cause a dramatic swelling of the lips, tongue, and throat. Both are described as **local reactions** because only the areas that contacted the food are affected.

When the swelling in the mouth is severe, there are often symptoms in more distant parts of the body as well, caused by food allergens that have entered the bloodstream. This is described as a **systemic reaction** because the body-system as a whole is affected.

The name used for systemic allergic reactions is **anaphylaxis** and, where it is severe enough to cause collapse, **anaphylactic shock**. It is important to be familiar with the symptoms of this (see p. 58) because it can kill remarkably quickly. Recognizing the problem at an early stage, and taking the right sort of action promptly, can prevent a death (see p. 98).

Anaphylactic shock is the most frightening of all sensitivity reactions to food. Because it is potentially fatal, many sufferers, or their parents, must live

Allergy not intolerance

Note that the next six pages deal with classical IgE-mediated food allergy, not with other immune reactions to food (see pp. 68–73) or with food intolerance (see pp. 74–7).

in a state of perpetual vigilance to avoid eating the food by accident. This is particularly difficult when extremely small amounts of the food provoke a full-blown anaphylactic reaction. Fortunately, the proportion of allergy sufferers who develop severe food allergies of this kind is relatively small.

One reason that doctors dislike the use of "food allergy" as a loose term for food intolerance is that true IgE-mediated food allergy can be such a dangerous disease. Those affected by true food allergy need to be taken seriously (by cafeteria staff or waiters, for example), and it does not help if thousands of other people also claim to have "food allergy" on the basis of reactions such as headaches or diarrhea, which are certainly debilitating but not life-threatening.

Most food allergies begin during childhood, but there are also cases of adults suddenly developing an allergy to a food, such as cow's milk or sesame seeds, that had previously been eaten without trouble.

No one can react to a food the first time it is encountered: there has to be an initial contact to sensitize the immune system. But this initial contact can occur before birth (from food molecules reaching the fetus in the mother's blood), or during breast-feeding (from food molecules in the mother's milk), so a child can react to a food the first time he or she eats it. This is why women in the U.K. are now advised not to eat peanuts—a source of powerful allergens—while pregnant. However, further research into this aspect of allergy prevention is needed before it can be generally recommended.

Will it get worse or better?

There are several different patterns with food allergy:
- Assuming they eat the same quantity of the food, most sufferers get the same degree of reaction—whether mild, moderate, or severe—every time.
- Some children grow out of their allergy eventually, especially if it is to milk (80 percent of babies with this problem grow out of it) or egg (50 percent grow out of it). Allergies to nuts and fish are more likely to persist (see box on p. 23). However, an aversion to the food may persist, quite understandably, due to the child's unpleasant and frightening early experiences of the food.
- A few sufferers experience mild reactions (for example, itching and tingling of the mouth) at first, but then go on to more and more severe reactions. The escalation can sometimes be very fast: it is even possible, though rare, to have fatal or near-fatal anaphylaxis with the second reaction to the allergenic food. For this reason, caution is always the best policy with food allergies.

One group of food allergy sufferers rarely gets any worse: those with **Oral Allergy Syndrome** (OAS). This is a tingling and itching sensation in the mouth on eating certain fruits and vegetables, caused by a **cross-reaction** from either pollen or latex (see box below). Oral Allergy Syndrome does not usually progress beyond mild reactions in the mouth. (What is more, simply cooking the fruit or vegetable substantially changes the characteristics of the allergen and this usually eliminates the reaction.)

However, there can also be severe anaphylactic reactions to some fruits and vegetables. This is particularly true of kiwi fruit (an increasingly common source of allergy), and celery. Severe reactions have also occurred with carrots, apples, plums, peaches, cherries, and apricots.

Pollen and food

Pollen is the primary sensitizer in many cases of Oral Allergy Syndrome. Birch pollen is a common offender, and the plant foods that cross-react with birch are very diverse, ranging from apples and cherries to spinach and carrots. Anyone allergic to ragweed pollen may have cross-reactions to melon, watermelon, chamomile, bananas, or sunflower seeds. *Artemisia* plants (common names include mugwort, wormwood, and sagebrush) produce pollen that can cross-react with celery, carrot, apple, spices, melon, and chamomile. Fortunately, these cross-reactions are usually very mild, but occasionally severe anaphylaxis can occur, as with a little boy allergic to mugwort pollen, who reacted to his first-ever cup of chamomile tea and almost died as a result.

Latex allergy, seen mostly in medical workers, can also generate cross-reactions to fruits and other foods (see p. 15).

Which foods can cause food allergy?

The range of foods that can cause food allergy is huge. But there is also a huge difference in the numbers of people affected—for every person allergic to garlic, fenugreek, or buckwheat, there are thousands allergic to cow's milk or peanuts.

This means that many doctors only come across patients who react to common food allergens. As a result, some nonspecialists may know little or nothing about the more exotic food allergies.

Why are certain foods more likely to elicit allergic reactions than others? In the case of cow's milk, the early exposure of the fetus to large doses of milk allergen (carried in the mother's bloodstream), followed by feeding with cow's milk formula, may make the development of allergic reactions more likely.

Frequency of eating the food also seems to have some influence. For example, rice allergy is very rare in Europe and North America, but frequently seen in Asia. In the Western world, the foods most likely to provoke IgE-mediated food allergy include several staples such as wheat, egg, milk, and, increasingly, soy (now widespread in processed food).

Finally some foods, such as peanuts, may behave like *agents provocateurs* and actually antagonize immune cells, so that IgE is produced rather than more innocuous antibodies (see p. 12). The same may be true of other nuts, sesame seeds, and poppy seeds. The frequency with which fish and shellfish provoke allergies is probably explained in a similar way.

Unusual forms of food allergy

"I visited friends one evening and they cooked moussaka. I enjoyed the meal, caught the train home, and went to bed," Chris recalls. "Then I awoke some time after midnight—about five hours after eating the meal—feeling ill. I vomited continuously until my stomach was completely empty and continued to retch even when there was nothing to bring up. During this violent retching, I lost control of my bladder. I ended up in an exhausted state, sitting on the bathroom floor, barely able to move. Eventually I crawled to my bed. I awoke a few hours later with bad diarrhea. No one else who had eaten the meal was ill. Then I recalled that the only time I had vomited before—in my adult life, at least—was after eating eggplants. They were something I never usually ate. I resolved to avoid them in future."

"Since then, I have been ill in this way three times, though never quite as badly. On each occasion, this has been some hours after a restaurant meal, and subsequent inquiries have revealed that the food did indeed contain some eggplant. The last time it happened, after I'd finished vomiting, I was aware of what felt like an enormous lump in my throat, making swallowing difficult. It was a bit frightening, as it appeared so suddenly. Swallowing was painful, and it took several days to subside. I have mentioned these incidents to my doctor, but I don't think he knows what I'm talking about. It was only from reading a book that I found out you can be allergic to the digestion products of certain foods."

For Chris, and others who react to a digestion product of the food rather than to the food itself, it may take many years to get an accurate diagnosis. Like all rare conditions, this one is very likely to be overlooked, misdiagnosed, or simply dismissed as "psychosomatic." This unusual form of food allergy seems to be particularly common with soy allergy.

Some people only react to their food allergen if they also exercise soon afterward—one form of exercise-induced anaphylaxis (see p. 59). An allergic reaction to food can also vary with emotional stress, alcohol, or a virus (viral) infection, but this is unusual.

Some people with food allergy do not react to the allergen when it is cooked. This happens frequently with fruits and vegetables, and occasionally with eggs, tuna, and salmon. Note that eggs must be very thoroughly cooked to become harmless). Much more rarely, cooking creates an allergen (see box on p. 186).

Most allergens are proteins, but a recent report describes allergy to a starch called inulin, found in Jerusalem artichokes. This starch is also widely used as an additive, and the unfortunate allergy sufferer had experienced reactions to a number of different foods, including margarine and desserts.

Diagnosis

Diagnosing true food allergy is usually very easy because the reaction is so prompt. Even so, your doctor will probably want to confirm your suspicions with skin-prick tests.

If you are extremely sensitive to your culprit food, you could experience an adverse reaction, even anaphylaxis, to a skin-prick test. There are no recorded fatalities, but caution is still advisable. Resuscitation equipment should be on hand. The test solution should be greatly diluted, not used at its normal strength.

Skin-prick tests always require some careful interpretation (see p. 91). A positive test does not necessarily mean that there is an allergic reaction on eating the food. In other words, the rate of **false positives** (see p. 91) is quite high.

Some allergists maintain that the rate of false negatives is, on the other hand, very low—so that a negative test result rules out the possibility of food allergy. This may be true for some allergens, such as peanut, but the picture is less clear for other allergens. Some doctors think that false negatives do occur reasonably often and they are concerned about patients being told, very firmly, that they are "not allergic" to a particular food, despite repeated bad experiences after eating it.

Not many people find themselves faced with this problem, so don't worry about it unless you have already had a negative skin-prick test. If you are in this situation, what do you do? The problem for the doctor is that some people do develop a psychological aversion to food that will produce exactly the same pattern—the patient says there are terrible symptoms from eating it, but the skin-prick tests are negative. The only way to show that this is not what's happening for you is to undergo a food challenge test, where you eat the food in a disguised form (a double-blind trial—see p. 90).

Diagnosing food allergy in babies

In contrast to food allergy in older children and adults, where symptoms usually affect the lips and mouth, the symptoms for babies tend to be in the lower parts of the digestive tract (vomiting and/or diarrhea—sometimes with blood and mucus). Atopic eczema may also be among the symptoms of true food allergy for some children (see p. 68).

Anaphylaxis is less common in babies than in older children or adults with food allergy, but it does sometimes occur.

The diarrhea produced by food allergy in babies can induce secondary lactase deficiency (see p. 79), which adds to the symptoms. Even when the allergen is removed from the diet, the secondary lactase deficiency may persist for a while, until the lining of the digestive tract recovers.

The allergen is usually cow's milk protein for bottle-fed babies. For those being breast-fed it may be any food that the mother is eating: tiny amounts get through into the milk. Common allergens such as cow's milk are the prime suspects.

For confirming true food allergy and identifying the culprit food, skin-prick tests may be useful in infancy, but there can be false negatives (a negative test despite a genuine reaction). False positives (a positive skin-prick test but no actual reaction to the food) are relatively rare in babies.

As a rule, the disease is more likely to be IgE-mediated if the symptoms occur very rapidly after a feed. It may help the doctor with the diagnosis if you have made a careful note of the timing of symptoms and any other details that seem relevant. Only IgE mediated allergies will give a positive skin-prick test.

Some babies with colitis (characterized by diarrhea with blood and mucus) are reacting to food. Such infants may be diagnosed as having **food-induced colitis.** This is a form of true food allergy, and skin-prick tests should show which foods are at fault. The colitis will probably clear up in time, but other classical allergic diseases, such as asthma, may follow.

Diagnosing food reactions in babies is especially difficult because there are so many different kinds of food sensitivity in this age-group—many of these are not true food allergy, but another kind of immune reaction (see pp. 68–73). Immune sensitivity to milk and soy proteins, causing vomiting and diarrhea, are common until age 2 or 3 (see protein enteropathy, p. 73). Often it is impossible to discover exactly what is going wrong, or to give the disease a name.

Alternative formula for babies

The ordinary brands of infant formula are made from cow's milk and will affect babies with any kind of sensitivity to cow's milk, including those who are unable to digest lactose (see p. 79). The alternative infant formulas described here are not only useful for babies with true food allergy, but also for those with other forms of sensitivity to cow's milk.

Many different types of alternative infant formulas are now available:

Lactose-free formula for those with lactase deficiency. Infant formula is also available that is both lactose-free *and* suitable for babies with cow's milk allergy—ask your pediatrician or pharmacist about this.

Soy-based formula, which often helps babies at first, but can create more problems in the long run because soya itself is a potential allergen. The parent of a child with soy allergy faces a lot of difficulties because soy creeps into just about everything these days—once the child is weaned, you will be slavishly reading labels and discovering that almost every ready-made packaged food is out of bounds. One of the other alternative formulas is therefore a better choice.

Hydrolysates, which are derived from cow's milk but with the proteins (i.e., the substances that provoke sensitivity reactions) partially broken down by a cunning processing technique that mimics digestion. The effect is to destroy most of the potential for provoking either allergy or other forms of immune sensitivity. However, small pieces of the cow's milk proteins do survive the processing, and the occasional baby will react to these because the piece that survives happens to contain the epitope (see box on p. 15) to which the baby is sensitized. A baby may react to one brand but be fine with another, so it is worth experimenting. Your pharmacist can show you various brands of hydrolysates.

Amino acid formula is the most drastic of the alternatives. Rather than taking cow's milk proteins and breaking them down, the approach here is to take the constituents of the proteins—amino acids—and mix them up in the right proportions to get the nutritional equivalent. Amino acids are too small to evoke a reaction from the immune system, so these really are foolproof, unlike hydrolysates. Unfortunately, some of the amino acids taste diabolical, so this is the least palatable option. Amino acid formulas are sold under various brand names.

These alternative infant formulas can be used for both diagnosis and treatment. If there is some doubt about the existence of the sensitivity to cow's milk, your doctor might prescribe one for a while, just to see what happens. Ask to try a second brand if the first does not help your baby.

Treatment
Emergency treatment

For first-aid treatment of anaphylaxis, see p. 98. Remember that emergency hospital treatment is also vital, even if injectable adrenaline is available and has been given.

Just occasionally, a severe allergic reaction to food can appear to be over, but the symptoms then recur between four and eight hours later. This is called **biphasic anaphylaxis** and you should be kept in hospital for several hours in case it happens. Some deaths have occured when people were sent home prematurely.

Routine treatment

Food allergy can only be treated at present by strict food avoidance—and strict means *strict* here (see pp. 110–11). This really could be life or death.

For a few very sensitive individuals with food allergy, even inhaling airborne molecules of the food is sufficient to spark a reaction. Someone opening a jar of peanut butter nearby, or a package of peanuts, can do it for those with peanut allergy. So can the smell in a fish market, or the cooking fumes from fish or vegetables for those with the appropriate sensitivity. This can be alarming, but be reassured by the fact that no fatal reactions have ever been recorded from airborne food.

If you have ever suffered a systemic reaction (anaphylaxis—see p. 58) or have been diagnosed as being potentially anaphylactic, you should be carrying injectable epinephrine (see p. 150) for emergency use, when the offending food is eaten by mistake. Make sure you get this *and that you know how to use it properly*—one Canadian study has shown that the training given by some doctors and other professionals is far from adequate (see p. 150).

An epinephrine inhaler, available in the U.S. only, may be useful for those whose throat swells, or who also have asthma as well as systemic reactions to food—they should use it *in addition to* an epinephrine injector (see p. 98).

Conventional immunotherapy (allergy shots—see pp. 164–9) is not used at present for food allergy, mainly because of the risk of an anaphylactic reaction during the treatment. The protection given is also far from certain, and there is concern about giving sufferers a sense of false security.

All this may soon change, as new vaccine-type treatments, using modified food allergens, become available. These are intended to produce good tolerance of the allergen without serious risk of anaphylaxis during treatment (see p. 169).

Drug treatment offers limited protection in true food allergy, unfortunately. Although sodium cromoglycate, which blocks the degranulation of mast cells, may reduce sensitivity, the risks of it not working when needed far outweigh the advantages.

The exceptions to this rule are those difficult cases involving multiple nonanaphylactic IgE-mediated food allergies and delayed reactions such as diarrhea (which may be reactions to digestion products of the food—see p. 64). For anyone with problems of this type, life can be tough, especially if new allergies develop at regular intervals. The symptoms can sometimes be eased, and the rate of development of new allergies reduced, with the judicious use of sodium cromoglycate (see p. 148). Careful food avoidance is still needed, but the reactions to accidental ingestion are less severe. Some people who suffer with this type of problem also seem to benefit from treatment to improve the balance of the gut flora (see pp. 204–5), but there is no strong evidence to support this.

Mimicking food allergy

Two different conditions produce symptoms that look just like true food allergy: false food allergy and histamine poisoning.

False food allergy involves mast cells but is produced without any allergic reaction (that is, without the involvement of the allergy antibody, IgE). It is due to substances found naturally in foods that can trigger mast cells directly.

Some of these substances bind to the IgE receptors on the surface of the mast cell, so cross-linking the receptors and making the mast cells degranulate (see box on p. 12)—it is the immune equivalent of picking a lock.

The symptoms of false food allergy are indistinguishable from true food allergy because the same basic mechanism—release of histamine by mast cells—is involved. However, it is unknown for this reaction to be fatal. False food allergy is generally regarded as less common than food allergy itself.

Some people are far more susceptible to false food allergy than others, for reasons that are not yet understood. As regards diagnosis, skin-prick tests are usually positive, but do not distinguish false food allergy from true IgE-mediated food allergy. A modified form of the RAST (a blood test—see p. 92) can distinguish the two.

Food avoidance is the only treatment. The usual culprits are beans, strawberries, tomatoes, fish, pork, chocolate, egg white, and tartrazine (a food additive used for its yellow color). Pineapple and papaya, which contain powerful protein-digesting enzymes, may also trigger mast cells directly.

Histamine poisoning is another reaction that can resemble a true allergy to food. Fish such as mackerel and tuna, if stored badly before eating (or before canning), can have a very high histamine content, due to bacterial action. Histamine is histamine, whether it comes from a mast cell (see box on p. 12) or is consumed with food, so the fish evokes a severe and unpleasant reaction. This is referred to as **anaphylactoid shock**, to distinguish it from true anaphylactic shock (see box on p. 59). It can be fatal, so watch out for fish that looks slightly discolored and has a sharp, peppery, or metallic taste. If you've only eaten a mouthful, you should be fine—it's the quantity consumed that counts here.

Other foods, such as well-ripened cheeses, also contain histamine, but in much smaller amounts. Most people can happily eat such foods, detoxifying the histamine in the liver. A few people seem to lack this power to break histamine down and may be badly affected by these foods. Sometimes this can cause chronic urticaria or other symptoms. A low-histamine diet may be worth trying (see p. 200).

Food sensitivity
IN ASTHMA, ECZEMA, AND OTHER ALLERGIC DISEASES

In 1995, medical researchers in North Carolina asked over a hundred dermatologists how they treated atopic eczema. All used standard treatments such as moisturizers and steroid creams, but only 14 percent mentioned the possible role of food to the parents of children with eczema.

Between them, the dermatologists in this study treated about 17,000 children with atopic eczema per year. Using the most widely accepted estimates for food sensitivity in atopic eczema—38 percent of eczematous children are sensitive to food—one can calculate that there were over 5,000 children in this study area who might perhaps have benefited from avoiding a problem food, but whose parents were never told about this treatment option.

North Carolina is by no means unique. The situation is much the same in other parts of the world, which adds up to *millions* of children and parents not even being told about a treatment that is frequently effective.

Other allergic diseases can also be triggered by food, although the percentage of patients affected is much lower than for atopic eczema. Here too, many doctors are unaware of (or skeptical about) the possible role of food.

These reactions are best described as "food sensitivity." They cannot be called food allergy (see p. 62) if there are no symptoms in the mouth or gut and if skin-prick tests are negative—as is often the case. Negative skin tests suggest that the reaction is not IgE-mediated (see box on p. 121).

However, in some children with atopic eczema, the skin-prick tests to culprit foods are positive. When these foods are eaten after a period of avoidance, such children sometimes suffer an immediate reaction, with symptoms typical of true food allergy. For these individuals, their atopic eczema seems to be a symptom of IgE-mediated food allergy.

How can an atopic eczema reaction in response to food be IgE-mediated in one individual and not in another? Research is finally beginning to answer this question (see pp. 18–19).

The allergic conditions that may sometimes be induced, or simply aggravated, by a *non-immediate* reaction to food are:

- atopic eczema (atopic dermatitis)
- asthma
- perennial allergic rhinitis (constantly blocked or runny nose)
- chronic sinusitis
- secretory otitis media ("glue ear")

In all of these conditions, many other causes exist. Except in the case of eczema, *the other causes are far more likely* than sensitivity to food. This fact will weigh heavily with your doctor, whose instinct, quite sensibly, is to look for likely causes first.

Taking asthma as an example, food sensitivity is relatively unusual as a primary cause, whereas allergy to airborne items, such as pollen or dust mite, is very common. Food probably affects only 8–10 percent of asthmatics overall, but is much more important for those with brittle asthma (the most severe and unstable form), affecting as many as 60 percent, in a recent study.

The pollen connection

People who suffer from both birch-pollen allergy and atopic eczema may have worsening eczema when they eat certain fruits and vegetables, e.g., apples and carrots. These same foods cause Oral Allergy Syndrome (see box on p. 63) in some with birch-pollen hay fever, but they can aggravate eczema *without* causing Oral Allergy Syndrome.

Diagnosis

Consider other likely allergens first. Look at p. 28 for the airborne allergens that could play a part in perennial allergic rhinitis, chronic sinusitis, secretory otitis media ("glue ear"), and asthma. Only in the case of children with atopic eczema is food a prime suspect (between 38 percent and 69 percent of children with atopic eczema are affected by food), but even here there are a lot of other factors to consider (see pp. 43-4).

If you do decide to investigate the role of food, don't abandon basic treatments in the meantime. By neglecting these, you could make the whole problem a great deal worse.

There are various clues that food is at fault:

- If you have other symptoms that suggest food intolerance (see p. 76). These problems often seem to go together with food-induced asthma or rhinitis.
- If you have noticed that a particular food makes your symptoms worse. Where there is intolerance to one food, there could well be intolerance to another, which you have not noticed.
- If you have exercise-induced asthma (see p. 41) and sometimes respond severely to exercise but sometimes have little or no reaction. Sensitivity to a food or foods may be instrumental in changing the response to exercise.
- If you have brittle asthma—but you must get your doctor's consent for an elimination diet. *Foods must be tested under medical supervision as severe life-threatening asthmatic reactions can occur on testing.*
- If there are also digestive problems such as diarrhea, vomiting, or belching. This is a strong clue in the case of children with atopic eczema. Symptoms such as diarrhea frequently *precede* atopic eczema, and it seems likely that a reaction to food in the gut increases the leakiness of the gut wall, allowing more food molecules through to the blood.
- If there is pronounced eczema around the mouth in children (but this can also be due to constant licking, or irritation by acidic or spicy foods touching the skin).
- For adults with atopic eczema, if there is a persistent rash on the hands, or the lips. Where there is a blistering rash on the hands that erupts at regular intervals, food may be the problem—or it may be metal contaminants of food such as nickel (see p. 55). In general, food sensitivity is rarer among adults with atopic eczema than it is among children.

Prick-puncture tests (see p. 91) for commonly eaten foods are worth trying in all the diseases—a positive result should be noted, but a negative one does not necessarily mean that food is inno-

cent—it could be the cause of a reaction with a non IgE-mediated mechanism. The many alternative tests being marketed (see p. 93) are highly inaccurate and unlikely to help.

Research from Tampere University Hospital, in Finland, suggests that babies are much more likely to give false-negative prick tests for food than older children and adults with atopic eczema. The Finnish researchers found that 52 percent of babies with atopic eczema give a negative skin-prick test despite having a genuine reaction when tested by food challenge. In an attempt to tackle this problem, they have devised a patch test, similar to those used for contact dermatitis. The patch test, in which food is applied to intact skin and left there for two days, gives false negatives in only 39 percent of babies.

The best way to detect food-sensitive eczema, according to Dr. Erika Isolauri, who heads the Finnish research team, is to use both tests, and take note of a positive reaction to either. This combined approach detects 80–90 percent of eczema-causing food reactions in infants.

Few other doctors are currently using patch tests for atopic eczema, because so much controversy surrounds this topic, and no standardized method has yet been devised.

To confirm the role of particular foods in atopic eczema, a food challenge test is essential, having first avoided the food carefully for two weeks. Great care is needed in testing (see p. 198).

If you cannot get suitable tests done, a simple elimination diet will be needed (see p. 198).

Treatment

There is a choice here, between avoiding the offending food or eating normally and controlling the symptoms with drugs.

The difficulty comes when parents have to make this decision on behalf of their children. Unfortunately, there is insufficient evidence as regards the consequences of this decision. Treating food sensitivity can reduce the eczema symptoms substantially in the short term, but it does not necessarily improve the long-term prospects for the child.

Mainstream doctors tend to think that eating a normal diet is much better for a child nutritionally and socially.

Doctors with a special interest in food sensitivity generally believe that treating the problem at source, rather than just suppressing the symptoms with drugs, must take the pressure off the child's immune system and give the child a better chance of growing out of sensitivity reactions in the long run.

The decision is yours—but it is vital that the diet is not more of an encumbrance than the disease itself and that the child's interests come first (see pp. 170–71). Whatever you do, don't allow a child to become malnourished (see p. 198).

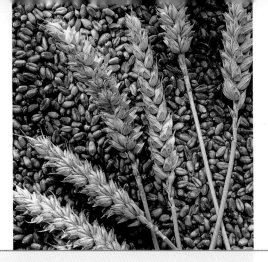

Celiac disease

During World War II, there was no bread to be had in the Netherlands and people were forced to eat tulip bulbs. "My mother roasted them," one survivor recalls, "and they tasted delicious then, because we were so hungry I suppose. I cooked some years later, just to taste them again, and they were absolutely disgusting."

While most of the population was thin and unwell on this starvation diet, a few children were actually healthier than before. An observant Dutch doctor noted that these were the children who, before the war, had suffered from constant diarrhea, fatigue, poor growth, and muscle wasting. They were suddenly stronger and, his inquiries revealed, their diarrhea had vanished. But when the food situation improved at the end of the war, all their old problems returned. By carefully experimenting with the diet of these patients, the doctor discovered that eating wheat and rye caused the symptoms. Subsequent research has revealed that both contain a collection of proteins, referred to as **gluten**, which are the source of celiac disease.

Belly disease

Celiac disease is an old name that simply means "belly disease." It is derived from the Greek word for "belly" *koilia*. Once the cause of the symptoms became understood, a new name was devised—**gluten-sensitivity enteropathy**—but it has not really caught on. Other terms that you may come across are **nontropical sprue** and **celiac sprue**, based on the close resemblance of the symptoms to those of tropical sprue. This disease, found in those who live or have lived in the tropics, is probably caused by bacterial infection. There is no causal link with celiac disease.

Symptoms

The symptoms of celiac disease are:

- Diarrhea, with pale, bad-smelling stools
- In a few patients, constipation rather than diarrhea, but this is very rare.
- Bloating and gas
- Damage to the lining of the intestine. This is of a characteristic type: the complex folded structures (the **villi**) of the intestinal lining are destroyed. Additionally, huge numbers of immune cells are present.
- The loss of the villi results in failure to absorb nutrients from food (**malabsorption**) causing poor growth in babies, and weakness and weight loss in adults.
- Poor appetite, especially in babies. This can greatly reduce the diarrhea.

Celiac disease usually appears in babies during weaning, a few weeks after cereals are introduced, but it can also begin for the first time in adults. The tendency to celiac disease is genetically inherited, so it runs in families.

Where celiac disease runs in the family, another disease, **dermatitis herpetiformis**, is also likely to occur. Dermatitis herpetiformis has the same basic mechanism as celiac disease but very different symptoms:

- An intensely itchy rash, sometimes with tiny blisters; the rash is symmetrically distributed on the buttocks, shoulders, scalp, and the outer surfaces of the knees and elbows
- The same characteristic damage to the lining of the intestine as seen in tests for celiac disease, though generally less severe
- Diarrhea, in some cases, but not all

About 5 percent of those with celiac disease actually go on to develop dermatitis herpetiformis. Most people have either one or the other.

Both diseases are caused by the same gene, which results in sufferers developing antibodies against one of their own proteins, an enzyme called tissue-transglutaminase. The job of this enzyme, which is found in the intestines, is to assist with the breakdown of gluten.

If no gluten is present, the enzyme does not arouse the interest of the immune system. It is the process of gluten digestion, in which a particular peptide is produced from gluten, that provokes the autoimmune reaction. (A **peptide** is any short length of protein chain, obtained from the complete protein chain by digestion.)

What seems to trigger the autoimmune reaction is this enzyme-peptide combination: the offending peptide, newly produced and still attached physically to the enzyme. There is something about the particular "chemical picture" that this combination makes which outrages the immune system of individuals with a particular genetic makeup.

The impact of this autoimmune reaction on the intestinal lining is severe in celiac disease, less so in dermatitis herpetiformis. What causes dermatitis herpetiformis is a particular type of antibody, called dimeric IgA, which is transported by the bloodstream from the gut to the skin. It is deposited in the skin all over the body, but for some reason only provokes inflammation in certain areas.

In rare cases, an IgE-mediated food allergy to wheat can coexist with celiac disease, making reactions more severe.

Secondary problems

Paradoxically, while the damaged gut lining of untreated celiac disease makes a poor job of absorbing specific nutrients (iron and vitamins, for example) in a form that the body can use, it also lets through far more intact, or partially digested, food molecules. These get into the bloodstream in such numbers that they can lead to idiopathic food intolerance (see p. 74). Sensitivity to soy is a common problem, because it is so heavily used in gluten-free bread and other prepared food. Those with celiac disease who have not improved fully, despite a strict gluten-free diet, often benefit from an elimination diet (see p. 194). This must be done under medical supervision.

Another possible effect of the intestinal damage is lactose intolerance (see p. 79), producing a sensitivity to milk.

The frequency of schizophrenia is higher among those with celiac disease than among the general population (and see p. 81). Celiacs not following a strict gluten-free diet are also vulnerable to other psychological problems. These might be linked to the effects of food-derived exorphins (see pp. 76–77) and other peptides on the brain. The increased permeability of the gut could play a part in this, allowing more exorphins to reach the bloodstream.

Diagnosis

A biopsy (see p. 92) is the only really reliable form of diagnosis. ***It is crucial that this is done before removing gluten from the diet,*** because the damage is repaired if gluten is avoided and the healing process is fairly rapid for some people (though in others it takes many months). If the intestinal lining reverts to a normal appearance quite quickly, an accurate diagnosis is never obtained, which can have serious consequences: if you or your child are celiac, you need to know.

New blood tests can also be helpful in diagnosis, but they do not give the unequivocal result obtained with a biopsy.

U.S. research suggests that celiac disease is under-diagnosed in some countries compared to others—for example, Italy screens children routinely but the U.S. does not. Some authorities suspect that there is a great deal of "hidden" celiac disease in the U.S. and this could be true in other countries as well.

The symptoms of celiac disease are not always distinctive. Many cases are first detected when patients with rather nonspecific symptoms are discovered, by a blood test, to be anemic.

Treatment

There are no drug treatments for celiac disease and avoiding gluten religiously is the only way to remain well. Those who are lax about their gluten-free diet may be more vulnerable to certain cancers of the digestive tract.

A strict gluten-free diet is not easy to follow (see p. 177). The most severely affected celiacs are so sensitive to gluten that they react violently to even a tiny amount: this is known as **celiac shock** and can be fatal.

A gluten-free diet is also the treatment for dermatitis herpetiformis, but at the outset the rash can be controlled with the highly effective drug, dapsone.

Other immune reactions to food

"When I finally found someone who could say what was wrong with me, it was such a relief. I can't tell you how much ill-health and pain and misery I'd had up to that point. I'm immensely grateful to the doctor who sorted the problem out for me. My life has been transformed."

Richard has eosinophilic gastroenteritis, one of the rarer immune reactions to food. Like all rare diseases, it can escape diagnosis for a long time. IgE (the allergy antibody—see box on p. 12) is sometimes involved in eosinophilic gastroenteritis, but it is not an essential part of the reaction. Those who, like Richard, do not make IgE antibodies to the problem food will not give positive skin-prick tests. For them, the possibility of food being responsible for their symptoms may well be overlooked.

Another difficulty for patients such as Richard is that most of the non-IgE immune reactions to food (other than celiac disease) affect babies and children only. A few of them can also occur in adults but this is very rare, so it's not something that automatically springs to mind when the doctor is searching for a diagnosis.

Eosinophilic diseases

The key event in these diseases is the arrival of large numbers of immune cells called eosinophils (see p. 19) in the walls of the digestive system. If the eosinophils converge on the tube leading down to the stomach (the esophagus), the disease is called **eosinophilic esophagitis**, and the symptoms include reflux (regurgitation) of food, occasional vomiting, refusing food (in babies), stomach pain, and disturbed sleep.

If the stomach is the focus for the eosinophils, this is **eosinophilic gastritis**, and there is vomiting, pain, poor appetite, and therefore poor growth. There can also be obstruction of the stomach outlet, which may, in a few babies, produce pyloric stenosis (the main symptom is projectile vomiting).

When eosinophils flock to the intestines as well as to the stomach, the disease is called **eosinophilic gastroenteritis**. In terms of symptoms, the picture is not much different from the previous condition, but there can be diarrhea as an additional symptom, and babies may be irritable and puffy in appearance.

These conditions are most common in babies, but sometimes they continue through childhood. Only eosinophilic gastroenteritis is known to occur in adults too.

Heiner's syndrome

This disease affects babies only and is very rare. It is a severe form of cow's milk sensitivity leading to wheezing and hemosiderosis (bleeding into the lungs). The child usually seems sickly, growth is slow, and there may be recurrent bouts of pneumonia. A full diagnosis requires blood tests to check for anemia and antibodies to milk, examination of sputum under the microscope, and a biopsy or lavage (see p. 92) from the lung. The only effective treatment is to completely remove cow's milk from the diet. Needless to say, this must be done under full medical supervision.

Other reactions to food

The cause of these diseases is not fully understood, but the immune system is clearly involved.

Dietary protein enterocolitis syndrome

In babies, the symptoms begin with general irritability and vomiting between one and three hours after a feeding. Unless the offending food—usually cow's milk—is withdrawn promptly, there will be bloating, diarrhea (usually containing blood), anemia, and poor growth. Older children have similar symptoms, while adults suffer terrible nausea, plus stomach pains and vomiting.

Nickel in food
Nickel and other metals in food may cause immune reactions for those with sensitivity to such metals (see p. 55). The symptoms are usually in the skin, but there can be a few digestive symptoms too.

Dietary protein enteropathy
Cow's milk and soy protein are the most common causes, and some babies are sensitive to both. The main symptoms are diarrhea and cramps, usually very severe. This reaction is often delayed, beginning 12–24 hours, or even days, after ingestion. Some babies vomit their feeding as well. Most have little appetite, and if the offending food is not withdrawn, they suffer from poor growth, anemia, and other signs of malnutrition. This is because damage to the lining of the gut prevents nutrients from being absorbed properly. Older children show similar symptoms, but the condition often remits by ages 2–3.

Dietary protein proctitis
This is a far less severe problem. The babies with this disorder look healthy, but there is inflammation in the bowel and small amounts of blood are passed with the feces.

Diagnosis
There are two aspects to diagnosis. First, what kind of disease is it? Second, what food or foods are causing the reaction? Your doctor will probably try to answer the first question by looking inside the digestive tract with special equipment (endoscopy) and by taking a small sample—a biopsy (see p. 92).

A blood sample may also be taken to look for raised levels of immune cells and antibodies. Skin tests or RAST tests (see pp. 91–2) will be tried to rule out the possibility of true food allergy—and because IgE can play a small part in these other forms of food sensitivity (as in the eosinophilic diseases, for example).

Often the tests yield no very clear answers, especially in babies, and an exact diagnosis is not possible. But failure to answer the first question does not mean that the second question should be ignored. Pinpointing the culprit food or foods is vital.

Identifying the food is easier the younger the child, simply because the range of foods eaten is so much smaller. Cow's milk is the most common offender when the disease affects young children—particularly bottle-fed babies, since standard infant formula is made with cow's milk. Your doctor will prescribe an alternative formula (see box on p. 66) for you to try. For older children and adults, an elimination diet will probably be required to identify the food concerned. Among young children, likely offenders include soy, egg, wheat, rice, chicken, or fish. A simple elimination diet, similar to that used for atopic eczema (see p. 198) may be adequate. You must have full medical supervision for this.

In the case of eosinophilic reactions, skin-prick tests may help identify the foods concerned, but are usually of limited value, so an elimination diet is again necessary. Where adults are affected by eosinophilic diseases, sensitivity to several different foods is likely, so identifying the offending foods usually requires the most exacting form of elimination diet, using an elemental diet for the exclusion phase (see box on p. 196). The symptoms are very slow to disappear: it can take up to 8 weeks of avoiding the foods.

Treatment
Avoidance is the only way here. Special infant formula (see box on p. 66) is required for cow's milk sensitivity in babies.

In the case of eosinophilic reactions, some doctors may use steroid tablets as an additional treatment, just for a few weeks, to get the inflammation under control.

Controversial topics
According to some doctors, a reaction to food may, on rare occasions, produce **vasculitis** (inflammation of the blood vessels).

Vasculitis itself is a well-recognized condition. The blood vessels are damaged by inflammation and become more leaky. Symptoms often begin with a general swelling (angioedema) and an outbreak of small red blotches deep in the skin—especially on the legs—where small amounts of blood have escaped. These blotches later turn purplish, then yellow, before fading. This type of rash is known as **purpura**. Sometimes there are larger emissions of blood, resulting in spontaneous bruising.

Many different medical conditions can cause vasculitis, but few doctors would agree that food sensitivity is one of them. Those who believe in the existence of food-induced vasculitis suggest that the inflammation could be caused by circulating immune complexes containing food antigens bound to antibodies (see p. 13).

Equally controversial is the suggestion that food sensitivity can be the cause of trouble for some children with kidney disorders. Some research groups have found that a few children with certain kinds of kidney disease recover on an elemental diet (see box on p. 196). All those affected have a classical allergic disease such as asthma or atopic eczema as well, and they tend to be sensitive to several different foods, plus pollen or other airborne allergens. Circulating immune complexes might be involved here, but no one is sure at present.

Some cases of food-related rheumatoid arthritis and palindromic rheumatism (see p. 76) could be due to immune complexes involving food molecules becoming deposited in the joints, but it is not the mechanism in all, or even most, of those affected.

Food intolerance

The comments of those who have recovered from food intolerance after many years of ill-health are always memorable. "It's like getting my life back again," said one woman. "I had actually forgotten what it felt like to be well," said another, "the effect of cutting out certain foods was just amazing."

For most of those with food intolerance, the disease begins very subtly and gradually—first one symptom (persistent and unexplained diarrhea, perhaps), then, some years later, another (migraine or headaches), and then, when a few more years have passed, another symptom (such as joint pain or muscle aches). Steadily increasing levels of irritability, "fuzzy-headedness" or inexplicable tiredness may accompany this decline in health.

Most patients have no idea that all these symptoms are connected until they try an elimination diet, and everything clears up at once, quite dramatically. As one former sufferer described it: "Some of the stuff that got better—well, I'd been like that so long I thought it was just the way I was—grumpy and exhausted, and feeling terrible if I didn't eat meals on time. It was an absolute revelation to feel completely OK again."

What does "food intolerance" mean?

In this book, **food intolerance** means any reaction to food where the immune system has no proven central role.

All the people whose comments are quoted above have **idiopathic food intolerance**, which means *food intolerance with no established mechanism*—in other words, doctors can't say exactly how it is caused. This is a highly controversial area.

The definition of food intolerance used in this book means that it also includes **metabolic abnormalities**, which have a well-established cause. These are due to defective enzymes (see upper box on p. 75).

The question of what words mean is a key part of the debate over idiopathic food intolerance. At one extreme, you may come across doctors who call this problem "food allergy," using the original meaning of the word "allergy" (see p. 6). (Some of these doctors use terms such as **delayed food allergy** and **masked food allergy**, to point up the distinction from true food allergy, but not all do.) Using the word "allergy" in this context causes a lot of aggravation and confusion, so the term "food intolerance" has, for a long time, been widely accepted as a useful one that avoids unnecessary conflict.

You will also hear the term "food intolerance" used to mean idiopathic food intolerance only—this is probably the most common usage. When the term is used in this way, metabolic abnormalities are being thought of as a separate entity altogether.

In the medical wilderness

The main text of this article is about idiopathic food intolerance, a disease with a distinctly dubious reputation among doctors. Because it is so controversial, few doctors actually look at the evidence that it exists—which is in fact quite strong (see box on p. 77). Such evidence is simply ignored in most of what is written by the major medical organizations debunking idiopathic food intolerance.

Failure to recognize the existence of idiopathic food intolerance also plays into the hands of those offering bogus diagnostic tests and phoney treatments, often at a very high price. These practitioners—who have moved in to fill the gap left by conventional medicine—are a considerable part of the problem, helping to give idiopathic food intolerance a bad name.

The waters are muddied even more by the fact that some people who believe themselves to have food intolerance are actually suffering from psychological problems, which they prefer to attribute to food. Such patients are a good source of revenue for the less scrupulous fringe practitioners and are unlikely, therefore, to be discouraged from their beliefs.

Fortunately there are enough conventional but open-minded family doctors who have come to realize, through experience with their own patients, that elimination diets have a remarkable curative effect for some people. The ones who benefit are often the doctor's "old faithfuls"—those with long-term multiple symptoms, who have been referred to innumerable specialists and treated with all kinds of drugs, but who never get much better. The conventional view of such patients is that they have psychological problems that are being expressed as physical symptoms. This may well be true for some of them—but others have idiopathic food intolerance.

The major issue now, in relation to idiopathic food intolerance, is the frequency with which it occurs. Is it just the occasional patient who suffers from this problem, or is it a common disorder that goes undiagnosed?

One of our enzymes is missing

Metabolic abnormalities are a distinct type of food intolerance. Unlike other kinds of food intolerance, metabolic abnormalities have a clearly understood cause: an enzyme that carries out a crucial task in the body's metabolism is either missing or inept. The problem is generally caused by a defective gene and is therefore inherited.

The most common metabolic abnormality is **lactase deficiency** leading to lactose intolerance (see p. 79)—this may or may not be inherited. Other metabolic abnormalities include:

trehalase deficiency, lack of the enzyme that breaks down a substance in mushrooms and most other fungi, including yeast.

galactosemia, a defect in the enzyme that processes galactose, one of the sugars found in milk (cow's or human). This is a serious disease and sufferers must avoid milk scrupulously.

fructose intolerance, which is extremely rare. Those affected have an unpleasant taste in the mouth on eating fruit and other sources of fructose, so avoidance is no particular problem.

phenylketonuria, also very rare. Those affected are usually identified early in life, by a routine blood test.

Is it just placebo effect?

Doctors who doubt the very existence of idiopathic food intolerance will say that people who recover on an elimination diet are just experiencing **placebo effect**—a psychological response that operates with any treatment, whether effective or ineffective, simply because people believe that the treatment will work. But this is to ignore certain facts:

• Placebo effect produces a fairly small improvement in most people—you have to be very suggestible to feel enormously better. By contrast, when people respond to an elimination diet (the standard method for diagnosing idiopathic food intolerance, see p. 194), they usually have a sudden and dramatic improvement.

• Most of those with idiopathic food intolerance have had it for years and tried all sorts of treatments. They have often experienced some small benefit from these, probably placebo effect. When they try an elimination diet, they have a response that is in a completely different league.

• The idea that all the different symptoms are linked has never occurred to many people who try an elimination diet—they are often trying it for just one symptom and are staggered when everything clears up. Placebo effect relies on expectation.

• Placebo effect doesn't last very long—it fades over the ensuing weeks and months. Avoiding the culprit food usually produces a lasting improvement for those with idiopathic food intolerance.

Symptoms

The symptoms of idiopathic food intolerance come on slowly after eating the offending food, and the foods to blame are often those eaten very regularly, such as wheat or milk. Consequently, the symptoms from one meal tend to overlap with those from the previous meal, and people with idiopathic food intolerance are more or less unwell for most of the time. It is usually not obvious that food is at fault.

All the symptoms of idiopathic food intolerance are common ones that can be caused in other ways. And no two patients have exactly the same set of symptoms, which makes both diagnosis, and a clear definition of the disorder, very difficult.

These are some of the symptoms commonly reported:
- headache or migraine
- diarrhea, sometimes with bloating and wind; this is often diagnosed as irritable bowel syndrome (IBS)
- in children, stomachaches
- occasionally constipation
- nausea and indigestion
- joint pain
- aching muscles
- a constantly runny or blocked nose (this could be perennial allergic rhinitis linked to food—see p. 68)
- glue ear (see p. 29)
- fatigue and a general feeling of vague ill-health

Asthma and eczema, triggered by specific foods (see p. 68), can also be part of the picture.

In babies, colic may be caused by food intolerance, including foods the mother is eating that come through into the breast milk in tiny amounts (see p. 202).

Less common symptoms include:
- recurrent mouth ulcers
- stomach or duodenal ulcers
- chronic urticaria (see pp. 50–53)
- swelling (angioedema)

The following diseases have also been linked to idiopathic food intolerance in some patients:
- Crohn's disease
- palindromic rheumatism (intermittent episodes of joint inflammation)
- rheumatoid arthritis

Psychological problems such as depression, anxiety, or hyperactivity in children can sometimes be due to food (see p. 80), but it is rare for such psychological effects to occur without any physical symptoms.

Remember that every single one of these symptoms and conditions can be caused in some other way. However, the constellation of migraine/headache, joint pain, and diarrhea is highly characteristic of idiopathic food intolerance.

How might intolerance be caused?

No one knows how idiopathic food intolerance is caused. There are probably many factors involved, with a slightly different mix of factors in each patient. This would help to explain why the symptoms are so extraordinarily varied, with no two sufferers exactly alike.

Although symptoms accumulate over the years, some people can in fact pinpoint the moment when their problems began. "I had this terrible bout of diarrhea from eating too much melon. I lived near a farm and they were free, because of a glut, so I just gorged myself on them. Although I was over the diarrhea in a couple of days, I was never what you'd call 'regular' after that, and the least thing would upset me. Eventually the doctor said it was irritable bowel syndrome. When the other problems began, ages afterward—headaches and hypoglycemia and fatigue—it seemed like something quite separate. I never associated them in my mind with the diarrhea."

Bad diarrhea can clear the intestines of their beneficial bacteria, known collectively as the **gut flora** (see p. 204), and this is probably what initiates food intolerance in such cases. Large doses of antibiotics (as are sometimes given before an operation, for example, a hysterectomy), or prolonged and repeated courses of antibiotics, given for glue ear or acne, can also disrupt the gut flora and lead to food intolerance. A study of hysterectomy patients has shown that antibiotic treatment before the operation tends to result in irritable bowel syndrome—a common symptom of idiopathic food intolerance—afterward.

A few interesting observations suggest that minor metabolic abnormalities—a defect in certain detoxification enzymes—may sometimes play a part in idiopathic food intolerance. This is especially likely where there is intolerance to food additives, or where there are behavioral symptoms (such as hyperactivity) or symptoms involving the nervous system (such as migraine).

A third factor that could play a part for some patients are **food-derived exorphins**. These are fragments of proteins (called **peptides**) produced by the digestion of food proteins. They happen, probably by pure coincidence, to resemble the substances called **endorphins** that we all produce for ourselves. Endorphins are our internal painkillers. They modify nerve impulses in the body and brain, reducing sensations of pain and improving the sense of well-being. The receptors to which they bind are the same receptors that bind morphine and heroin—it is the intensive stimulation of these receptors that makes these drugs so effective.

Food-derived exorphins may sound like the stuff of science fiction, but they have actually been demonstrated in the digestion products of wheat and milk. They may exist for other foods as well. They are nowhere near as strong as morphine, but do seem to improve mood.

These exorphins may explain the strange observation that patients with idiopathic food intolerance often eat huge amounts of their offending food, and "can't live without it." Often they eat the food several times a day, sometimes at every meal. With a ubiquitous ingredient like wheat or milk, this is not particularly difficult—wheat cereal and milk for breakfast, a cheese sandwich at lunchtime, pasta with a creamy sauce for supper, a milky drink and biscuits at bedtime.

Any of these abnormalities is likely to be just one factor in a multifactorial disease.

Diagnosis

Unfortunately there are no simple accurate tests for idiopathic food intolerance. The kind of tests you may see offered commercially (in advertisements in health magazines for example) are very inaccurate and a waste of money. Consequently, the only way to diagnose idiopathic food intolerance is through an elimination diet, in which you cut out all the foods you commonly eat and then—if you get better—test them one by one.

It sounds easy but it isn't, so make sure you read all the instructions for doing the diet before you start (see pp. 194–7). You should also see your doctor and get his or her approval. Some symptoms—such as severe diarrhea or headaches—should be investigated by conventional methods first, in case there is some serious underlying cause.

The first step in diagnosis is to decide if a food really is the cause of the symptoms, and the second step is to identify the food or foods concerned.

The first step is crucial. One of the problems with the diagnostic tests that are advertised—such as those using samples of hair or blood—is that they begin with the second step. In other words they assume that food is the problem (see p. 93).

When it comes to the second step, remember that although common foods are often the culprits, almost anything that is eaten can cause idiopathic food intolerance. Every patient with this problem is different in the foods they react to.

Treatment

Avoidance of the food is usually the best treatment for idiopathic food intolerance—however most people do not have to avoid their problem foods for ever. After a while—it could be six months or it could be three years—you can usually go back to eating it again, but in moderation. You must never start eating the food in large amounts again, and it is best not to eat it every day—certainly not at almost every meal, which is the usual pattern for cow's milk and wheat in the Western diet.

The patients who should avoid the culprit food indefinitely are those with Crohn's disease and rheumatoid arthritis: a severe and irreversible relapse can occur otherwise.

The evidence

The evidence for idiopathic food intolerance is more substantial than its opponents would have you believe.

One very well conducted and interesting study involved children with severe migraine who were investigated by a research team at Great Ormond Street Hospital in London. These are children who are very difficult to treat successfully by normal means. On an elimination diet, 88 percent of those children got better—an astonishing number. Not just their migraine, but all sorts of other symptoms as well, including aching limbs, runny noses, asthma, eczema, diarrhea, gas, mouth ulcers, and hyperactivity. Some of these children also had epileptic seizures, and even this symptom cleared up on the diet, recurring when culprit foods were tested.

A notable feature of this study is that, of the five researchers involved, four were deeply skeptical at the outset. Their report notes that they "embarked on this study believing that any favorable response, such as that claimed to substantiate the dietary hypothesis, could be explained as a placebo response. The positive double-blind controlled trial…provides clear evidence that a placebo response was not the explanation."

Other studies with good scientific credentials have demonstrated a role for idiopathic food intolerance in adults with migraine and for sufferers from irritable bowel syndrome and Crohn's disease. There are also good studies of individual patients with rheumatoid arthritis and palindromic rheumatism (an episodic form of inflammatory arthritis) who have responded dramatically to avoidance of a particular food. Some of these patients were given several double-blind challenges and showed changes in certain immunological tests, as well as joint symptoms, when challenged with the offending food. This suggests that the immune system could be playing some part in these food reactions.

Colic

A baby who wails loudly for hours every day, for no apparent reason, is enough to shatter the nerves of any parent. Occasional crying can be expected: it is a baby's way of registering needs and discomforts—hunger, tiredness, wet diapers, boredom, or a need for comforting. Lengthy spells of uncontrollable crying are another matter. To most people in those circumstances, it is clear that the baby is in acute distress, and that they should seek medical advice. Colic may be the final diagnosis, but other causes—inadequate feeding, overstimulation, or illness—must be ruled out.

If an infant draws up its legs and goes red in the face when crying, the cause may well be infantile colic. A lot of crying babies have colic—one in 10 infants suffer from this condition, generally thought to be due to a spasm in the intestines. The cause of this painful spasm is unknown, but one school of thought is that it is due to food intolerance.

If a food is the cause, sort out the diet and the crying often stops—provided, of course, that the baby has the other basics of infant life, such as warm dry clothing, enough food, plenty of cuddling, reassuring skin contact, and a reasonably consistent and predictable environment.

Colic is often called "3-month colic" because it tends to clear up when the baby is about 10–12 weeks old. One explanation of this spontaneous improvement dismisses the whole idea of colic—something being physically wrong with the baby—suggesting instead that the newborn baby is merely picking up on the mother's anxiety, and expressing this anxiety with crying. According to this theory, all mothers automatically become less anxious when the baby reaches 3 months and the babies stop crying accordingly. Another scenario, which is backed up by a certain amount of evidence, is that the baby's system partially adapts to the problem food at 3 months and stops responding with the acute symptoms of colic.

But while the colic abates, the baby continues to react to the food in other, more subtle ways. Eczema may begin soon afterward or there may be diarrhea or other symptoms. Some of these children go on to develop a persistent and troublesome allergy to the food in question.

Overcoming colic

Stage 1: Stop smoking
If you smoke, stop now. Your partner should stop too. Babies with smoking parents are much more prone to colic.

Stage 2: See the doctor
Ask your doctor to examine the baby for intestinal obstruction and for acid reflux (stomach acid coming up into the esophagus). If there are no serious problems such as these, talk to the doctor, in general terms, about the possibility of a reaction to food. It is useful at this stage to have some idea of how your doctor reacts to such ideas. If you get a hostile or dismissive reaction, go very gently and be diplomatic. You need to keep the doctor on your side. Make it clear that you are not fixated on the idea of food as the problem, but have an open-minded approach.

Stage 3: Could the problem be caused by lactose?
All milk, whether human or animal, contains a virtually tasteless sugar called **lactose.** This sugar should be digested in the intestines by an enzyme called **lactase,** and then absorbed into the bloodstream. If there is too little lactase, a lot of the milk sugar remains unabsorbed, to the delight of some of the bacteria found naturally in the baby's gut. They have a big party on the excess milk sugar, causing colic and/or diarrhea. This condition is known as **lactose intolerance.**

All babies produce the enzyme lactase, except for the few who are unlucky enough to suffer from **primary lactase deficiency.** This rare condition, in which little or no lactase is produced, is usually detected soon after birth because the child gets severely ill on any kind of milk. (Note that some babies are diagnosed as having primary lactase deficiency when they actually have a sensitivity to the proteins in the milk—see page 202. This may be the explanation if the baby does not improve even on a lactose-free formula.)

Children who stop having dairy products once they are weaned lose the capacity to produce lactase. In the Far East, where milk is not part of the traditional diet, older children and adults get diarrhea if given milk because they have no lactase. But a regular intake of milk may eventually induce tolerance.

Lactose intolerance in adults
Lactose intolerance affects older children and adults as well as babies. If you have primary lactase deficiency, you need to avoid lactose completely, or take a lactase replacer (see p. 205). If you have secondary lactase deficiency, due to an infection, or to some other form of food sensitivity that has caused diarrhea, then you need to avoid lactose until you are better.

Even regular milk drinkers can find themselves without enough lactase after a bout of diarrhea, because the lining of the intestine is depleted and takes a while to recover its ability to make lactase. Known as **secondary lactase deficiency,** this problem can affect people of any age. So if a baby has an infection that causes diarrhea, drinking milk during or just after the infection can lead to further diarrhea and/or colic.

Finally, it is possible that some babies have enough lactase to cope with an ordinary feeding, but their lactase capacity is overwhelmed by a very large feeding. This may be why they suffer colic more in the early evening, which is when the king-size morning feeding reaches the intestine.

Armed with these facts, you are in a position to investigate lactase deficiency:

- Babies who have suffered severe symptoms from birth should be tested by the doctor for primary lactase deficiency. There are sophisticated tests that can distinguish between primary and secondary lactase deficiency—ask if these can be carried out. The routine tests do not make this distinction, which can lead to misdiagnosis (see p. 202).
- If your baby has recently had diarrhea, suspect secondary lactase deficiency. Babies who are being bottle-fed can switch temporarily to formula feeds that are free from lactose. Ask your doctor or pharmacist about these. Mothers who are breast-feeding should continue to do so, even though their milk contains lactose, as breast milk contains antibodies that fight disease and is therefore the best option on balance.
- Where colic occurs at any time of day, try giving smaller feeds more frequently. The baby may have enough lactase to cope with small feeds only.
- Evening colic can often be relieved by making the morning feed smaller. If you are bottle-feeding, this is no problem. If you are breast-feeding, try any of the following:

1 Express some milk before the feed and freeze it for later.
2 Give a little boiled water first to help fill the stomach.
3 Feed from one breast only and then from the other, rather than switching sides several times.
4 If your milk is abundant, feed from one breast only in the morning. Note that this will reduce your total supply of milk.

Stage 4: Investigating other possible causes
Should there be no improvement during the first three stages, then it is time to think about a different type of sensitivity reaction – one involving the proteins found in milk or other foods (see pp. 202-3).

Psychological reactions to food

In his book, *Not All in the Mind*, Dr. Richard Mackarness tells the story of a former colleague, a psychiatrist, who attended one of his lectures on idiopathic food intolerance. Dr. Mackarness mentioned that severe fatigue could be a symptom of food intolerance, and that people with food intolerance often experience a craving for the offending food. The psychiatrist had suffered serious fatigue for some time and medical investigations had revealed nothing. He was profoundly skeptical about food intolerance, but prepared to give anything a try. The only food he ever craved was bacon, so it was easy enough to give this up.

The result astonished him. After feeling worse for a few days, he improved—in fact his fatigue lifted completely. Of his colleagues, all but Dr. Mackarness himself reacted with utter disbelief to this news. Intent on proving that the whole thing was **placebo effect**—an outcome of wishful thinking on his part—the skeptics secretly asked the hospital cook to slip some slivers of bacon into the steak pie she was making for lunch.

The unsuspecting psychiatrist began his lunch, but halfway through his head started to nod. Pushing his plate aside, he laid his head on the table and fell fast asleep.

As Dr. Mackarness recalled: "The doctors who were in on the experiment were impressed and some of them even admitted that there might be something to it after all."

Dr. Mackarness's book was published over 30 years ago, but its message has made little headway—the idea that sensitivity to food can cause psychological symptoms is still deeply unacceptable in medical circles.

Crying and epilepsy

Occasional reports linking psychological symptoms to food reach the medical journals. One was of a patient with epilepsy induced by beef. The reaction occurred reliably in a double-blind placebo-controlled trial (see p. 90) and could be recorded objectively with an EEG, which measures electrical output from the brain.

A patient who reacted with violent crying fits after consuming milk was tested with the same type of rigorous double-blind trial. In this case, giving the drug sodium cromoglycate beforehand stopped the reaction. Sodium cromoglycate blocks the firing of mast cells (see p. 148), so this suggests that a true allergic reaction was taking place.

In both these cases, the very careful testing that was done places the role of food beyond doubt. However, those conclusions are applicable to those particular patients only, not to others with epilepsy or crying fits. And most doctors would consider these cases to be highly atypical and extremely rare.

Exactly how rare they are is a subject worth discussing. If doctors and psychiatrists believe that food sensitivity is extremely rare in patients with psychological symptoms, they don't go looking for it. So the odds of a patient getting the kind of intensive and careful testing used for the two described above is exceptionally remote. Without such rigorous testing, any link with food would be considered highly implausible. In other words, the fact that such reports are very rare tells us little about how rare the phenomenon itself might be.

Having said that, absolutely no one would argue that cases like this are either common or typical. Psychological symptoms, which affect a great many people in our society at some time in their lives, mostly have psychological causes (see p. 236).

The links with food

It is very unusual for food sensitivity to generate psychological symptoms alone—eating the culprit food almost always produces some physical symptoms as well.

A link with food has sometimes been observed for the symptoms listed below. In addition, psychological symptoms are occasionally a feature of celiac disease, and food has been cited as a possible cause in Chronic Fatigue Syndrome (CFS) and autism (see p 85).

The associations discussed on this page remain controversial and mostly unproven. It is difficult to gather scientific evidence to confirm this type of link because many of the complaints are subjective and not easily measurable.

Depression and anxiety

Some patients who recover from physical symptoms during an elimination diet also experience a lifting of their former depression. This seems to be more common when the depression is accompanied by excessive fatigue.

Anxiety can sometimes be a symptom of idiopathic food intolerance. Too much caffeine (from tea, coffee, and cola) can also induce anxiety and other symptoms. Hyperventilation—breathing too quickly—may play a part in anxiety, and this is especially likely if there are panic attacks (see p. 227). Sometimes there is a complex interplay between idiopathic food intolerance and hyperventilation, with the culprit food contributing to the hyperventilation. Caffeine can also trigger hyperventilation.

Minor mental symptoms

Among the symptoms that have cleared up during an elimination diet and have recurred on food challenge are: tension, nervousness, insomnia, dizziness, confusion, memory lapses, mental fatigue, and poor concentration.

Bed-wetting

If children over the age of six wet the bed, the cause is usually a psychological one. But some children who begin following an avoidance diet for other symptoms—ordinary physical symptoms in most causes—stop wetting the bed when on the diet and start again if they eat the offending food. This may be a direct effect on the muscles of the bladder. It is most unlikely that bed-wetting would occur alone, without any other symptoms typical of idiopathic food intolerance (see p. 76).

Schizophrenia

There are occasional reports of patients with a long history of complex psychological problems improving remarkably on an elimination diet and then falling ill again when given their food in a disguised form. Such patients have usually been given various psychiatric diagnoses, including schizophrenia.

When gluten-free diets (or gluten-free, milk-free diets) have been tried for schizophrenic patients, a small minority respond well. Some researchers believe that exorphins or other peptides produced from the wheat or milk (see p. 76) may be at fault here.

Attention Deficit Disorder (ADD)

This problem is also called hyperactivity or Hyperkinetic Syndrome. The problem mostly affects children, but can continue into adulthood and typically includes:

- short attention span and poor concentration
- impulsive, fidgety, restless behavior; irritability
- sudden mood changes, outbursts of crying or temper
- frustration at any difficulty or obstacle
- clumsiness and lack of coordination
- difficulty in sleeping

The potential causes of this problem are many. Because drug treatment (notably with methylphenidate—Ritalin) has helped many children (or at least helped their parents), it is widely assumed that ADD is a disorder of the brain chemistry. But Ritalin increases concentration and mental focus for anyone, including perfectly normal adults, and the fact that it improves matters for these children proves very little. A percentage of children with ADD do appear to have some kind of subtle damage to the brain or a deficit in brain function, which could be inherited.

It seems likely that many different causes can produce symptoms that earn the diagnosis of ADD. Some children with this label may simply be exceptionally lively children. Others may have genuine behavioral problems that can be traced back to difficulties within the family, or lack of attention from one or both parents. Or there may be other psychological problems of the child that are not directly related to current circumstances.

The potential role of food or food additives in ADD is a highly contentious issue. After several decades of work in this area, the collective experience of doctors suggests that a few children with ADD have idiopathic food intolerance and improve on an elimination diet. They are likely to have other symptoms suggesting food sensitivity as well, such as asthma or eczema induced by food (see p. 68), or some of the typical symptoms of idiopathic food intolerance (see p. 76).

Despite all the publicity given to the Feingold diet, food additives do not seem to be especially important in ADD—only a few children with ADD are genuinely sensitive to them. However it is still a possibility that is worth investigating as part of a general elimination diet.

"Candida"

Spores of the fungus *Candida albicans*, a focus of medical controversy.

"As a small child Jason was plagued with ear infections that led to many courses of antibiotics," Hannah Mitchell recalls. "Eventually he started to get symptoms such as an upset stomach, itchy bottom, flulike symptoms, and extremely itchy eyes. The doctor prescribed eyedrops and when I put them in, Jason screamed his head off. In the morning every single eyelash had fallen out. Jason's health deteriorated and a few months later his eyebrows started to itch. Within two days every single eyebrow hair had fallen out. His eyes were worse and I was offered steroid eyedrops again. Reluctantly I accepted.

"Putting the drops in caused Jason extreme pain. The red patches of skin around his eyes spread and the itching increased. I was at the end of my tether when I came across a book in the library about food-related illness... "

What Hannah discovered from her reading was that, for some with diarrhea, bloating, gas, and an itchy bottom, the cause is attributed to an overgrowth of yeasts in the gut, caused in part by repeated courses of antibiotics that kill off friendly gut bacteria in the **gut flora** (see p. 204) and allow yeasts to flourish. This is not mainstream medicine, which is why none of the doctors who had seen Jason mentioned the possibility of yeast overgrowth.

Yeasts are microscopic fungi, so antifungal drugs are needed to kill them. However, reducing the intake of sugar in the diet is also very effective because yeasts living in the gut thrive on sugar. Hannah took matters into her own hands and tried out a diet containing no sugar and no yeast. (The reason for avoiding yeast in food is discussed below.) There was some improvement and, encouraged, she went back to the doctor and asked for antifungal drugs.

The doctor agreed, and to Hannah's immense relief, the combination of diet and drug treatment worked for Jason—it cleared the diarrhea, gas, and itching and eventually allowed his eyelashes and eyebrows to grow back. (Note that few other patients with yeast problems suffer hair-loss—this is a very exotic symptom—but yeast overgrowth can produce some other quite unusual reactions.)

The elusive culprit

So far, you will notice, I have not mentioned *Candida*. Among those doctors who study and treat this condition, this particular yeast was once considered the prime suspect. Indeed, the disease itself was called "candidiasis." But the role of *Candida* is now considered doubtful by many.

British researchers such as Dr. John Hunter, of Addenbrooke's Hospital in Cambridge, have tried to find *Candida* in their patients without success. "I think now we have to reject the idea of *Candida* causing the symptoms," says Dr. Hunter. "But I do believe that there is an imbalance in the gut flora—the microorganisms that live in the gut. I believe that's at the root of so-called 'candidiasis'." This new evidence has not yet affected beliefs about "candidiasis" and "Candida" in the complementary health field.

The fact remains that antifungal drugs have proved very helpful to many patients with the typical cluster of symptoms—diarrhea, gas, bloating, and an itchy anus—that were previously attributed to *Candida*. Given the effectiveness of these drugs, it seems probable that yeasts of some kind are playing a large part in this condition. So the term "yeast overgrowth" is being used, rather tentatively at the moment, as a label for this condition. The yeasts concerned have not, as yet, been identified. Nor has there been any large-scale scientific trial to establish, beyond doubt, that yeast overgrowth can cause these symptoms.

The facts about *Candida*

This box is about *Candida* as understood by conventional medicine, rather than "Candida" and "candidiasis" as understood by alternative medicine.

The yeast known as *Candida* lives naturally in the gut, usually causing no trouble. Problems are usually caused by *Candida* only when it sets up home in the throat, vagina, or penis ("thrush" infections). Such localized infections have well-defined symptoms and, in most cases, are easily treated with antifungal drugs. Patients with damaged immune systems, caused by anticancer drugs or AIDS, often develop more widespread *Candida* infections, but this *never* happens to people with a normal immune system.

Inhaling steroids and not rinsing out the mouth afterward can make asthma sufferers more susceptible to *Candida* infections in the throat (see p. 145).

Other symptoms claimed for yeast overgrowth are:
- fatigue
- poor concentration
- irritability, depression, and confusion
- headache or migraine
- severe premenstrual problems
- recurrent cystitis
- skin rashes
- aching muscles
- chronic urticaria

Sometimes there is constipation rather than diarrhea. Recurrent vaginal candidiasis—a genuine *Candida* infection—can also be a feature of this problem. Occasionally allergic symptoms such as asthma seem to get worse with yeast overgrowth.

Is there an allergic reaction to the yeast?

Those with symptoms typical of yeast overgrowth may give a positive prick-puncture test (see p. 91) to *Candida*, but what this means is debatable. For one thing, not everyone with this condition gives a positive test. For another, some entirely healthy people give a positive prick-puncture test to *Candida*. To complicate matters, there are a lot of cross-reactions (see p. 14) between different kinds of yeasts and molds, due to similarities in their chemical constituents. So the positive skin-prick test does not mean that *Candida* itself triggered the original IgE-response.

The question of whether some kind of sensitivity reaction to yeasts is occurring in those with yeast overgrowth, and contributing to their symptoms, is an interesting one. The benefits from avoiding yeast in food (see Diagnosis and treatment) suggest that it may be—but this is a question that cannot be answered at present.

Diagnosis and treatment

Unfortunately, this is one of those "try-it-and-see" conditions, where diagnosis and treatment are the same—you try the treatment for yeast overgrowth, and if it works you assume that the disease is, or was, yeast overgrowth. This is far from satisfactory, but is the best that can be done at present.

It is only worth trying this treatment if you have quite a number of the symptoms listed. Bowel problems and an itchy anus are characteristic, and if you have neither of these it is unlikely the treatment will help you.

A key part of the treatment is a no-yeast-no-sugar diet (see p. 205). This diet has been developed on a largely pragmatic basis, and seems to work—but why? The rationale for cutting out sugar is clear—it feeds yeasts in the gut. But why avoiding foods containing yeast should help is uncertain. Possibly the yeasty food supplies some special nutrient that benefits the yeasts living in the gut. Alternatively, there might, for some people, be a sensitivity reaction to the yeast in food (see left).

If it seems that you are on the right track, because there is some improvement with this diet, discuss antifungal drugs with your doctor. If prescribed, you should take these in addition to the diet. Nystatin (see box below) is very safe for most people, since it is not absorbed from the gut. Probiotics (see p. 205) may also be a useful part of treatment.

Try to avoid doctors and alternative therapists who are part of the "Candida" craze and think that "candidiasis" explains a huge variety of illnesses. You may not have yeast overgrowth at all, so you need someone with an open mind.

Eczema and yeasts?

Doctors have found that some children whose eczema looks very red, and is not responding to treatment, have IgE in the blood against a range of yeasts and other fungi (*Candida, Trichophyton, Saccharomyces* and *Pityrosporum*). Given the tendency to cross-reactions among fungi (see main text), it is not clear exactly what these reactions indicate. A proportion of these children get much better on antifungal drugs, including a drug called nystatin, which is not absorbed through the gut wall—so cannot reach the skin. The eczema improves and at the same time there is a fall in levels of antifungal IgE in the blood. In other words, a treatment that can only affect fungi living in the gut benefits the skin. Exactly what is going on here is unknown, but the important point is that the treatment seems to work. This is a controversial topic, but since nystatin is an extremely safe drug, your doctor may be prepared to try it out. A course of 3–4 weeks is the minimum needed.

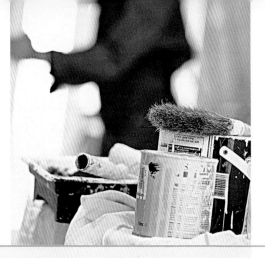

Chemical intolerance

"To start with, I just used to get this irritation in my throat when I was reading a magazine. Over the years it got much worse, and there was a dreadful burning feeling, not just in my throat now, but also in my eyes and nose. Sometimes I could scarcely breathe. My doctor said it couldn't be magazines and diagnosed asthma. Twenty years on, I can't look at a magazine, even for a few minutes, and other things affect me now too. If I go in a room with a photocopier running, I start to choke and can't breathe. Whenever I describe this problem to anyone—apart from a doctor, that is—they almost always say they know someone else who has a similar problem. But the doctors still say that what happens to me can't happen."

Mary has chemical intolerance, which is also known as chemical sensitivity, environmental illness, or idiopathic environmental intolerances. It is a condition that arouses more passionate controversy than any other described in this book. Many believe that it simply does not exist, or rather that people who claim to have chemical intolerance are actually victims of psychological problems, which express themselves as physical symptoms. Careful studies show that, while some people with supposed chemical intolerance do fall into this category, others do not—they have no psychiatric problems, but they do appear to have valid symptoms when exposed to certain synthetic chemicals.

"People with MCS are desperate. They will go to great lengths and do almost anything to find a doctor, anyone, who believes them." So speaks one sufferer from MCS (**Multiple Chemical Sensitivity**,) the most extreme form of chemical intolerance. It is often severely disabling, with symptoms such as exceptional fatigue, nausea, headaches, poor memory and concentration, dizziness, muscle aches, joint pain, chest pain, and digestive problems. Those with MCS react to a very wide range of chemicals, and very often to foods and food additives as well.

These severely affected patients are a small minority, however, and many more people are like Mary, with sensitivity to just one or two types of chemical exposure. Surveys in the United States suggest that about 30 percent of the population are affected in this way. The authors of one such survey note that "the widespread idea that chemical sensitivity is a condition of educated, urban housewives was not supported by our study. The region surveyed was rural…and individuals who reported chemical sensitivity were found in all age, gender, income, race, and employment groups."

The chemical exposures that are identified as triggering symptoms include:
- perfumes
- pesticides
- cigarette smoke
- paint fumes
- gasoline
- exhaust fumes
- cleaning products
- newspaper ink
- plastics, especially those with a strong smell
- glossy paper (for example, in magazines)

Typical symptoms, in those with sensitivity to just one or two chemical products, are:
- a blocked or runny nose
- sore throat
- irritation of the eyes
- sinus pain and congestion
- headache
- breathlessness and wheezing
- nausea
- skin rashes
- extreme fatigue
- dizziness

How does chemical intolerance begin?

For some of those with MCS, the problems began with a sudden overexposure to a toxic chemical, such as a chemical spill, or pesticides from a crop-spraying plane. Others are first affected by regular doses of pesticide at lower levels, such as spray drift from nearby fields or from a neighbor's garden. It seems as if, for these people, their inborn ability to detoxify both natural and man-made toxins is overwhelmed by an unusually heavy exposure and never fully recovers. Although there have been no systematic studies of this—it is difficult to imagine how they could be done—there is a large body of well-documented cases. And studies of those exposed to high levels of pesticides in accidents at work support the idea that this can cause lifelong sensitivity to *very small* doses of some synthetic chemicals. Sensitivity to alcohol and caffeine usually increases enormously too.

In some cases, classical allergies also feature in the range of symptoms for those with MCS. If they had an allergic tendency before the accidental exposure to pesticides, this is especially likely: after the accident, along with chemical intolerance, they have far more pronounced allergic reactions to common allergens.

There is speculation that the loss of tolerance to everyday chemicals may be related to some kind of damage to the enzymes in the liver that carry out the important task of detoxifying toxins that enter the bloodstream. This detoxification system evolved to deal with natural toxins, such as those in plant foods, and those produced by bacteria living naturally in the gut. These enzymes can also detoxify the widely used synthetic chemicals, when these are encountered in relatively small amounts, but the enzymes are overwhelmed by large doses.

Chronic fatigue syndrome (CFS)

This is a disease that probably has multiple causes rather than a single cause. The main symptom is fatigue that is not relieved by rest. Many people with CFS also have a slightly raised temperature, problems with concentration and memory, headaches, sore throat, and swollen lymph nodes ("swollen glands"). The lymph nodes are part of the immune system, so this symptom suggests some immune involvement. Other findings, related to immune cells in the blood, also support this idea. However, there are often minor abnormalities in the brain as well, with some loss of the insulating material around the nerves (myelin).

For many patients, the disease develops in the wake of a viral infection, but for others the origin may be unclear. Whatever the origin of the disease, avoiding synthetic chemicals is very helpful in many cases. Some sufferers also find an elimination diet helpful (see pp. 194-7). Doctors working in this area say that there is no sharp demarcation between patients with Chronic Fatigue Syndrome (CFS) and those with MCS.

Autism

In the search for a cause of autism, many possibilities are being investigated. The consensus now is that there is a genetic predisposition which, when combined with certain trigger factors, leads to autism.

Some researchers suggest that autistic children are sensitive to synthetic chemicals, both in food and the environment. The suspicion is that these chemicals affect the developing nervous system.

Other researchers pinpoint food as the culprit. They believe that children who develop autism are affected by exorphins (see p. 76) and that these damage the child's developing nervous system. There are claims that a dairy-free and gluten-free diet can help, but that it must be ultra-strict to work, and may need to continue for at least 6 months before any improvement occurs. Consult your doctor before trying this approach.

Before starting them on such a diet, some doctors also give a course of antifungal drugs to those autistic children who have been treated repeatedly with antibiotics. This combined treatment is reported to have very good effects for some children. These treatments are highly speculative and have not been tested properly. It is not known if they would benefit the majority of autistic patients.

Treatment

Assuming that you really do have chemical intolerance rather than some deep-rooted psychological problem—and you have to be honest with yourself here, because otherwise you will never get better—then careful avoidance of the offending synthetic chemicals is the only effective treatment. If you have eliminated everything that obviously affects you and are not much improved, then try tackling common indoor pollutants (see pp. 128-30) as well.

Such measures are of value to some with chemical intolerance but may not be adequate for those most severely affected. If you need to take more radical steps, you may benefit from the bedding, paints, and other household items manufactured for those with chemical sensitivity. Once you reduce the level of synthetic chemicals in your everyday environment, you may find that you can tolerate occasional exposures much more.

Some doctors recommend taking supplements of vitamins and minerals to speed your recovery. These (especially antioxidants—see p. 206) may be helpful for some people, but be sure to get nutritional advice from someone with good medical qualifications, rather than a self-styled "nutrition therapist".

Neutralization therapy (see p. 211) has been proposed for people with chemical intolerance, but this has not been scientifically validated as an effective treatment. Avoidance of the offending substances is still necessary. Hyperventilation (see p. 236) can make chemical intolerance much worse.

Chapter 3
medical help and self-help

The days when doctors wanted their patients to obey orders and ask no questions are largely gone. Patients with allergies and other forms of sensitivity—or their parents—have to play a key role in managing the condition. Most doctors now recognize this and encourage their patients to learn about their condition, its diagnosis, and its treatment, and to be partners in their own medical care.

Quite apart from this, there are aspects of allergy management in which few doctors can afford the time to become experts. The nitty-gritty details of dust-mite avoidance or food labeling practices are good examples. You can usefully supplement your doctor's treatment here by informing yourself.

But where should this process stop? That is a difficult question which doctors are increasingly forced to consider. One modern phenomenon, being discussed in many medical journals at present, is the abundance of medical information on the Internet. Some doctors dread the arrival of patients who have logged on the night before their appointment and are armed with a huge number of facts about their illness—some accurate, some utterly wrong, and some highly debatable. But other doctors welcome the fact that patients are actively interested in their health problems.

The reactions of doctors to "Internet patients" highlights an issue that also runs right through this book—that of medical orthodoxy. Who decides what is true and what is false in medicine, and how do they do it? Make no mistake—this is a deep and abiding problem that afflicts not just scientific medicine, but science in general.

If a doctor dismisses as "nonsense" a web page claiming that allergies are caused by space aliens intent on destroying Western civilization, he or she is not, strictly speaking, taking a scientific approach. In science, you consider all the different hypotheses.

In theory, science works by questioning everything and taking nothing on trust—but you can't make much practical progress if you stick rigorously to that approach. Neither scientists nor doctors start their careers by running experiments to establish the truth of everything they were ever taught. At some point in science, and in scientific medicine, you have to assume that certain things are probably true, and proceed accordingly. If you make significant progress working on those assumptions, then the chances are they were correct. But a good scientist always remembers that they are only assumptions.

Scientific medicine rests on a huge number of assumptions. Some of these are clearly accurate—for example, that eating wheat triggers celiac disease—and it would be a waste of time to argue about them. But this "fact" about celiac disease began as just a theory (see p. 70), and a highly debatable one. It has taken time for it to become substantiated by more and more evidence.

Some medical assumptions become enshrined as facts rather too quickly. Fifty years ago, orthodox medicine accepted as a "fact" that many asthmatic children had "intrinsic asthma," which was psychological in origin. Research since then has shown that there is usually an allergy underlying childhood asthma. Many other examples could be given of established medical "facts" that are overturned by subsequent research.

Doctors thirst for certainty, something that is quite understandable when they are faced with so much human need. A significant part of the healing power of medicine comes from the **placebo effect** (see

p. 233), and that relies on patients having faith in the doctor. The traditional way for doctors to cultivate that faith was by assuming an air of absolute certainty—about their diagnosis of the patient's illness, about the treatment, and about medicine in general. This need for certainty has always hastened the transformation of assumptions into facts.

The fatherly, authoritarian attitude of old-fashioned doctors was, in large part, a reflection of how little they had in the way of useful treatments and how much they relied on the placebo effect. Modern doctors have far more genuinely effective remedies to offer and can afford to take a different approach. Many now rely on a different kind of authority, one based on intelligence, flexibility, good information, curiosity, and openness. It's a form of authority that allows a doctor to say, "I could be wrong..." or "Let's try this and see what happens..." without losing face.

Unfortunately, there is another powerful force operating in this complex situation, and that is quackery—the age-old business of selling phony cures (see p. 209). Official bodies within the medical community try to curb quackery by weighing the evidence about novel treatments, coming to decisions on their validity, and providing information to the public. This information is now available on the Internet too, and it can be very useful. But in deciding what is not good scientific medicine, medical organizations always run the risk of mistaking their own unverified assumptions for facts.

Establishing criteria for good treatment is essential in medicine, but high standards should not develop into dogmatism. Among the treatments that are being dismissed as valueless today are several that deserve a fairer hearing.

Some of these treatments have been shown to work by the most excellent of scientific methods. The use of elimination diets in Crohn's disease is a good example—for some patients, there is a huge and sustained improvement, suggesting that their disease was caused, at least in part, by food sensitivity. The tactic used by those who want to reject this evidence is simply to ignore it. When scientific review papers (summaries of all the current knowledge and latest research) are written about Crohn's disease, the research on diet is usually not mentioned. Evidence that is routinely ignored in this way slips into oblivion because most doctors have time to read only the review papers, not the original research reports.

Occasionally—and this is even more shameful—good scientific evidence that goes against the grain of current orthodoxy is actually misreported in review papers. This happened with an impeccable scientific study showing the benefits of an elimination diet for some patients with rheumatoid arthritis. By omitting certain key facts, a review author managed to give the impression that the results of this study supported the conventional view on the subject (diet makes no difference to rheumatoid arthritis). In fact, the study actually disputed the conventional view.

New approaches to currently untreatable diseases such as autism and Chronic Fatigue Syndrome (CFS) are also subject to unthinking rejection. Such medical problems always attract experimental treatments, just as they always attract sheer quackery, and sorting out one from the other is not easy—it takes time and a clearheaded approach, not knee-jerk dismissal.

Finding the right doctor

Expertise is obviously a prime requirement of any doctor, but communication skills come a close second. This is particularly important with long-term health problems, such as allergies and asthma, where you—as a patient or a parent—shoulder a lot of responsibility for day-to-day management and treatment.

This is how researchers Noreen Clark and Molly Gong, from the University of Michigan School of Public Health, put it in a recent article: "The patient should be the primary manager of chronic disease, guided and coached by a doctor or other practitioner to devise the best therapeutic regimen. The practitioner and patient should work as partners, developing strategies that give the patient the best chance to control his or her own disease and reduce the physical, psychological, social, and economic consequences of chronic illness."

So does your doctor work as a partner with you? That approach requires a particular attitude toward patients which comes more easily to some doctors than to others. Fundamental elements in that attitude include:

• respecting your intelligence, and your particular viewpoint on illness and treatment
• taking the time to listen to your concerns
• understanding your priorities in relation to health issues, and planning the treatment program accordingly
• being flexible and open-minded as regards treatment

Another important quality in a doctor is empathy. The National Eczema Association in the U.S. advises its members: "Providers who dismiss eczema as being a 'minor problem' or 'just a skin rash' may give your condition minimal attention when you go to them for help. Find someone who takes your condition seriously."

A doctor who is located close to your home—whether a primary care doctor or a specialist—has advantages over one that is a long journey away, and this is something worth factoring in when making a decision. Anyone with a medical condition that has big ups and downs, such as asthma or atopic eczema, benefits greatly from having quick and easy access to their doctor.

In the U.S., some kinds of health insurance effectively limit your choice of doctor (see p. 96–7). So choosing a doctor and choosing medical insurance may have to go hand in hand.

Recommendations are often the best way to find a good doctor. These are some of the approaches you could take:

• Find other patients or parents in your area who are dealing with the same medical problem, and ask which doctor they use and if they are satisfied. In the case of a commonplace problem such as asthma or atopic eczema, you could ask people at your workplace, school, social clubs, or place of worship. Don't rely on just one person's opinion. With a more unusual problem, such as food allergies or chronic urticaria, you may get better help from a patient support organization (see p. 255)—there will probably be other members in your area who are able to recommend their doctors.
• If you are moving, and feel happy with your current doctor, ask if he or she knows a colleague near your new home who has a good reputation.
• Once you have a shortlist of possible doctors, call them to arrange a "get-acquainted" appointment, so that you can talk over your medical concerns, see for yourself what facilities are available, and judge how well you and the doctor get along. During this visit, ask the doctor how much experience he or she has with the particular health problems facing you and your child. Ensure that the doctor knows the reason for the appointment so that he or she schedules sufficient time.

Choosing a primary care doctor

Your primary care doctor could be

- a family physician—someone who can care for the basic needs of the whole family and refer you to specialists when this seems necessary. These doctors have the advantage of knowing your family as a whole and can build up a valuable understanding of your needs and priorities.
- for children, a pediatrician—someone with specialist training in children's health.
- for adults, a general internist—someone with specialist training in internal medicine. (Internal medicine is general nonsurgical medicine of adults, encompassing cardiology, pulmonary medicine, gastroenterology, endocrinology, infectious diseases, and geriatrics, to name a few.) They are particularly good for older patients with complex health problems.
- for women, a gynecologist-obstetrician.

Choosing a specialist

If you are happy with your primary care doctor, or another doctor you are seeing, ask his or her advice about finding a specialist. For example, your pediatrician may be able to recommend a good allergist when you need one.

Alternatively, start with a professional organization that represents specialists of the kind you are seeking—for example, the American Academy of Allergy, Asthma, and Immunology, or the Canadian Society of Allergy and Clinical Immunology. These can be located via the Internet, or by mail (see p. 255). They may be able to give you details of their members practising in your area.

Before you begin this process, consider whether you really need to see a specialist, or whether your primary care doctor can deal with your allergic symptoms.

Asthma

Research shows that when asthma patients are cared for by asthma specialists, they have fewer symptoms, need emergency treatment less often, and feel significantly better. You should definitely be seeing a specialist if:

- you have ever had a life-threatening asthma attack
- your asthma is not under control despite following your treatment schedule carefully (see pp. 40–41)
- you have chronic sinusitis or repeated chest infections
- you need high-dose inhaled steroids
- you sometimes need steroid tablets
- the diagnosis of asthma is uncertain
- you require frequent emergency room visits, or have recently been hospitalized for asthma
- you require supplemental oxygen

Chronic sinusitis

Specialist help, of a really expert kind, is required here. In the U.S., try to find someone who is board-certified (see box below) in both allergy and otolaryngology (the treatment of the head and neck, especially the ears, nose, and throat). Ask how much experience they have with chronic sinusitis.

Hay fever and perennial allergic rhinitis

Mild cases can generally be dealt with adequately by primary care doctors. Look for a specialist if there are additional problems such as "glue ear" or chronic sinusitis, or if you want allergy shots.

Food allergy and insect-sting allergy

If you have ever suffered anaphylaxis, especially anaphylactic shock (see p. 58), you should be seeing an allergist.

Atopic eczema

Except in very mild cases, specialist help is probably advisable. But should you see a dermatologist or an allergist? Depending on which type of specialist you see, the emphasis of the treatment could be very different (see pp. 42–9).

Overall, a combined approach to atopic eczema—tackling allergies, calming inflammation, restoring skin structure, and treating infections—is undoubtedly the most helpful. In the U.S., the best kind of specialist in atopic eczema would probably be someone who is board-certified in both dermatology and allergy.

Contact dermatitis

You should be seeing a dermatologist if you think your problem could be work-related or if you have severe symptoms that are not responding to treatment.

Checking credentials

Any specialist you see should have advanced training in a particular discipline (allergy and immunology, for example, or dermatology).

In the U.S., a medical board, such as the American Board of Allergy and Immunology oversees this training. If you want to check that a doctor is really board-certified, the American Board of Medical Specialties (ABMS) runs a Certified Doctor Verification Service (see p. 255 for contact details).

In Canada, professional examinations are set by the Royal College of Physicians and Surgeons of Canada, and only a certified specialist (fellow) may use the designation FRCPC (Fellow of the Royal College of Physicians of Canada). You can verify specialists' credentials by contacting the Royal College of Physicians and Surgeons or by checking the Canadian Medical Directory at your local library.

Accurate diagnosis

The simplest and most certain test for any sensitivity reaction is to expose the person concerned to the substance under suspicion and see what happens. This is known as a **challenge test**. With true allergies, challenge tests are powerful tools, but they are also alarmingly close to reality. The risk of provoking a severe reaction requires a very cautious approach.

By comparison, an indirect test—a roundabout way of seeing how the body responds, such as the prick-puncture skin test (see p. 91)—has the advantage of rarely producing dangerous reactions. The downside is that indirect tests can be misleading, precisely because they are *not* like the real-life situation. No indirect test is perfect—there are always false positives and false negatives (see box on p. 91).

Challenge tests

If you undergo a challenge test with food or an airborne allergen, you will also be given dummy challenges with an innocuous substance that is indistinguishable from the item being tested. Neither you, nor the tester who is scoring the reaction, should know which is which. This is called a **double-blind trial** because both of you are in the dark, to eliminate all possible bias. (The full name is "double-blind placebo-controlled trial"; the dummy challenge is also called a "placebo challenge" or "control challenge.")

The double-blind trial is a standard procedure and does not imply that the doctors think you are faking symptoms. Psychological forces are powerful—and just thinking that you might react to a test can be enough to produce a reaction. The process that generates such symptoms is largely unconscious.

Food challenge

A food challenge—eating the food that is under suspicion—is a key test for food intolerance (see p. 197). It is sometimes used for food allergy and other forms of food sensitivity too, as a follow-up to skin tests. Some allergists use a food challenge only if the skin test is at odds with actual events reported by the patient. Other allergists use food challenge more readily, to confirm skin test results, and to assess the severity of the reaction.

Extreme caution must be exercised with immediate food allergy, because of the considerable risks involved. *For anyone with a positive skin test to the food, the test must be done under medical supervision with resuscitation equipment at hand*. A challenge test should *never* be done for true food allergy without some careful preliminary tests on the face and lips (see p. 23). Even if these tests produce no reaction, only tiny amounts of the food should be eaten to begin with.

Bronchial challenge

This type of test involves inhalation of the airborne allergen—such as pollen or animal allergens—suspected of causing asthma. Bronchial challenge carries the risk of provoking a severe asthma attack, and few doctors use it unless there are compelling reasons to do so.

Prick-puncture tests

This family of tests, which are indirect methods of detecting true allergic reactions, includes the following:

- skin-prick tests or prick tests
- puncture tests
- scratch tests

For the **skin-prick test**, a small drop of liquid containing an allergen, such as ragweed pollen, is placed on your arm. The doctor makes a small prick in the skin, under the drop of liquid, allowing a minuscule amount of the allergen to get into the skin. A positive reaction is recorded if a red bump develops soon afterward. For accuracy, the bump must be compared to positive and negative controls (see below).

The **puncture test** is very similar to the skin-prick test but uses a slightly different technique for breaking the skin. In this book, **prick-puncture test** is used as a collective term to cover both techniques.

With the **scratch test**, the skin is scratched lightly, and the allergen solution is then applied over the scratch. This method is going out of favor because it gives less consistent results than prick-puncture testing.

It is important to include a **negative control** in the test—a prick or puncture test with plain salt-water (saline). This should not produce much of a bump—if it does, the skin is clearly overreactive and the tests more difficult to assess.

The doctor should also include a **positive control**—a prick or puncture test with histamine, the substance that plays a central role in allergic reactions. This should always produce a bump. If it does not, the skin is decidedly under-reactive, and the tests are invalid.

Taking antihistamines will make the skin under-reactive, and you should stop taking them before the testing, for a period ranging from a day to several weeks—it varies depending on the particular antihistamine. Ask your doctor for specific instructions about stopping these and other drugs.

People with dermatographism (see p. 51) have skin that tends to be over-reactive to testing. Blood tests known as **RASTs** (see p. 92) are needed for anyone with this condition. Eczema sufferers with a rash over large areas of the body may also require blood tests, simply because there is too little clear skin for testing.

Prick-puncture tests can produce both false positives and false negatives (see box below). Some allergic diseases will give a lot of false negatives and relatively few false positives, while for others the reverse is true.

The allergen itself influences the rates of misleading reactions: for example, tests for soy allergy are notoriously unreliable, whereas those for peanut are far more accurate. The age of the person being tested also makes a difference. With all these influences at work, interpreting the test responses is a real art, and the doctor's experience counts for a lot.

All sorts of different people offer skin-prick tests, including a few alternative practitioners. Get them done by a qualified doctor, preferably by an experienced allergist, who will know how to make sense of the reactions.

The safety record of skin-prick tests is very good. Occasionally a systemic reaction (anaphylaxis) occurs with these tests, but there are no records of any deaths. Nevertheless, if you have severe asthma or have experienced anaphylactic shock in the past, it is advisable for the doctor to have resuscitation equipment available. Taking beta-blockers (see p. 150) increases the risk of a life-threatening reaction.

False positives and false negatives

Apart from direct challenge tests, none of the tests used for allergy work with one hundred percent accuracy. Most tests give both false positives and false negatives.

A **false positive** means that there is a positive test but no actual reaction when the allergen is encountered (for example, eaten or inhaled).

A **false negative** means that there is a negative test result despite a genuine reaction (as shown by a challenge test, for example).

A test that gives relatively few false positives has **good positive predictive value**—in other words, if it suggests you are allergic to something, you probably are.

A test that gives relatively few false negatives has **good negative predictive value**. If it comes up negative, you are probably not allergic to that allergen.

Intradermal tests

These tests (also called "intracutaneous tests") put allergen more deeply into the skin than prick-puncture tests. The skin tends to react more when penetrated to this depth so the test is more sensitive, but there are more false positives. There is also a greater risk of a serious reaction that may require emergency resuscitation. Therefore intradermal tests are usually performed only if skin-prick tests have been performed initially, and are negative. Intradermal testing is not generally used for food allergy testing, because there are too many false positives, as well as a higher risk of anaphylaxis. Don't undergo these tests if you are taking beta-blockers (see p. 150).

Radioallergosorbent tests (RAST)

A blood sample is required for this kind of test. It is sent to a laboratory that uses a very accurate test for IgE (the allergy antibody). Specific types of IgE are measured—for example, IgE against cat allergens, cow's milk, or birch pollen.

Research shows that RASTs are no more accurate than prick-puncture tests in confirming real-life allergic reactions. They are also a great deal more expensive. However, they are useful for patients who can't discontinue their antihistamines without suffering severe symptoms, and for those with dermatographism or very bad eczema (see p. 91).

Patch tests

These tests, used primarily for contact dermatitis, are similar to straightforward challenge tests, because the suspect substances are applied directly to the skin. The test substances are placed on the skin—usually on the back—in small chambers. They are held in place with sticky tape and left for several days. Ideally, the reaction of the skin should be checked three times: after two days, again the next day, and again the day after that. It really is worth going back for all these separate visits, because the accuracy of the test increases greatly with repeated checking.

The items chosen for testing are a standard set of antigens that most commonly cause contact dermatitis. This standard set of tests will pick up 60–80 percent of all sensitivity reactions in contact dermatitis. If you have items that you suspect may be causing symptoms, such as cosmetics, the doctor can usually test for these too.

You should not be tested while you still have a rash, as the testing will probably make the existing rash flare up, even though the test patches are applied well away from that area.

Steroid creams and any light treatment (including exposure of the back to ordinary sunlight) must stop at least a week before testing starts, otherwise the results will not be accurate.

Interpreting patch tests requires a huge amount of skill, plus extensive knowledge of the details of the test substances. You need a dermatologist with considerable experience in this area.

False positives (see box on p. 91) can occur, especially if you react very strongly to one of the items tested—some people develop what dermatologists call an "angry back," which generates false positives to various other substances being tested. Should you be told that you are sensitive to many different things, you may want to query this reading of the test. Ernest N. Charlesworth, an allergist and dermatologist at the University of Texas, describes patients who "develop into environmental cripples," after being told—on the basis of misinterpreted patch tests—that they are definitely sensitive to multiple antigens.

False negatives (see box on p. 91) are also possible, even with very careful testing. Should this occur, a type of challenge test known as a ROAT (Repeat Open Application Test) is possible. The suspect substance is applied to the inner fold of the elbow twice a day for a week. Get your doctor's agreement, and detailed instructions, before trying this test.

Endoscopy and biopsy

Miniaturized cameras and sophisticated fiber optics have allowed modern doctors to do something that their predecessors could never have imagined possible—look right inside the human body. This procedure is called **endoscopy**, and it has a useful role in a few sensitivity reactions.

Looking inside the sinus cavities can assist in understanding exactly what is going wrong in chronic sinusitis. Inspecting the digestive tract can be valuable in several of the non-IgE immune reactions to food, such as celiac disease (see p. 70) and eosinophilic gastroenteritis (see p. 72).

A **biopsy** is often carried out at the same time as endoscopy. This involves taking a small sample from the affected area, such as the lining of the gut, and studying it under a microscope.

One purpose of a gut biopsy is to look for characteristic types of damage to the lining of the gut—such as the distinctive changes produced by untreated celiac disease. A biopsy may also be studied to see what kind of immune cells are present. Abnormal numbers of certain immune cells, for example, eosinophils (see p. 19), may suggest a particular diagnosis.

Another way of looking at what kind of immune reactions are going on, used for lung diseases, is a **bronchoalveolar lavage**— literally a "washing out" of the airways and lungs, allowing immune cells to be collected and studied. This diagnostic technique is used for Heiner's syndrome (see p. 72).

Tests for food intolerance

The only really effective way of testing for food intolerance is an elimination diet (see pp. 194–7). This is the gold standard. However, it is neither easy nor quick—which has led to a constant search for alternative tests.

The proposed alternatives are all indirect tests, that is to say, non-dietary. The results of the tests are used as a basis for an avoidance diet. In other words, the foods that give a positive test result are avoided.

Some of these tests use samples of hair or blood, others use pulse testing, pendulums, Vega machines, or muscle strength tests ("applied kinesiology"). Most of these tests have not been evaluated objectively.

Of those that have been evaluated, a few do show some promise. A blood test called the "lymphocyte transformation test," for example, can give a general indication of sensitivity reactions—sometimes. However, even in the most expert hands, these do not give a result that is accurate enough to be useful.

Many of these tests are advertised directly to the public, and one of the problems with this approach is that the testing company starts by assuming that food is the problem. The same is usually true of "dietary therapists" and others in the alternative health field offering tests of this kind.

Almost everyone who undertakes an alternative test is given a fairly long list of foods that came up positive in the tests. This does not fit with the evidence from medical trials in which a group of people with irritable bowel or migraine (typical food intolerance symptoms) undertake an elimination diet. *A significant proportion of them always find that they do not have food intolerance.* Of the rest, many find that they react to one or two foods only. The long lists of foods issued to *everyone* by the commercial tests are, to put it mildly, implausible.

For tests requiring a sample of blood, sending two blood samples from the same person, under different names, is a simple way of assessing the validity of the tests. This exercise has been tried several times with different testing companies, and every time two completely different lists of foods have been drawn up—for the same person.

Covert studies of this kind have also shown that the tests overlook genuine reactions. In one alarming case, a woman with a true allergy to peanuts was assured by a "dietary therapist" that she really could eat peanuts safely.

Many people with food intolerance will tell you that they did well after following a diet based on such tests—and they may well have done. Given that common foods such as wheat and milk are regular offenders in food intolerance, and that these foods very frequently feature on the lists of positive test results generated by commercial testing companies, quite a few people should do well. The problem is that these people may also be avoiding many other foods quite unnecessarily.

Furthermore, if people have sensitivities to some other foods that are *not* on the list, they will be missing out. They could enjoy a far better level of health if *all* the foods causing symptoms were identified and removed from their diet.

In the end, an elimination diet is both cheaper and far more likely to give the right answers.

Testing for IgG antibodies

In diagnosing food intolerance, some doctors offer tests for a type of antibody called IgG. This antibody is formed to any food molecules that get into the bloodstream after a meal—and some do, even in entirely healthy people. So finding IgG antibodies to food molecules is not indicative of *any* disease at all. They are perfectly normal.

Nevertheless, some doctors feel that by measuring the level of IgG antibodies to foods, they can get a general idea of the permeability of the gut wall (which might *possibly* be true), and of particular foods that could be causing intolerance reactions (very doubtful—the tests just tell you what you eat most, and you know that already).

This test does have a genuine basis—it is measuring something real, unlike some of the alternative tests for food intolerance. But the relevance of what it measures to the health of the individual concerned is partial and indefinite. These tests seem to be very poor value for money, and potentially misleading, whereas an elimination diet is a far more precise and reliable way of pinpointing food intolerances.

Taking care of yourself

You can successfully manage your allergies and ensure that they interfere with your life as little as possible. For this you need good information and advice, optimal treatment with drugs and/or allergy shots, and careful avoidance of your allergens.

Quite often, however, people have all the information and drug treatment they need, but they still don't stay on top of their health problems. For some people this is due to the severity of the disease itself, but for others it is because they are not following their treatment program properly.

There can be two distinct reasons for this: either they are not wholehearted about wanting to be well (ambivalence)—or they have never really accepted that they are ill (denial).

Ambivalence

Sometimes being ill has certain benefits—or being entirely well has certain disadvantages. Our state of health determines how people treat us, especially within the family, and the expectations people have of us. It may be comforting to be ill, because others are more supportive then, or it may be less risky because we are not forced to try things (such as physical activities) at which we might fail. Being ill as a child often sets up a pattern for how we interact with the world.

These habitual patterns can survive in the mind long after any real advantages have evaporated. Many people become stuck with a way of thinking and living in which ill-health is a cornerstone of their existence.

If any of this rings a bell with you, try to tackle the problem at source. Such mental blocks are not immovable. Indeed, simply recognizing that the block is there can start to change things for some people. Others may need professional help to overcome these long-standing habits of mind. Counseling or cognitive therapy can be very valuable, and your doctor may be able to help in locating a suitably qualified person for this.

Denial

At the opposite end of the spectrum are people who want to deny that they have any kind of health problem. Often these people cannot quite accept that they have a long-term disease, such as eczema or asthma, and this makes them "forget" to take their medication. Ironically, these people frequently wind up having far more trouble with their allergies than they need to, because they neglect preventive treatments.

To be really well, you first have to admit that you do have allergies and then sort out your conflicting feelings about what this means. Again, some form of counseling, cognitive therapy, or some other kind of psychotherapy can be helpful.

Making use of this book

As everyone knows, a little knowledge is a dangerous thing. You can use the information in this book to help yourself, but it's important to remember that there is no substitute for the comprehensive understanding of the human body that your doctor gained during many long years at medical school. Always check with your doctor before changing your diet, stopping your drugs, practicing breathing exercises, taking a nonprescription medicine, or trying any other experimental treatment.

The information about disease, diagnosis, and treatment in this book falls into four categories:
- basic information that no doctor would disagree with
- the findings of new research, or research that is not widely known, but which falls within the accepted medical model of the disease. Your doctor may not know about some of this research (there is a *terrifying* amount of new information bombarding doctors every week, and no one can keep up

with it all), but he or she won't find it unbelievable.

• evidence from research that is entirely valid but which is widely ignored because it falls outside the accepted medical model of the disease concerned (see p. 86–7).

• information based on the repeated observations of doctors or patients. This does not amount to scientifically valid evidence, but it's included here if it seems plausible and if it could be useful to some readers.

You should be able to tell, from the context in which it is presented, which category any item of information falls into. When talking to your doctor about items that belong in the last two categories above, be prepared for a certain amount of skepticism.

The important thing to ask the doctor is whether there is good reason not to try the suggested measures, in addition to your usual treatment—is there any *risk* involved, given your particular state of health?

Playing safe with allergens

For people with a tendency to allergies, the dangers of heavy exposure to potential allergens—those you are *not* allergic to at present—is something to bear in mind. People with relatively mild allergy symptoms, such as hay fever, can develop asthma and severe allergies to molds or dust mites as a result of renovating old houses or damp basements. Sleeping on an old sofa, or on a bed with an ancient mattress or eiderdown comforter, can have the same effect, due to the huge dose of dust-mite allergen inhaled.

Managing asthma

Of all the diseases described in this book, asthma—especially severe asthma—is among the most difficult to live with. Learn to recognize asthma symptoms before they get out of hand, and take immediate action.

Studies of patients who die from asthma attacks find that the deaths could, in almost all cases, have been prevented. Factors contributing to fatal attacks include: heavy exposure to allergens, smoking, and failure to use preventer drugs.

For the day-to-day management of asthma, you should have a written **management plan** prepared by your doctor.

This should tell you how often to take your drugs under normal circumstances and what to do if your symptoms change or you develop a cold or chest infection. The brand names of your drugs (or the color of the inhaler) should be included on the management plan. If you have a peak flow meter, specific peak-flow values should be included on your management plan, with instructions for how to respond if your peak flow falls to these levels.

Your plan should tell you how to recognize a severe attack coming on and what to do at the various stages of the attack.

A key part of asthma control is having everything with you that you need in case of an attack. It's tedious, but you have to do it. You should take your reliever inhaler with you wherever you go. Those with severe asthma can also benefit from carrying a compact spacer (ask your pharmacist or see p. 255).

For a long day out or a stay away from home, check that you also have your management plan, your peak flow meter, your preventer inhaler, steroid tablets, if you sometimes need these, and your doctor's phone number

Peak flow meters

A peak flow meter can detect narrowing of your airways—the beginnings of an asthma attack—before there are any obvious symptoms. The signs of worsening asthma include:

• a morning reading that is less than 80 percent of the evening reading

• average readings less than 80 percent of your best-ever reading. (If they get to less than 50 percent of your best reading, this is a severe and possibly life-threatening attack.)

You must learn how to use a peak flow meter from your doctor, who should also check your technique regularly—it is very easy to get into bad habits.

Standing up for your rights

People with allergies and asthma are covered in the U.S. by the Americans with Disabilities Act (ADA), even if the symptoms are under control. The act states that you cannot be discriminated against in education (see p. 105) or employment, nor be excluded from public places such as hotels, restaurants, theaters, stores, or museums. Human Rights legislation in Canada provides similar protection. Check with your provincial or federal Human Rights commission.

If something in the air affects you badly—such as molds or strong-smelling cleaning fluids—then you have a right to clean air that you can breathe safely.

Emergency alerts

An emergency alert bracelet or pendant should be worn by anyone who

• is allergic to latex rubber, or to drugs such as penicillin

• has a severe allergy to insect stings

• suffers from exercise-induced anaphylaxis, or anaphylactic shock as a result of food allergy

• has very severe asthma attacks

Key information is engraved on the bracelet, along with a telephone number that gives medical staff access to a computer database containing vital medical data about you. This valuable service is provided by a nonprofit company called MedicAlert. For contact details, see p. 255.

Choosing medical insurance

If you have allergies, choosing medical insurance or, in Canada, supplemental medical insurance (see p. 97), needs special care.

The traditional form of medical insurance is called **Indemnity Insurance**. With this kind of policy:

- you can choose any doctor or hospital
- your insurance company pays a fixed proportion (70, 80, or 90 percent) of the cost. The part the patient pays is called the **coinsurance**. There is usually a limit on the total you must pay in the event of a major illness.
- if the fee charged by the doctor or hospital is higher than the "Usual and Customary" fee in your area (as defined by the insurance company), you have to pay the difference in full.
- there is usually a fixed sum—for example, the first $1500 of medical costs a year—that you have to pay in full. This is called the **deductible**.

This type of insurance gives you a lot of freedom, but can be expensive, in terms of both the premiums, and—if you fall seriously ill at some stage—the coinsurance payments.

In an attempt to keep premiums down and to control costs for the medical insurance companies, a variety of different plans have been devised that are known collectively as **Managed Care**. All the plans of this type revolve around a group of doctors and hospitals that have contractual arrangements with the health plan. The plans vary in the extent to which you, as a patient, are restricted to this group of doctors and hospitals. Some types of plan allow you to go to doctors outside the plan and still be partially reimbursed, while others offer no financial help in seeing doctors outside the plan.

The earliest version of Managed Care was the **Health Maintenance Organization** or **HMO**, in which

- you choose a primary care physician (PCP) from a list of those who are part of the plan. This doctor could be a family physician (general practitioner), an internist, or—for your children—a pediatrician.
- your primary care doctor decides when you should see a specialist, and makes the referral.
- you pay a fixed amount each month
- you then, in some plans, have unlimited access to all medical care. In other plans you have to make a small payment each time you use the service—for example, $10 for a visit to the doctor and $5 for a prescription. This is known as a **co-payment**. Unlike coinsurance, it is a fixed amount, which makes health care costs far more predictable.
- if you want to see any specialist who is outside the HMO, you have to pay the full cost yourself.

Under an HMO plan, you don't have to fill in claims forms, and the amount of paperwork involved is greatly reduced. There are also few exclusions—for example, preventive care, checkups, convalescent care, and routine dental and eye care, are usually covered. Some or all of these may be excluded with Indemnity Insurance, although the policies vary a great deal.

There are two forms of Managed Care that aim to give you more flexibility than you get with an HMO.

A **Point of Service** plan (POS) is like an HMO with two additional features:

- Your primary care doctor can refer you to a specialist or other medical provider who is outside the plan, if he or she feels that the circumstances merit this. The insurance company covers most of the cost.
- You can refer yourself to someone outside the plan, and get more limited help with the cost.

A **Preferred Provider Organization** (PPO) goes one step further in loosening up the restrictions of Managed Care. It does not require you to choose a primary care doctor and it gives you complete freedom to make your own referrals to specialists. There are two basic options when you need medical help.

- Consult a doctor, hospital, or other medical service that is part of the plan, and pay a small fixed charge.
- Refer yourself to someone outside the plan, in which case the rules are the same as those for Indemnity Insurance.

From the point of view of allergy sufferers, there may be downsides to some Managed Care plans. For example, the number of allergens treated with allergy shots may be limited by cost restrictions, which, for some patients, can reduce the effectiveness of treatment. The type of diagnostic tests that the health plan covers may be limited—they may not pay for RAST tests (see p. 92) except in particular situations, for example; but this is a reasonable restriction since, in most circumstances, skin tests are just as accurate and a lot cheaper. Drug costs are sometimes limited too, but research suggests that doctors usually find a way to give their patients the treatment they need, whatever the restrictions of the health plan may, in theory, dictate.

Overall, research into the effects of Managed Care suggests that it makes doctors more cost-conscious without seriously affecting the quality of care. However, some U.S. allergists are concerned that they are not able to provide an adequate level of treatment under Managed Care.

Most insurance plans, of whatever type, also exclude "experimental treatments." Find out exactly what counts as an experimental treatment and consider how this might affect you now or in the future.

Three levels of insurance in Canada

Medicare in Canada provides extensive medical coverage but it does not cover the cost of drugs, medical devices, experimental therapies or diagnostic procedures, or complementary medicine. Outside of basic coverage, each province varies somewhat in what is covered. Patients on social assistance do have extensive prescription drug coverage under other programs.

Short-term Supplemental is recommended if traveling outside Canada because Medicare reimbursement rates may be much lower than the fee charged by the country you are visiting. Check the terms of the policy as regards pre-existing conditions, and ensure that you are covered for your asthma and allergies.

Long-term Supplemental for Non-Medicare Services: usually a comprehensive package that covers prescription drug costs, travel medical insurance, and some other services, for example, physiotherapy and psychology, some complementary medical services, dental and vision care, and medical devices. Deductible and co-insurance (see p. 96) often apply, and it is important to clarify coverage of preexisting conditions. The majority of prescription allergy, eczema, and asthma medications are covered, but because most antihistamines are nonprescription, you will have to pay for these yourself. Epinephrine autoinjectors are non-prescription, but drug plans usually reimburse for these.

Buying a health plan

It is usually best to get a health plan through your job, or the job of a family member, if you can. When insurance companies sell to a large group of people—all the employees of a big company, for example—they are spreading their risk across a wider base, and can offer lower premiums. If your employer does not offer a health plan, it may be possible to get one through a labor union, professional organization, or club.

Check the details of what is offered by a group plan, as described below for individual plans. Also talk with your employee benefits office. There may be a choice of plans available. Talk with others who have allergies and are already part of the plan—are they happy with their treatment?

Buying a health plan as part of a small group—a company with fewer than 50 employees, for example—means that you may not get such a good deal. Buying as an individual is also difficult and requires special care. It is best to buy through an independent broker, who can describe a range of different plans and give you impartial advice, based on your particular health needs.

Those with severe long-term health problems sometimes find it difficult to get medical insurance at all—or the premiums may be unaffordable. This is more likely to be the case with individual policies or those purchased by a small group. In the U.S. legal reforms are under discussion, with the intention of eliminating such situations. In the meantime, if you are faced with a refusal, get the advice of an independent insurance broker. You may also want to check, with the Insurance Commissioner for your state, that the insurance company's refusal is not breaking state rules regarding medical insurance.

Key questions to ask

You can telephone the health plan with questions. These are some of the things you may want to ask:

- Will it be necessary to change from my current primary care doctor, allergist, pediatrician, or other specialist?
- Is renewal of the policy guaranteed?
- How does the plan cover, or provide for, emergency medical care? This is particularly important for anyone with asthma, true food allergy, or allergy to insect stings. Ask how the plan provides access to care outside your own geographic area, such as during travel and vacation.
- Does the plan offer help from a nutritionist or dietitian for those needing such help—such as those with food allergy or other form of food sensitivity, and on a restricted diet?
- Is there a special program for asthma? Is full preventive treatment for asthma covered?
- How long do patients generally wait for an appointment with an allergist, or other specialist?
- Are other ancillary services offered or covered, such as physical therapy, nebulizers and/or home oxygen if required for asthma, and rehabilitation services after hospitalization?

In the U.S. a prime source of objective information about Managed Care plans is the National Committee for Quality Assurance (NCQA). By means of the NCQA web site (see p. 255), you can find out how a particular plan compares with others.

Don't let your coverage lapse

If you have allergies, these will be considered as "preexisting conditions" by a health insurance company. In other words, you had allergies before taking out the health plan. Given a free choice, companies selling health plans would like to exclude all preexisting conditions from coverage, at least for a while after the policy begins. Under a U.S. law passed in 1997, a health plan cannot exclude the treatment of preexisting conditions if you were insured with another company throughout the previous 12 months. So when you change plans, your coverage continues.

If you allow your coverage to lapse, even briefly, you will face restrictions when you start a health plan again. Treatment of your allergies, and any other long-term health problem, will not be covered for a time—usually 12 months, but it varies from plan to plan.

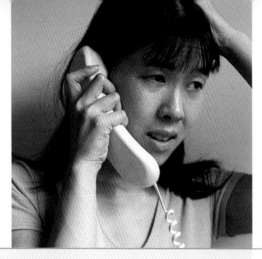

Dealing with emergencies

Let's hope it never happens—but if it does, knowing what to do could make the difference between surviving and not surviving. The sensible thing is to read these pages—or whichever parts are relevant to you or your child—*before* you encounter an allergy-related emergency. It is often helpful to rehearse the procedure in your mind and actually imagine yourself going through the actions described here.

Find out in advance what the local ambulance service is like, and ask your primary care doctor for advice about who to contact in an emergency. These are the options:

• Call your primary care doctor. If the doctor is nearby and the hospital or ambulance a long way off, this may be the best decision. Doctors in rural areas may have supplies of epinephrine for emergency treatment and oxygen for those suffering a severe asthma attack.

• Call an ambulance. If the ambulance is carrying oxygen and epinephrine and is staffed by paramedics, this is the best option.

• Go by car or taxi to the nearest hospital emergency department. This is not usually a good plan, because your condition may quickly get worse, and you have no emergency treatment available. But there may be situations in which it is a sensible decision.

Remember that emergencies can occur when you are away on vacation or on business. Never stay anywhere without a phone—and check that it is working as soon as you arrive. Make sure you know where the nearest hospital is and that you have the phone number of a local doctor. A remote vacation cottage can be a dangerous place to develop an asthma attack or anaphylactic shock.

Anaphylactic shock

This is an emergency requiring *immediate medical help*. The signs of anaphylactic shock are listed on p. 58. In the case of food allergy, there are additional signs in the mouth (see p. 62).

Use epinephrine (see p. 150) right away if you have it—**but get emergency medical help also**. With injectable epinephrine, remove the cap and push firmly into the outer thigh, going straight through any thin clothing if it cannot be easily removed. Never inject into any other part of the body—this can be dangerous.

Epinephrine inhalers are available, as an additional treatment, in the U.S., but not Canada. If you have an epinephrine inhaler, you can use this first to treat symptoms in the throat and airways, then use the injector if you still have symptoms. For those who have relatively mild reactions normally, this is a good approach. (Improvise a spacer—see p. 100— if there is difficulty in inhaling the epinephrine.)

If your reactions tend to be severe, use the injector first and follow up with the inhaler if needed.

Overdosing with epinephrine is possible, **and can be fatal**, but using the inhaler as well as the injector is safe as long as you don't have a heart condition. (Don't exceed the maximum number of puffs allowed for the inhaler, because the propellant can cause problems.)

If you do not improve after using the injector, a second one can be used, 10–15 minutes later. In situations where medical help is not yet available and the symptoms are not abating, another shot of epinephrine can be given every 15–20 minutes. But the maximum number of shots recommended by your doctor, or by the manufacturer, should **never** be exceeded. Keep count of how many you've had, and tell medical staff.

An asthmatic who does not have an epinephrine inhaler can use a beta-2 reliever inhaler such as Ventolin (see p. 152) as well as the epinephrine injection, although it probably won't help very much.

Suppose you know for sure that you have encountered your allergen, but you don't have any symptoms yet? Most doctors say go ahead and use the epinephrine injector if you have reacted very badly in the past. In general, for people with no other health problems, it is better to give an epinephrine injection which *isn't* needed than to delay giving one that *is* needed.

Following anaphylactic shock, you should be kept in the hospital for several hours even when everything seems fine. Attacks can recur as much as 8 hours later. Corticosteroids may reduce the chance of this happening—ask if these have been given. If you are being discharged early and it is a long journey home, consider waiting in the hospital, or nearby, until 8 hours after the original reaction.

First aid for anaphylactic shock

A badly swollen tongue or throat can cause suffocation. If there is visible swelling and the person is unconscious or turning blue, try to keep the top of the trachea (the main airway leading from the throat) open. Bend the base of the neck (where it meets the shoulders) forward, and tilt the head slightly backward.

If there is swelling in the throat and difficulty breathing, a sitting position is better than lying down.

A first-time attack

The first allergic reaction you ever experience can be very mild—maybe no more than tingling or itching of the mouth in the case of food allergy. Stay near a phone for an hour or so, in case you need to call for medical help. Often the symptoms just wear off, and that's it. Keep well away from the food, insect, or whatever, read pp. 58–9, and see your doctor soon. If symptoms worsen, and if they affect the body as a whole (for example, widespread hives), or if your breathing is affected, then you need emergency medical help.

A person who is losing consciousness should be put in the standard recovery position (see any first-aid manual) to reduce the chance of them inhaling vomit—a particular risk with food allergy.

Insect-sting allergy

If you don't have an epinephrine injector, get medical help immediately.

If you've had a **cutaneous systemic reaction** (widespread hives—see p. 60) in the past, use the epinephrine injector if there is any difficulty in breathing, hoarseness, stomach cramps, diarrhea, nausea, faintness, dizziness, or confusion. If you are unsure, remember that, unless you have a heart condition, it is usually better to overreact (use the epinephrine unnecessarily) than underreact.

If you've had a **severe systemic reaction** (anaphylactic shock) in the past, use an epinephrine injector at the first sign of any reaction other than immediately around the sting.

If there is a honeybee stinger left in the skin, scrape or flick it out sideways, using a fingernail, knife blade, or credit card—*the venom sac is attached and will go on injecting venom for up to 10 minutes if you leave it there. Don't try to get hold of the stinger and pull it out*—this squeezes the venom sac and pumps more venom into the skin.

Get emergency medical help, and follow the other measures for anaphylactic shock (see left).

Don't go alone

If you suffer vomiting or diarrhea during anaphylaxis, and have to go to the bathroom, tell someone to call an ambulance *and take someone else with you*. Do not go in alone and lock the door, in case you collapse.

Asthma attacks

Even those with mild asthma, who have never had a serious attack before, can quite suddenly get into difficulties and require emergency treatment. Don't be overanxious about this, because it is unlikely to happen—but do be prepared. Not having your reliever inhaler with you when a severe attack starts is a recipe for disaster—*always take it with you*, wherever you go.

Deal with an attack promptly. The sooner you act, the fewer drugs you'll need in the long run to control the attack. Most asthmatics wait too long and then under-treat their asthma.

The important thing is *recognizing* an asthma attack and knowing when it is getting out of control. Not all attacks are the same—some come on fast, some come on slowly.

Rapid asthma attacks come on in a matter of hours. You may have been fine all day, but then start to feel very breathless and wheezy, or begin coughing badly. Less than an hour later, despite using the reliever, the breathlessness is worse and it is a struggle to speak or walk across the room, or a bluish tinge is noticed on the lips or fingernails. *This is a severe attack: don't delay in getting emergency medical help.*

Slow asthma attacks come on over a period of days. At first you are more breathless and wheezy than usual, and your reliever inhaler is not helping much. Asthma wakes you up at night, and you are far more breathless than usual in the morning. This could be the beginning of a severe attack, so don't delay in getting medical help. If you get to the point where your asthma is disturbing your sleep every night, and in the morning you have difficulty in speaking or walking around, this is a very serious situation—*you must see your doctor or go to the hospital now.*

A few asthmatics have great difficulty recognizing when they are increasingly breathless, and for them, using a peak flow meter

Recognizing an asthma attack in a very young child

With a young child, these signs indicate a severe asthma attack:

- The nostrils are flared.
- The shoulders are unusually high.
- The child can say only one or two words between breaths.
- The ribs are pushed out, and the spaces between the ribs, and below the chest cage, are sucked in during breathing.
- You can hear wheezing (a whistling noise).
- The lips, tongue, or fingernails are blue.

If wheezing stops, without any other apparent improvement, this is a very bad sign—it may mean that the airways are now so narrow that no air is passing through them. This is called a "silent chest," and indicates an *urgent* need for medical attention.

(see p. 95) every day is essential. Indeed, most asthmatics find that monitoring peak flow is a valuable way of spotting attacks in advance. However, if your peak flow seems normal, and yet you feel breathless and have a tight feeling in your chest, *pay attention to your symptoms* and get medical help.

Your response to your reliever inhaler is another helpful sign in assessing asthma attacks. Things are serious if

- the reliever inhaler does not seem to be working at all within 10 minutes of taking a puff
- it does not work as well as usual
- it works, but the effect wears off in less than 3 hours

If you have an asthmatic child, give *everyone* who normally takes care of the child, detailed written instructions for recognizing and dealing with an asthma attack. People forget verbal instructions, especially in an emergency. A child who is exhausted or upset by an attack should always be given medical care.

Taking action

If your reliever inhaler is not working well (see above), take another puff to open up your airways—*and then take further action,* as described below.

If you seem to be in the early stages of a slow asthma attack, check your management plan and if the peak flow has fallen below the recommended level, double the dose of inhaled steroids (twice as many puffs each time) now. Add any other medicines (for example, steroid tablets) as recommended by the management plan.

Those who don't have a peak flow meter or management plan should double the dose of inhaled steroids and make an urgent appointment to see the doctor.

If you are suffering a rapid attack, or a slow attack that has gotten out of control, you need emergency medical help. Phone for an ambulance, phone your doctor, or go to the hospital—the ideal course of action will vary, depending on where you live and what the local services are like (see p. 98).

Use your reliever inhaler until medical help arrives. You can take one or two puffs every 5–10 minutes if needed, but keep a count of how many puffs you've had, and stop after 30. Some doctors suggest taking up to 30 puffs all at once. (If you have a heart condition, this dose might be dangerous: follow your doctor's advice carefully.)

If it is difficult to inhale, use a spacer—this can make all the difference, especially for children. You can improvise a spacer from a plastic cup, a plastic bottle, or a paper bag. Make a hole in the bottom of the cup or bottle, or in one corner of the paper bag, and insert the mouthpiece of the inhaler here. The open end

The six golden rules for asthma attacks

- Breathe as slowly as possible and concentrate on breathing out, not on breathing in. Exhale as fully as you can and your in-breath will follow automatically.
- Never panic—if you do, you may start hyperventilating, and this make matters much worse (see p. 226). Panicky parents are the worst possible thing for an asthmatic child during an attack.
- Adopt a position that makes breathing as easy as possible. Propping your arms up at about shoulder height can help—for example, sit back-to-front on a dining chair, with your arms folded and resting on the back. Or put pillows on a table, sit in an upright chair, and rest your head and arms on the pillows. Don't lie down, as this makes matters worse. Open a window, as long as the air outside is not cold, polluted or loaded with pollen.
- Avoid factors that can make an asthma attack worse, for example, vigorous activity, cold air, irritants and allergens.
- Drink plenty of water, fruit juice, or other liquids as a lot of water is lost through the surface of the airways during an asthma attack, and you can become dehydrated.
- Don't take anything to help you sleep, even herbal pills. If your asthma gets worse during the night, you need to wake up so that you can get more air.

of the cup, bottle, or bag goes in or over the mouth (you have to bunch up the bag and hold it around the mouth). Squirt the inhaler repeatedly into the improvised spacer, while breathing steadily in and out.

After an attack

Asthmatics who have suffered a severe attack are occasionally sent home from the hospital before they are completely better. Some of them die as a result. So if you feel breathless or otherwise unwell after you leave the hospital, don't hesitate to go back—or seek other medical help.

See your primary care doctor or specialist within a few days of any emergency treatment. Don't be overconfident just after a severe attack—this can be a very vulnerable time. Get more rest than usual, and drink plenty of fluids, as you may be dehydrated. Keep taking your preventer inhaler at the increased dose—reducing the dose now could lead to another severe, possibly fatal, attack. Keep taking steroid tablets if you have been given them.

If you produced a lot of mucus during the attack, try to clear it, but without violent coughing. Mucus can sometimes form solid plugs that block small airways. Expectorants—drugs to help bring up mucus—may be tried, but are rarely helpful. Don't take ordinary cough medicine (see p. 163). There are also some breathing exercises that can help move mucus (see p. 231).

An asthma attack represents a chance to learn more about preventing asthma—so think about what went wrong. Had you forgotten to take your preventer inhaler regularly? How long is it since you had your medicines reviewed by the doctor or asthma clinic? Have you been using your peak flow meter daily? Were you exposed to a high dose of allergen or an irritant?

A reaction to aspirin-like drugs

Aspirin sensitivity can begin quite suddenly in someone who has previously taken aspirin without trouble. If you have unexplained chronic urticaria, or polyps in the nose, plus asthma and/or rhinitis, the development of aspirin sensitivity at some time in the future is a distinct possibility (see p. 151).

A sensitivity reaction to aspirin or aspirin-like drugs usually begins between 30 minutes and 2 hours after the drug is taken. You will have some or all of these symptoms:

- a runny or badly blocked nose and red eyes
- a feeling of warmth, flushing, and sweating
- a general rash
- a sensation of tightness in the chest, a dry cough, increasing breathlessness
- malaise and exhaustion
- vomiting or diarrhea
- swelling (angioedema) and/or hives (urticaria)

If you have such symptoms, **_get emergency medical help immediately_**, because the reaction can quickly develop into severe asthma, shock, collapse, and unconsciousness.

If you have asthma, use your reliever inhaler as much as required (up to 30 puffs of the inhaler) until medical help arrives. Anyone who has an epinephrine injector or epinephrine inhaler (see p. 150) can use this also. Tell the ambulance crew and doctors exactly what you have taken.

Helping children to cope with their illness

Suffering from a long-term illness, especially if it is severe and sometimes limits activity, can easily make a child feel different from other children, and "not good enough." Children with allergies, especially those with severe asthma or food allergies, may also be very frightened and anxious. At the same time, such children often feel that they have to protect their parents by not revealing their fears.

Children may think that their illness is a punishment for something they have done wrong. Their guilty feelings can be so powerful that they may not tell their parents without lots of encouragement and sensitive discussion.

One of the most valuable things you, as a parent, can do for children with allergies is to build up their self-esteem. This is especially important when they start school, because they have to adjust to other children and learn how to deal with questions about their illness, as well as some unkindness.

For children whose allergies limit what they can do physically, or restrict some normal activities, try to find other interests and hobbies that the child can do well. When talking with the child, always emphasize the positive things—the difficulties that you have overcome together in the past, the measures the child can take to keep the symptoms under control (such as stopping scratching, applying creams, or using a preventer inhaler), and the areas of life in which he or she is particularly successful. As the child gets older, introduce the idea that coping with illness makes you a stronger, kinder, and more resolute person, who can cope with any of life's challenges. Show the child how much you value their maturity and perseverance.

Pay attention to what the child's friends are saying—a bit of eavesdropping is allowed—and be prepared to counteract any negative messages. Teach your child to be strong and confident about choosing his or her friends, and to prefer those who are sensible, understanding, and supportive. Ask casually what schoolteachers and other adults say when you are not around, because they can, without meaning any harm, undermine a child's confidence with thoughtless remarks.

For children with problems that are potentially life threatening, such as true food allergy, your natural anxieties as a parent can lead you to be overprotective. This can make the child feel smothered, but letting go is not easy. You have somehow to find a middle path that works for you both.

With asthmatic children, focus on letting them live as normal a life as possible. Avoid saying "no" automatically to things that might induce an asthma attack—such as running around outdoors in cold weather. Take some small risks, and let the child make the decision sometimes—he or she will gain a lot from taking the responsibility, *especially* if the decision is the wrong one.

This is the only way for children to learn how to manage their own condition and make sensible choices. The sooner you can begin letting go, the better the child will cope in his or her teenage years, when it really will be necessary to make some difficult decisions without your help.

A pitfall for parents

In bringing up a child with allergies, remember that there should never be any "secondary gain" from illness—absolutely no advantages to having the eczema get worse (easily done by scratching) or starting an asthma attack (some children can bring one on by breathing in a particular way). If your child has to take time off from school because of ill-health, ask the teacher for work that can be done at home, and check that it really is done. Children who are allowed to benefit from being ill can establish an unhealthy pattern for dealing with life's difficulties (see p. 94), which may be long-lasting. Such a mind-set can seriously limit a child's development.

Incidentally, the "secondary gain" from illness may be quite altruistic in nature. It can include stopping parents from arguing, or from nagging a naughty brother or sister, as well as more obvious things such as getting a parent's attention—so be aware of all the circumstances in the family that are affecting the child.

Sometimes a child realizes, unconsciously, that attending to illness gives a parent a welcome distraction from emotional problems and a comforting feeling of being needed and useful. The allergies can become part of the structure of a family, the glue holding everyone together.

Conversely, long-term illness can tear families apart: research shows that divorce is more common in families where a child suffers from severe asthma. Doctors frequently notice that severe eczema can also create a lot of tension in the home. If you feel that a child's illness is affecting the family badly—in whatever way—talk to your doctor, or someone else who you trust. You may need the help of a counselor or family therapist to sort things out. Local allergy support groups can also be very useful.

Children and medicines

Parents often feel very anxious about all the medication an allergic child uses. On the whole, the drugs prescribed for allergy are very safe, and only children with severe disease are at risk of significant side effects. These children will be carefully monitored by the doctor.

Needless to say, if you can cut down on the drugs by reducing allergen exposure, avoiding irritants (for example, tobacco smoke and indoor pollutants – see pp. 128–30) and implementing some of the other measures described in this book, you should do so. But if the child still needs drugs to control the symptoms, it is far better to accept them than to let the child struggle with all the discomfort, limitations, and distress that the illness imposes.

Parents who are very concerned about drugs should talk openly to the doctor about their fears. If there are differences of opinion about drugs within the family, try not to expose the child to the disagreements. Decide on a joint policy in advance and present a united front to the child; otherwise he or she may feel confused and anxious about the situation—or even learn to manipulate it.

Coping with food allergy

The following concerns true food allergy (see p. 62), which can be life-threatening, not idiopathic food intolerance (see p. 74).

Protecting a child with severe food allergies is a major task. You will find it enormously helpful to be in contact with other parents who are facing the same challenge. The practical details are everything here, and you can benefit from other people's ingenuity in solving day-to-day problems. Several support groups exist (see p. 255), offering a wealth of advice.

For very small children, the main task is to make sure that everyone who looks after the child understands exactly what can and can't be eaten. Child-care workers and babysitters should spend time with you seeing what is involved in preparing food for the child—this is *far* better than just giving verbal instructions. Also make sure that everyone knows how to use the epinephrine auto-injector (see p. 98).

Once children start going to parties, you should always stay at the party for the whole time and supervise your child closely. Take food with you that your child can safely eat, but which other children can also share. Some parents put a label on toddlers warning other adults that certain foods are taboo; for children under reading age this is probably acceptable and does allow you to relax

The asthmatic child
Children with asthma should have a management plan (see p. 95) and may benefit from using a peak flow meter (see p. 95). Once your child is old enough to understand the difference between preventers and relievers, explain that using the preventer regularly keeps asthma under control, which means no sudden attacks and less need to use the reliever inhaler in public—something that most children find intensely embarrassing. You should oversee the child's treatment closely until the age of seven or eight, then gradually let the child take over some of the responsibilities.

a little, but with older children, the dangers of being teased or stigmatized should always be borne in mind.

Plan ahead all the time. Keep a snack box in the car containing food that the child can safely eat. Whenever you go on a trip, however short, have some safe foods with you, in case you get stuck somewhere and the child gets hungry. If you go out to eat, exert maximum caution about the restaurant food (see p. 111). Some parents take along a super-delicious sandwich or guaranteed-safe burger, and ask the restaurant to warm it up in a microwave (where appropriate) and serve it when they bring out the other food. If you do this, be sure the staff understand that the brought-from-home food must not touch any other food (for example, cheese for a milk-allergic child).

At home, some parents opt for everyone eating the same allergen-free food, on the basis that this makes for being "a real family." Others, finding this too problematic or expensive, make a virtue out of the allergic child having a different meal. "I try to make her feel special about having her own food. The allergen-free dinner or pastry always looks and tastes really good."

As children get older and more independent, you need to educate them thoroughly about avoiding the offending food. Equip them for difficult situations by role-playing. Act out being offered a tempting item of food by another child and being jeered at for refusing. Act out suffering an allergic reaction to food and getting help quickly, even though other people don't understand and are uncooperative.

Allergies and schools

When your child starts at a new school, nursery school, or kindergarten, request a meeting with staff and teachers to talk about the child's allergies. Do this well before your child starts at the school so that any necessary changes can be made. If your child has a serious food allergy or severe asthma, you may have to make several visits, because there are usually a number of different people you need to meet and follow-up sessions may be required with some staff. If all this sounds daunting and "not my style," you need, for the sake of your child, to develop your skills in dealing with people and being assertive. Talk to a psychologist, or look for suitable training courses.

In addition to ensuring that the school takes good care of your child's health (see below), you should also discuss wider issues of adjustment to school life. Teasing or bullying can be a problem for children with any kind of health problem. Ask the teacher to keep an eye on your child and make sure that he or she is coping well—for example, that there is no difficulty about using an inhaler in front of other children when it is needed.

Eczema

Make sure that all staff realize that the skin rash is not infectious and that they communicate this to other children. The appearance of the skin can create a lot of problems with classmates, and teachers need to be alert for taunting remarks or nicknames.

Unfortunately, children with eczema are very susceptible to infections caught from others, such as impetigo (see p. 44); but you can't really protect children from such infections without isolating them socially. The best way to tackle this problem is to deploy every available treatment so that your child's skin becomes stronger and more resistant.

Asthma

If your child has asthma, ask what arrangements are made for inhalers. Children who can take responsibility for their own treatment should keep their inhalers with them. For younger children, the inhaler should be in the classroom and easily accessible (*never locked away*) and should be taken along during breaks and mealtimes. The child must always be able to get to the inhaler quickly: even a small delay in using it when an attack occurs can have dire consequences. Make sure everyone at the school understands this and knows how to recognize an attack and how to react. Assure the teacher that there is little danger of an asthmatic child overdosing, and that if other children take a few puffs they will come to no harm.

If the teacher seems to believe that asthma is a psychological problem (some still do), go and see the principal. Suggest that a local doctor comes in and talks to the school about asthma.

Make sure that the teacher knows about the effects of cold air and exercise on asthmatics. Talk to the phys ed teacher or athletics coach, and the playground attendants. It is vital that the phys ed teacher is encouraging but understanding toward asthmatic children. They should never be told to continue exercising if they feel breathless.

Food allergy

If your child has a food allergy, go and see the cafeteria manager personally. It may be helpful to take some printed material on food allergy with you, plus lists of synonyms for food ingredients (see pp. 172–4) where appropriate. Concentrate on building up a good relationship with the kitchen staff, while ensuring that they understand how dangerous certain foods can be to your child. (A ruling by the USDA Child Nutrition Division does oblige schools to provide suitable meals for allergic children, on receiving written instructions from a doctor, but obviously it's better to work by cooperation rather than coercion if you can.) The Canadian School Board Association and Health Canada have published a resource manual for schools to help them develop policies to protect anaphylactic children. The Food Allergy Network in the U.S. has a similar manual.

Many parents feel more relaxed if they supply their child with a packed lunch that they know is allergen-free. This is often a good strategy, but don't be complacent. Most allergic reactions in schools involve food given or traded by another child with entirely good intentions. Some schools with food-allergic children have set up a "no trading food" policy, which seems to work well. Other schools establish milk-free or nut-free tables in the cafeteria, so that friends can sit together and trade food safely. (The mothers of the other children sitting at these tables need to be well-versed in food avoidance, of course, so that their packed lunches are as safe as your own.) Some North American schools have banned nuts or peanuts altogether, where there is a nut-allergic student. Many Canadian schools have established a "nut-free" policy in any class with nut-allergic children in the lower school grades, as recommended by the Canadian Society of Allergy and Immunology (also endorsed by the American Academy of Allergy, Asthma and Immunology).

Some parents prepare a printed information sheet about their child's food allergy, with a photograph of the child, and put these up at stategic points in the kitchen and cafeteria area. This information can include instructions on how to deal with anaphylactic shock (see below) and whom to contact in an emergency.

Finally, include the art teacher in your rounds—foodstuffs are often used in art and craft projects.

Anaphylaxis

For children with severe food or insect-sting allergies that can lead to anaphylaxis, check that everyone at the school understands the potentially fatal nature of this condition. Key staff must know how to recognize anaphylactic shock and exactly what to do: show them how the epinephrine injector kit works. You could take along an old one so they can practice, or purchase a trainer (see p. 150). Injector kits and epinephrine inhalers must be within easy reach for adults, **never locked in a cupboard**. Repeat this educational process at the beginning of each new school year, and before school trips. As an additional precaution, your child should wear a bracelet or pendant (see box on p. 95) that informs medical personnel about his or her allergies—this is also vital for children with latex or drugs allergies.

Parents may be requested by the school to sign a waiver. You should sign a waiver allowing the school to inject epinephrine if needed, but *don't* sign a waiver absolving them from any responsibility if the epinephrine injector was *not* used.

Allergens and irritants in school

Schools today often have carpeting and other fabric furnishings, and these may be full of dust mites. If your child is allergic to mites, and if allergy symptoms are frequent at school, have a look around the classroom and see if this might be the cause. Before discussing the problem with the school, learn all you can about dust mites (see p. 114–117), so that you can assess whether proposed solutions to the problem would actually work.

Pets are sometimes kept in elementary school classrooms and can cause allergic reactions in sensitized children. Molds flourish in many school buildings, and will affect a child with mold allergy. Portable classrooms may become contaminated with molds that generate airborne toxins, causing respiratory irritation. Poor ventilation is sometimes a major problem in school buildings, especially those where windows cannot be opened. The School Board can arrange for air quality and mold spore testing.

Irritants in school air include glue, paint, the solvents from markers, disinfectants, air fresheners, and the fumes produced during science classes. Make sure the science teacher is aware of the risks and always uses a fume cabinet if irritant gases such as nitrogen dioxide are likely to be given off during an experiment.

Applying sunscreens to children's skin, especially very young children, is now routine in many schools and preschools. Teachers probably won't think to ask permission, so if your child is sensitive to any common ingredients of creams or sunscreens, let the teacher know in advance.

The rights of children with allergies

The Americans with Disabilities Act (see p. 95) prevents schools, daycare facilities, and preschools—public or private—from refusing to enroll a child because of allergies. They must accept children with allergies unless their presence fundamentally alters the program or poses a threat to others. If taking your child means that the catering arrangements are affected, staff have to learn to give epinephrine injections or use nebulizers, or the insurance premium goes up, these are things that the school or preschool just has to accept.

If children or older students are affected by items such as perfume, staff and other students should be asked not to apply any scented product before class. Likewise, children affected by insecticides and cleaning fluids should be catered to, and the air in a school should be free from these and other irritants.

The Asthma and Allergy Foundation of America can advise you if you need help in establishing your child's rights to equal treatment. For contact details, see p. 255. In Canada, check with your provincial or federal Human Rights commission for information about your child's rights.

Allergies and pregnancy

Great care is taken in prescribing drugs during pregnancy. This is something that doctors are now exceedingly cautious about, but do tell the doctor *as soon as you decide to try for a baby*. The fetus is most vulnerable to damage by drugs during the first three months, and especially the first few weeks after conception.

Your prescription will be changed if the drugs you are currently taking could pose any threat to the unborn child (see right).

If you are already pregnant as you read this, don't worry too much. With a few notable exceptions—certain antihistamines and antibiotics—most of the drugs used for allergic diseases do not pose any major risk to the unborn child. See your doctor as soon as you can—and talk to a pharmacist, in the meantime, if you are concerned.

Some nonprescription medicines are best avoided during pregnancy. Read the package carefully, and talk to your pharmacist if you have any doubts.

Allergy shots and skin testing

Allergy shots should not begin during pregnancy, because of the risk of anaphylaxis (see p. 107), but pregnant women who are already undergoing immunotherapy can continue. The safety procedures described on p. 167–8 should be followed with meticulous care during pregnancy.

Most doctors continue allergy shots at a steady "maintenance dose" because there is always a small risk of anaphylaxis with allergy shots when the dose is increased. Some doctors are even more cautious and reduce the maintenance dose during pregnancy, but give more frequent injections—this minimizes the chance of bad reactions.

Some doctors do not give skin tests for allergy during pregnancy, as these also carry a very small risk of anaphylaxis. If you do have skin tests, there must be resuscitation equipment available. Intradermal tests (see p. 92) are best avoided.

Allergy drugs

The U.S. Food and Drug Administration classification system for allergy drugs and pregnancy (also used in Canada) has come under fire from many doctors. The categories are as follows:

- **FDA Pregnancy Category A**
Scientific studies in humans show no risk to the fetus during the first three months of pregnancy.
- **FDA Pregnancy Category B**
Either: Animal studies show no risk to the fetus during pregnancy, and no human studies have been done or: Animal studies showed a risk but human studies did not.
- **FDA Pregnancy Category C**
Either: Animal studies have shown a risk to the fetus during pregnancy, and no human studies have been done or: neither animal nor human studies have been done.
- **FDA Pregnancy Category D**
Human studies have shown some risk to the fetus, but the benefits may outweigh the risks in certain cases.
- **FDA Pregnancy Category X**
There is a definite risk that outweighs any possible benefit.

FDA guidelines recommend the use of group A and B drugs. The problem is that many drugs commonly used to treat allergies and asthma during pregnancy have a "C" classification—no scientific studies have been done on these drugs, but they have been used in pregnant women for many years and experience suggests that they are safe. Many doctors feel that the system causes unnecessary anxiety among patients, because the "C" rating implies that the drugs are far more risky than they actually are.

Severe allergic reactions (anaphylaxis)

Special care should be taken to avoid anaphylaxis during pregnancy, as this may increase the chance of a miscarriage.

Injecting epinephrine during the first three months of pregnancy *may* carry some small risk of malformation of the baby. But the evidence here is uncertain, whereas the danger to your own life, if you don't use epinephrine when you need it, is both certain and substantial. The best policy is to be ultracareful about avoiding your allergen, so that anaphylaxis does not happen.

Women who suffer from **exercise-induced anaphylaxis** (see p. 59) generally play it safe by exercising less strenuously while pregnant. The problem can get worse during pregnancy, but it does not usually do so. Labor itself is very strenuous, but problems during the birth are uncommon. If anaphylaxis does occur, the reaction is usually quite mild—just hives—and the baby is delivered alive and well. However, many women find that the attacks of exercise-induced anaphylaxis are more frequent and severe when they start exercising again after the baby is born. It is best to resume exercise very gradually.

Eczema and other skin problems

Atopic eczema may improve during pregnancy, probably because the body produces slightly more of its own natural steroid, hydrocortisone. Contact dermatitis may either improve or flare up.

Stretch marks often itch a great deal, and widespread itchy skin, with or without a rash, is a common problem. These are not usually allergic reactions, and no cause can be identified in most cases. The itching should subside a few days after the birth.

If there is itching in the vulval area, this could be due to a *Candida* infection (your doctor can prescribe a safe treatment), or it might be just another of those unexplained itches of pregnancy.

Hay fever and other nasal allergies

The natural hormone changes of pregnancy can make your nose more blocked. If you have allergic rhinitis, this will add to your woes. Make sure that your drug treatment is adequate (see p. 29). The nose-clearing exercises on pp. 230–31 might also help.

Asthma

Severe asthma can be bad for both the pregnant mother and the unborn child because it can reduce the supply of oxygen to the baby. Uncontrolled asthma increases the risk of the baby being born prematurely—and premature babies are more likely to develop asthma themselves. The death rate for newborn babies is also higher if the mother has poorly controlled asthma.

Treating a severe asthma attack promptly helps to prevent any damage to the baby, so don't hesitate to call an ambulance— and tell the operator you are pregnant. The ambulance should be carrying oxygen, which will help the baby through the attack.

If you have asthma, *don't stop using your drugs or reduce the dose* unless advised to do so by a doctor. Because it is so important to keep asthma under control during pregnancy, your doctor may want to add, or increase, preventer drugs (see p. 152). It also makes sense to monitor your peak flow twice a day (see p. 95) so that you have advance warning of serious attacks.

Some asthmatics—usually those who have severe asthma— get much worse during their pregnancy. In such cases, careful monitoring and increased use of preventer medicines are essential. The symptoms usually increase from week 24 to week 36 of the pregnancy. The last 4 weeks tend to be much better, and things are back to normal by about 3 months after the birth.

Some women with asthma have fewer symtoms while they are pregnant, and for others, their asthma stays about the same.

Asthma can also appear for the first time during pregnancy and may be quite severe. However, a relatively mild breathlessness can be due simply to the fact that, as the pregnancy advances, the chest cavity, and therefore the lungs, become compressed.

This simple physical effect can also add to the difficulties of women who were already asthmatic before becoming pregnant.

GER (acid reflux)—see p. 38—can contribute to asthma during pregnancy, and treating this problem may help.

During the birth itself, severe asthma attacks are very rare. But it is still important that all the medical staff in attendance know you have asthma. They should also be told if you have taken steroid tablets during the previous two years. A record of when you took steroids, for how long, and at what dose, will be valuable. You may need a low dose of steroid to get you through the physical stress of labor (see p. 142). Some doctors believe that patients who have been using high-dose inhaled steroids should be treated in the same way.

Smoking

Smoking is a bad idea if you have allergies or any allergic tendency in the family. Smoking is a very bad idea indeed if you are pregnant, or a parent. This is the moment to give it up.

Enlist your doctor's help, and ask if counseling, psychotherapy, or other forms of support are available. If you have tried all this before, and failed, talk to your doctor about the possibility of using nicotine patches, or other smoking cessation medication. Some doctors believe that, for pregnant women who smoke 20 cigarettes or more a day, the advantages of nicotine patches outweigh the risks to the fetus. Nicotine levels in the blood are lower with patches than with heavy smoking, and your baby is not enduring the hundreds of other toxins found in cigarette smoke.

Chapter 4
avoiding allergens and irritants

Many countries have special schools for children with severe asthma and other allergies. Italian children are sent to one in the Italian Alps, where there is no trace of pollen, dust mites, or animal allergens. After nine months these children are a great deal healthier and more active—all their lung function tests are vastly improved. Blood tests show that they are actually less allergic to common allergens than before.

You may not be able to do quite this well at home, but *all* allergens and irritants can be avoided to some extent. Even if you can't eliminate them completely, you can certainly reduce exposure.

Before you start, it is important to be clear about exactly what affects you; otherwise you will be wasting a lot of effort. For example, people who are allergic to dust mites often think that a dusty house will necessarily be worse for them than an apparently clean house, but this is not so (see p. 115). Or they may say, "Oh, I got asthma on my vacation, because the roads were so dusty and I'm allergic to dust," forgetting that only house dust contains dust mites. The road dust may have acted as an irritant and helped to spark the asthma attacks, or it may have contained pollen or mold spores—but it does not contain dust mites or their allergens. Blaming the wrong thing for the asthma attack means that the real culprit is not identified.

If you are not absolutely sure what causes your allergies, skin tests (see p. 91) can identify the allergen. These tests are especially recommended if your reactions to the presumed allergen are inconsistent, or if you don't respond to the anti-allergen programs described here. For example, a few people who react to house dust are not allergic to dust mites, but to something else in the dust such as wool fibers or mold spores, or particles from cockroaches, houseflies, carpet beetles, or a long-departed cat. Even pollen that has accumulated in house dust can provoke allergic reactions—if you are not an over-keen duster, it can still be there long after the pollen season.

If you have hay fever, knowing which pollens cause your symptoms (and learning to recognize the plants concerned) is useful. You will probably need skin-prick tests to be sure. "Hay fever" can even be a seasonal mold allergy in some people (see p. 27).

Tackling allergens is now big business. There are a lot of people out there competing for your money, and false claims are common, especially for anti-mite products. Only a few manufacturers are deliberately misleading, and most false claims probably stem from ignorance or wishful thinking, but be very sure you know the facts about your allergen before you buy.

Air filters are a good example. A really good quality air filter (called an HEPA filter—High Efficiency Particulate Air filter) is an expensive purchase and, as the advertising tells you, it takes out very small particles with staggering efficiency. But this is entirely irrelevant if the source of those particles is no distance at all from your nose—your mite-infested pillow, for example, or the cat on your lap.

Something else that advertisements for air filters rarely mention is that unless you take measures to reduce allergen production—tackling mold growth in the house, for example, or keeping the dog outside— the filter can't help much. In short, filters do have their uses for *some* allergens, but they can't work miracles.

The products mentioned here, if not available in your locality, can be bought mail-order from specialist suppliers of anti-allergy products (see p. 255). Note that some offer both very good products and distinctly doubtful products, so judge each item on its individual merits. Ask to see scientific evidence that it works.

Don't be taken in by vague statements such as "anti-allergenic"—get the facts. The "anti-allergenic" label is often used on pillows with synthetic filling, for example, and people assume that it refers to dust-mite allergy, whereas it simply means that the pillow does not contain feathers. But unless you are allergic to feathers, there is no reason to avoid feather pillows. (In fact, if not covered with mite-proof covers, synthetic pillows collect *more* dust mites than feather pillows, because the fabric cover is less tightly woven, and the mites and skin particles get in more easily.)

Bad advice is also a hazard. Some of it just wastes your time and effort, but some could actually increase your exposure to allergen. Advice to vacuum floors daily or to vacuum beds is common but this achieves little and it means breathing much *more* allergen unless you have the right kind of vacuum cleaner (see p. 117). One health magazine even advised its readers with dust-mite allergy to "air mattresses by regularly turning them." This will not affect mite numbers at all, but it will shoot *massive* amounts of mite allergen out of the mattress and into the nose and lungs.

Ridding your house of allergens and irritants is, in itself, a hazardous procedure because more of the offending substances will be released into the air during the work. If you take up carpets or remove mattresses, dust-mite allergens and mold spores will be churned up in the millions. Just bundling up blankets will produce invisible clouds of dust-mite allergen—and cat allergen, if your pet once slept on the bed.

Ideally, the allergic individual should not do the work, nor be in the house until it is complete *and* the house has been thoroughly aired. This is particularly important for those with chronic sinusitis and mold growth in the house, because of the risk of fungal infections in the sinuses (see p. 32).

If you are an allergy sufferer and have no choice but to do the work yourself, or to be present, then get a good-quality dust mask and wear it whenever you're indoors—take it off only when you go outdoors. Those with eczema and sensitivity to airborne allergens should cover their skin carefully—with clothing, not barrier cream.

Remember that an ordinary hardware-store dust mask is not adequate for most allergens—it takes out only really big particles and lets through all the common airborne allergens except pollen. You need a more serious kind of mask, designed for workplace use and conforming to official standards. Before buying one, ask what is the smallest size of particle that it filters out (at 90 percent efficiency, or better). Compare this with the particle size for your allergen. These sizes are given in the following sections of this chapter.

You must be able to breathe well through the mask even when physically active, and it must fit tightly against your face, forming a seal at all edges. Beards and mustaches prevent this, as does stubble.

Masks that combine an activated carbon filter with a dust filter will take out gases and chemical vapors as well as particles. Bicycle shops sometimes sell such masks, but an industrial supplier may offer them more inexpensively. Such a mask can be useful if you are affected by traffic exhaust or industrial pollution as well as an allergen, for example, or if you are exposed temporarily to wet paint or other fumes at home.

Some people who try the anti-allergen programs feel much better quite fast. But generally these are long-term strategies—you may not reap any benefits for a few weeks, and the improvement may be small at first. Sometimes it takes several months for the full effects to be felt, so be persistent.

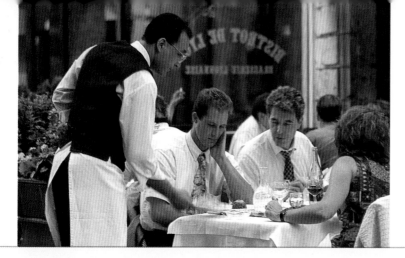

Allergens in food

Anyone with true food allergy or celiac disease needs to be very careful about avoiding certain foods. The information given here is aimed mainly at such people, rather than those with food intolerance (see p. 74), who can usually tolerate small amounts of their offending foods. However, some of the basic information given here is also relevant to those with food intolerance.

There are different levels of sensitivity, even among those with true food allergy. The "exquisitely sensitive" can react to unbelievably minute traces of the food, and for them life is especially difficult. The same is true of some celiacs, who can be affected by the tiniest quantity of gluten.

These people are a small minority. The level of vigilance required of such people will not be necessary for most people reading this book, so don't get things out of proportion. While it is vital to be sensible about avoiding your problem food, it is also important not to become overanxious.

Buying basic ingredients

People with true food allergy and celiac disease are safest when they cook for themselves. There are relatively few hazards, but do beware of well-meaning assistants in health-food stores who try to sell you some exotic package of grain or flour—spelt or kamut or triticale, for example—reassuring you that

it is "definitely not wheat." Be well informed about the different forms of your problem food and the names under which it is sold (see pp. 172–5).

Oils made from foods such as corn or peanuts sometimes cause concern. Ordinary refined oils have been so thoroughly processed that they actually contain no allergenic proteins. However, some doctors believe that, if you have an anaphylactic allergy, it is wise to avoid even highly refined oils, in case of a lapse in good manufacturing practice. The little bottles of gourmet walnut oil and almond oil are not refined at all and must be avoided if you have nut allergies. Sesame oil is not purified and can provoke serious reactions.

Those with allergy to tuna can usually eat canned tuna because the high degree of processing destroys the allergens. However, ordinary cooking may not make tuna safe. The allergens in fresh fruit and vegetables are generally inactivated by cooking, so jams, canned fruits, and well-cooked vegetables tend to be safe—but test very cautiously. Cooking does not have much effect on other food allergens, aside from eggs. In some cases, cooking can create allergens (see box on p. 186).

If you share your kitchen with others, and are highly sensitive, check that all cooking utensils are truly clean before use. Celiacs should watch out for breadcrumbs in the butter dish, jam, or toaster.

Genetic engineering and food allergy

Many people with food allergies are very concerned about the possibility that genetic engineering could introduce allergens from one plant species into another. This concern seems to be shared by government officials and those in the food industry, who are being extremely vigilant and cautious at present. As long as this attitude continues, there should be little danger to food allergy sufferers.

Finding food in funny places

If you are suffering some inexplicable reactions to nonfood items, it might, just possibly, be a food reaction. Some latex gloves contain the milk protein casein, for example, added as a manufacturing aid.

Where small children are allergic to a food, it may be best to keep the culprit out of the house entirely to avoid disasters.

Buying packaged foods

There are several different issues here:
- The need to read labels carefully for allergenic ingredients described by unfamiliar names (see p. 172).
- Errors in the packaging used (see pp. 174–5).
- Contamination by minute traces of a food substance due to processing machinery not being cleaned adequately. Cartons of fruit drink have occasionally been contaminated with traces of milk because the same production lines were used for packaging milk drinks. Tofu desserts made in ice-cream factories can also become contaminated with milk. These tiny traces of a food will affect only the most highly sensitive individuals, but contamination by nuts can involve large pieces and affect anyone with nut allergy (see p. 174).
- foodstuffs that are not an ingredient as such but are used as part of the production process (see p. 174).

Be very cautious indeed about ready-made food that is unlabeled, such as that from bakeries and farmers' markets. Egg is frequently used as a glaze on baked products; nuts may lurk within, and milk or wheat can turn up in the most unlikely places.

Restaurants, delis, and takeouts

The majority of fatal and near-fatal incidents involving true food allergy occur when people eat out. Fast food can also be a problem, except in the case of the large chains such as McDonald's, where ingredients are standardized and ingredient lists are published. It is alarming that highly allergenic foods (for example, peanuts) are sometimes used—yet far from obvious—in recipes and sandwich fillings where they would simply not be expected. Anyone with peanut or shellfish allergy should be ultracautious about Chinese, Thai, or Malaysian cooking—but those with milk allergy should find a haven here, because milk is not part of these culinary traditions.

The simplest solution is to eat very plainly when you go out—steak and salad, for example. Steer clear of casseroles and thick soups, where you can't see what's in it (the occasional chef throws in peanut butter to thicken the mix…). Things wrapped in pastry are best avoided for the same reason. Desserts are risky for anyone with nut, egg, or milk allergy.

You must insist on accurate information about the food before you taste it. If the counter staff, the waiter, or the waitress is unsure of the ingredients, ask them to check with the chef, or with the label on prepackaged food. Be persistent, and never eat anything unless you are sure. Make eye contact with the person concerned, and learn to be a good judge of character. Your life could depend on telling the difference between the waiter who knows the facts about the food and the waiter who is being blithely reassuring for the sake of a quiet life.

It is a great mistake to pick out the pieces of offending food—kiwi fruit from a fruit salad for example—and eat the rest. There is often enough allergen left behind to cause anaphylaxis in the highly allergic individual.

Those who are extremely sensitive to the offending food must also consider the problem of contamination in the kitchen. Grills, broilers, and fryers in restaurants and cafeterias can become contaminated with fish allergens or nut allergens and these can be transferred to fried potatoes or other foods, provoking anaphylaxis in the highly allergic individual. Sesame seeds can also contaminate equipment, work surfaces, or bakery counters.

Parties and buffets

Milk, egg, shellfish, or nut allergies can make it especially hazardous to eat buffet or party food. Regard everything with suspicion. Cocktail snacks with nuts or peanut paste hidden inside are a particular problem. Drinking alcohol may reduce your judgment regarding potentially allergenic foods. In addition, alcohol may mask the early stages of an allergic reaction, and lead to delayed treatment. It can also make allergic reactions more severe.

When fish allergy isn't fish allergy

Anisakis is a parasitic worm that infests fish and can sometimes survive the cooking process to infect humans. The worms are easily thrown off by the human immune system, but the body is primed to make IgE antibodies should it ever encounter *Anisakis* again. Another meal of parasitized fish—even if the *Anisakis* worms are all dead this time, and only the allergens remain—will provoke a massive IgE-mediated reaction, leading to anaphylactic shock. This problem is usually misdiagnosed as allergy to fish itself.

Other inconsistent reactions to food can be due to contaminants such as antibiotics, preservatives, other food additives, or (especially in the case of shellfish) naturally occurring toxins.

Stinging insects

"Know your enemy" is always a good motto, but particularly for those with insect-sting allergy. Being allergic to yellow jackets or hornets, for example, is enough of a problem without panicking every time you encounter a hover fly as well.

If your reaction to this is "What's a hover fly?" then you need a good field guide. These common insects, also known as flower flies, have yellow-and-black stripes to mimic those of vespids. This coloration gives the hover flies some protection against birds. They fool a lot of people also, but it isn't difficult to tell the two apart—hover flies are a different shape from vespids, hold their wings differently at rest, and fly in a completely different way (for one thing, they hover). Knowing one from the other will make life much more relaxing.

When you have an allergic reaction to an insect sting you may not see the insect that stung you. Ask the doctor which skin tests came up positive (see p. 61), and use a field guide to check exactly what the insect(s) looks like.

Besides knowing what your problem insect looks like, you need to know a little about its habits and tastes:

- The most dangerous thing you can do is to disturb the nest—all stinging insects go into attack mode when this happens. If there is a nest in or around your house, call in an expert to destroy it and stay well away while this is done. If you think there may be an insect nest on or around your property, call in an expert to do a survey. Regular annual examinations of the property are advisable if insects have nested before.
- Insect repellent works only for biting insects, such as mosquitoes. It does not repel stinging insects.
- Insecticide spray can be useful, but make sure the insect is really dead before you get close. A groggy poisoned insect may well sting. Even a recently dead insect can still sting.

- A small, thick blanket can be useful for catching bees or wasps that have flown into automobiles.

Honeybees and bumblebees

- When it stings, a bee usually dies, so stinging is a last resort. Most honeybees are not aggressive, and sting only if their nest is attacked or if they are threatened when feeding.
- Bees feed on nectar from flowers. They may be attracted by brightly colored clothes, especially red, and floral prints, mistaking these for flowers. Wear dull colors.
- Some perfumes, shampoos, and scented cosmetics may also attract bees. If bees do approach you, never swat at them, and don't panic. Just brush them away very gently.
- Bees often feed on clover, which grows in lawns, and it is easy to tread on them. Don't walk barefoot outside.
- Bees are attracted by water, including swimming pools.
- Although large, bumblebees are also very placid and rarely sting.
- Swarming bees are dangerous because they have the queen with them. If you see a swarm, keep well away.

Africanized honeybees

Africanized honeybees, which are hybrids between domestic honeybees and an aggressive variety of wild African bee, will sting with much less provocation. They are found in South and Central America. Swarms moved into Texas in 1990, then into Arizona and finally California. While they are much more pugnacious than ordinary bees, they are intent only on defending their hive and do not maliciously hunt people down, as horror movies have implied! They inject slightly *less* venom with each sting than a normal bee, but multiple stings are more likely because more than one bee is usually involved. Measures to stop their northward spread are being taken.

Wasps, yellow jackets, hornets

These closely related insects are known collectively as **vespids**.

• If you react to one species of wasp or hornet, you may well have a cross-reaction to other species in this group, so take care.
• Yellow jackets like sweet foods, so avoid taking jam, honey, cakes, or cookies on picnics. They will also crawl into open cans of beer or soft drinks—never *ever* drink straight from the can.
• In spring and early summer, wasps and yellow jackets collect protein-rich food for their young and may be attracted to meat. If eating outdoors, keep food covered.
• Yellow jackets are drawn to fallen fruit in the fall. They get very sluggish and bad-tempered late in the year and will sting with little provocation. They may crawl into crevices or hollow logs as winter approaches. Be very careful about picking up fruit or dead leaves. Wear thick gloves, long pants, and long-sleeved shirts when working outside.
• Yellow jackets are often on the ground, especially in the fall. Wear shoes and socks.
• Garbage attracts yellow jackets. Make sure your own garbage can has a tightly fitting lid, and that no garbage accumulates around it. Ask neighbors to do the same. Keep away from trash cans, especially at picnic sites.

Fire ants

These unwanted arrivals from South America build their nest mounds in lawns, meadows, golf courses, parks, and school playgrounds, especially near water. Sometimes they come indoors in search of food and water, particularly during hot dry weather. Very occasionally they make a nest in wall voids or rafters.

Fire ants will attack without much provocation. The fire ant hangs onto the skin with its jaws, while swinging its rear end around and making 7–8 stings in a circular pattern. The stings burn and itch intensely, even if you do not have allergy. Then a small blister forms, developing into a white pustule over the next 48 hours—this is all quite normal. So is localized hives. Don't break the pustule or it may become infected.

If you have fire-ant allergy, you will suffer symptoms away from the site of the sting, such as flushing, hives, swelling, chest pains, nausea, or breathlessness. Deal with this promptly (see p. 98), as fatalities have occurred.

Anyone with fire-ant allergy should always wear shoes (not sandals), socks, and gloves when gardening or working outdoors. Children with this allergy should be fully clothed when playing outside. They should be taught to look around for ants and never to disturb their mounds. Allergy shots are also advisable.

All fire-ant nests in the area should be destroyed—otherwise the problem only spreads. You have to kill the queen to destroy the nest. Poison bait, which the workers take to the queen, is the most effective and safest treatment, but it takes a few weeks to work. Very hot water, poured into the nest holes, is an alternative; you need to use 1–2 gallons (4–8 liters).

Cross-reactions between insect stings

There are cross-reactions between the venoms of wasps, yellow jackets, hornets, and related insects (vespids), so someone allergic to one may react to another. Cross-reactions are very unlikely between bee and wasp venoms.

Honeybees and bumblebees have very similar venom, and these cross-react (but honeybee allergy shots do not work for bumblebee allergy—see p. 168). Surprisingly, there is some cross-reaction between honeybee venom and snake venom.

The usual suspects

Wasps, paper wasps, yellow jackets, hornets, and bees are the most common source of allergic reactions worldwide. Fire ants are a particular problem in the southeastern United States and have even reached California.

A few people are allergic to kissing bugs (*Triatoma* spp.)—also called conenoses, "big bedbugs," or "Mexican bedbugs." They are found in rural areas of the southern states, especially where there are prickly pears. They also inhabit South and Central America. These large insects creep into beds and bite painlessly by night. The bite injects allergen and can cause a systemic reaction, even anaphylactic shock, though this is rare. Keeping an epinephrine injector (see p. 150) by the bed is advisable if you have had any kind of systemic reaction (symptoms distant from the bite) before.

Dust mites and cockroaches

Because dust mites are a major source of allergic reactions, they have been studied intensively, and various ways of killing them devised. But simply killing the mites is not enough. Their allergens will remain and continue to cause allergic reactions for years. The allergens have to be either removed or inactivated—that is, changed chemically so that they are no longer recognized by the immune system.

There are two major types of dust mites in North America, *Dermatophagoides farinae* (New World mite) and *Dermatophagoides pteronyssinus* (European or Old World mite). Both are a common cause of allergic reactions.

Tackling dust mites is easier if you know certain key facts:

1 Dust mites prefer humid conditions. They do not drink, but absorb water from the air. When the relative humidity falls below 50 percent, the mites gradually dry out and are killed.

2 Mites feed on our skin scales, but only if the scales have been broken down first by molds. High humidity (70–90 percent relative humidity) is a particular problem because it favors the mold that suits dust mites best.

3 Dust mites live inside mattresses, pillows, upholstery, and soft toys. The allergens are blasted out when you settle into an armchair, get into bed, or turn over in the night. This is when you inhale the biggest dose of allergen, or get the maximum dose to your skin. Carpets also contain dust mites, but the numbers are generally lower.

4 Dust-mite allergen is relatively heavy, compared to cat or mold allergens, for example. Little of it floats around in the air, and the most significant exposure is inhaling it close to the source—from a pillow, mattress, or teddy bear. This is why air filters are of little value against dust mites.

5 Dust mites are everywhere and are carried around in clothing. Even if you could eliminate all the mites from your house, new ones would soon appear. A new mattress will usually be colonized by dust mites within four months.

The size of the allergen particles

The droppings of the dust mite, not the mites themselves, are the main cause of symptoms. The droppings are 4–20 microns in size, but they can crumble into fragments of 1–3 microns, and the tiniest bits are only 0.5 microns across. The pores of mite-proof covers (which really means mite-*allergen*-proof) should be less than one micron across, and preferably less than 0.5 micron. Dust masks (see p. 109) should also filter out particles of this size to be effective. The mites themselves are much bigger, 200–300 microns long. (A micron is one thousandth of a millimeter.)

The basics of mite warfare

• A temperature just above boiling point kills dust mites and inactivates Der p1, which is the troublesome allergen for most asthmatics. However Der p2, the other mite allergen, is not affected by heat. (Note that the carpet treatments advertised as "steam cleaning" generally just use hot soapy water, not steam. Because they leave the carpet very damp, they can *increase* the numbers of dust mites.)

• Washing with detergent at 130°F (55°C) or above kills mites and removes the allergen.

• Cooler washes will not kill mites, but will remove the allergen. This can be useful if the mites have already been killed by some other means. Regular cool washes of clothing or sheets will also remove human skin scales, reducing the mites' food supply. (Doing this is beneficial if you have eczema, because flaking skin adds to the problem by giving dust mites even more to eat.)

• You can buy mite-killing substances (see p. 255) to add to cooler washes, so that the mites are killed—the chemicals are rinsed out at the end of the wash, so are pretty safe.

• Dry cleaning kills mites and it removes some of the mite allergen, but the amount removed is variable (20–70 percent).

• Freezing for more than 6 hours kills mites. Three hours' direct sunlight in dry air will kill mites living in rugs and blankets. Neither freezing or sunlight treatment removes allergen.

• Mites hang on to the carpet fibers when the vacuum cleaner passes overhead, and about 65 percent of them remain afterward. An ordinary vacuum cleaner sprays mite allergen into the air as it goes. The amount in the air—and available to be inhaled—is *three times higher* after vacuuming.

Combating mites

Bear in mind that mites are the enemy—not dust itself. A house may be thick with dust, but, if the windows are open a lot and the air is dry, it will have few mites. Another house may look perfectly clean but be seething with mites because it is thoroughly draft-proofed, warm, and slightly humid. The mites will be thriving in the carpets, beds, draperies, and upholstery. What is more, vacuuming and dusting every day, if done with an ordinary type of vacuum cleaner and a dry dustcloth, will stir up the allergens and ensure that the air is full of them. So a person with mite allergy would feel far *worse* in the apparently very clean house than in the dusty one.

One crucial aspect of a mite-reduction program is making the air drier—see p. 119 for the details—so that mites no longer flourish. Most of the other measures—described below—will involve stirring up dust-mite allergens, so the allergic person should not do the work, nor be in the house (see p. 109).

Too dry or too moist?

It is a well-established fact that the air in most modern houses is too humid, encouraging dust mites and molds. Yet many people install humidifiers because they believe that the air is "too dry" and that this irritates the nose. Some very good scientific studies have shown that it is indoor pollutants plus overheating that is the problem here, not dryness—even very dry air is not irritating, as long as it is clean. Should your nose feel dry and ticklish, try to reduce indoor pollution (see pp. 128–9).

It is true that during an asthma attack, dry cold air *does* make matters worse, so this should be avoided.

The bed

Begin with the bed, because this is the main exposure zone. A Danish study showed that just fitting mite-allergen-proof covers to the mattresses and pillows of dust-allergic children worked well. After 12 months the children were having much less asthma at night, using half as much inhaled steroid, and producing better peak-flow readings.

The best approach is to buy a new mattress and new pillows and then put anti-mite coverings on them. These covers keep skin scales and mites out, which should prevent a new mattress or pillow from becoming colonized. The modern covers have tiny pores that allow perspiration to evaporate—this makes them comfortable to sleep on. They should be zippered to fully enclose the mattress and pillows.

These pores are small enough (see box on p. 114) to keep any mite allergens inside, so they *will* also keep the existing allergen inside an old mattress. But the mites themselves will also thrive inside (there's enough old skin there to keep them in business for years) and there is always the risk that if a small tear develops, the abundant stores of allergen in the mattress will come pouring out again. So start with a new mattress if you can.

Another possible option is to arrange for a contractor to heat-treat the bed, the mattress, and all bedding. This is a new specialist treatment (see p. 255), in which the bed is enclosed in a plastic tent and heated to a very high temperature. It is designed to kill all mites, even those right inside the mattress, and inactivate the allergen. (The contractor can do your living room furniture at the same time.) This treatment is not yet available in all countries.

If the covers are for a small child, check with the manufacturer that they pose no threat of suffocation. Mattresses, pillows, and comforters with integral covers may be safer.

If you have a comforter, buy a new one (or wash or dry-clean your existing one) and put an anti-mite cover on it. Alternatively, buy a comforter and pillow that can be washed at 130°F (55°C) or more, and wash them every 2–4 weeks. You must have the use of a tumble dryer, because mites will flourish if bedding is not *completely* dry.

An upholstered box spring will have its own (much smaller) population of mites. Buy a simple wooden or metal bed if possible. Or you could enclose the upholstered base in a mite-proof cover, or in plastic sheeting completely sealed with heavy-duty tape.

Wash all sheets and blankets at 130°F (55°C) or more, or have blankets dry-cleaned—or buy new ones. From now on, wash sheets once a week and blankets once every two weeks. Get rid of any other bedding such as patchwork quilts or fleecy under-blankets unless you can wash or dry-clean them regularly.

Electric blankets can be cleared of allergen by washing them, and are very useful in keeping the bed free from moisture. This prevents mites from setting up home in the *outer* surface of your new mite-proof covers, so that you don't need to wash the covers, sheets, and under-blankets so frequently. After making sure there is no risk of fire, leave the electric blanket on during the day at a high setting, with the bed made, for at least 12 hours (monitor it regularly). *Note that some mite-proof covers might be damaged by this procedure*—check with the manufacturer. There are some made from Egyptian cotton that can tolerate this level of heat (see p. 255).

Consider purchasing a water bed, in which case anti-mite covers are not necessary (except for pillows). The bed surface will require regular damp-dusting and the sheets hot washing.

Children's beds and toys

Where children share a room, all the beds and bedding need dust mite control. Even then, an asthmatic child should never sleep in the lower half of a bunk bed, because mite allergens will shower down from above.

Once a week, all soft toys should spend at least six hours in the freezer, or go through a hot cycle in the dryer, to kill the mites. The first time, wash the toys immediately afterward to remove any existing allergen and dry thoroughly in a tumble dryer.

A hot wash or the freezing/washing treatment should also be used for "comfort blankets," dressing-up clothes, and dolls' clothes.

The next steps

Clothing is often full of mites; this is especially true of sweaters, coats, and woolen trousers. Dry-clean all such items, or wash using a mite-killing wash, then store them in a well-heated place so that they are always *very* dry.

Dandruff consists of skin flakes and may help to feed mites. Using an antidandruff shampoo reduces this possibility. Semen also gives mites nourishment, so use condoms, or launder sheets regularly.

From now on, be careful about exposing your airways to dust. Get someone else to empty the vacuum-cleaner bag—they should, of course, do it outdoors. If you are stripping wallpaper, wash it down first to remove dust. Going into the attic, spring cleaning, turning out closets and cabinets, or moving furniture should all be avoided—unless you have a good mask on.

Do not use fan-heaters or convector heaters, which churn up mite allergens from the carpet. Seal off any hot-air ducts from

What about sprays?

Chemicals that kill mites (known collectively as acaricides) are sometimes useful but have various limitations. They do not penetrate inside upholstered furniture, pillows, or mattresses, so make little difference to the total population of dust mites. Even on carpets, sprays won't reach most of the mites unless you rub the spray in really hard. (And "anti-mite" carpet shampoos are *completely* ineffective.)

The safest chemical is benzyl benzoate—so safe that it is used directly on the skin for treating scabies infections. It can cause skin irritation at these doses, but rarely does so at the concentrations used in anti-mite sprays.

However, the idea of constant spraying, over a period of months or years, is rather worrying. Doctors generally advise against spraying bedding, and carpets or furniture where babies or small children play, to avoid close and prolonged contact with the spray residue.

Even more alarming are sprays containing a pyrethroid (pyrethrum) compound. The latter is derived from a plant and is therefore sold as "natural," but pyrethroids are potentially toxic with prolonged exposure, and they quite often provoke allergic reactions, too. They should definitely be avoided.

Sprays that inactivate allergen (rather than killing mites) sometimes have their uses. There are two kinds, and both should work against a variety of allergens, not just dust mite. Polysaccharide sprays stick the allergen particles together, so that they don't float around and get inhaled. Tannic-acid sprays change the allergen chemically, making it nonallergenic. Because tannic acid is found in tea, it is assumed to be harmless, but the sprays vary a lot and often contain many impurities, so it is hard to be sure about their long-term safety. Don't use these sprays on bedding.

Carpets and bedding covers pretreated with pesticide are also available, but are probably best avoided.

central heating systems, as these blow mite allergens around the bedroom, and provide alternative heating.

If possible, invest in a central vacuum system, or in a vacuum cleaner that keeps in all the allergens, or vents them outside, rather than spraying them out into the air. Make sure that the vacuum cleaner you buy really does its job well—a lot of machines now claim to be "allergy" vacuum cleaners but they are not all equally good. Alternatively, cover the bed with a clean sheet and open the windows whenever you vacuum, leaving them open for half an hour afterward. After closing the windows, allow the dust to settle for another half hour, then carefully remove the dust cover from the bed.

For dusting, use a damp cloth to pick up dust rather than spread it around. Alternatively, use a special anti-mite dustcloth with an electrostatic charge that holds the dust.

Above all, keep the moisture levels in your house down. Ultimately, this is the key to eliminating dust mites. Look at p. 119 and check that you are doing everything possible.

The bedroom in particular should be kept dry. Air your bedroom whenever it's dry and sunny. Remove plants and fish tanks. Don't dry clothes in the room, and don't shampoo the carpet. Avoid using kerosene heaters, as these produce a lot of moisture. If your bedroom has a connecting shower, install a powerful exhaust fan, or open a window wide during and after showers— or just stop using this shower. Even a sink generates moist air.

Do you need to do more?

Give it some time before deciding if you have done enough. In one study, it took *eight months* for the full benefits of an anti-mite campaign to be seen. If you are still not as much improved as you hoped, you could try a more drastic mite-elimination program.

Thoroughly clean the bedroom, getting rid of any dust along baseboards or picture rails, on top of armoires, or behind other furniture. Remove anything stored under the bed, so that vacuuming is easier in future. During this cleaning operation, completely cover the bed.

Get rid of the bathroom carpet, if you have one. In the bedroom, either remove the carpet or buy a special anti-mite steam cleaner that kills mites in the carpet and inactivates the allergen. To work properly, the device must produce steam at a temperature *above* boiling point, by means of high pressure. Make sure you are buying the right kind of device.

If you take out the carpet, you will need to mop the floor, with a wet or oiled mop, several times a week, as the dust will quickly build up and is easily made airborne from an uncarpeted floor. One advantage of carpet is that it "holds" dust at floor level.

Wash the draperies, or dry-clean them, or replace them with blinds or shades of a kind that can be easily wet-dusted. If you have bought an anti-mite steam cleaner for the carpet, use this on the draperies every two to three weeks.

Remove dirty clothes from the bedroom, clean out drawers and shelves, and dry them thoroughly. Store only freshly laundered clothes in the room.

Remove all upholstered items from the bedroom, such as padded headboards, cushions, armchairs, or stools with padded seats. Fabric lampshades and anything in velvet should also go.

A different approach

If you are even more allergic to housework than you are to dust mites, consider buying a really powerful dehumidifier, especially designed for killing mites. This makes the air too dry to breathe (its relative humidity goes down to 25 percent), so you leave it on in the bedroom during the day, with the bedroom door closed. You must eliminate all sources of moisture that will counteract the dehumidifier and have fairly tight seals around your windows and doors for it to work. In the evening, turn the dehumidifier off and leave the bedroom door open for an hour before going to bed.

Of course, all the allergen that was already there in the bed, carpet, draperies, clothes, and soft toys will still be present. You need to either eliminate or inactivate this allergen using the methods described above. But once you have your daily dehumidifier routine going, you do not need to rewash everything regularly, because mites will be a thing of the past, so no new stocks of allergen will be produced.

The rest of the house

A completely mite-free house is hard to achieve, but if you are determined, you can come close. Everything so far described for the bedroom, such as reducing moisture in the air and dealing with carpets and draperies, is applicable to the rest of the house.

The exception—and the toughest nut to crack—is the upholstered furniture in the living room. Fixed upholstery (that is, everything other than removable cushions) is a safe haven for mites, which is especially hard to deal with.

One option is to give all such furniture a specialist heat treatment, if this is available locally (see p. 115). The mites inside will be killed and the allergen inactivated. If you drastically reduce moisture levels at the same time—with a powerful dehumidifier used at night, perhaps—you should avoid serious reinfestation.

Alternatively, you could replace all your existing upholstered furniture with leather-covered or vinyl-covered furniture. Both are impenetrable to mites. Furniture made of wood or bamboo with loose cushions and no fixed upholstery can also work. Fit the cushions with tailor-made mite-proof covers (hard to get, but ask around) when new. Then put the ordinary covers on top, and wash them regularly.

Cockroaches and other insect pests

Compared to the huge amount of research that has been done on dust mites, very little effort has gone into elimination methods for cockroaches and their allergens. This is a real tragedy, because these insects are responsible for a great deal of allergy, especially in urban areas of the United States. Several other countries, including Israel, South Africa, and France, have now recognized a problem with cockroach allergy.

In colder regions, cockroaches are usually killed by the winter weather. In spite of this, they may infest some high-rise buildings. Because numbers build up during the summer and dwindle in the winter, cockroaches may cause seasonal allergies that are often mistaken for hay fever.

Cockroaches are miniature six-legged vultures, feeding on our leftovers. The allergens are found in their sloughed skins, their droppings, and their saliva. To get rid of cockroaches, you must

- clear up all food scraps and crumbs promptly, and wash dishes right after each meal. Keep all food in cockroach-proof containers, and take garbage out daily.
- eat only in the dining area, and keep the floor there especially clean. Never eat in the bedroom.
- eliminate any pools or drips of water that the roaches can drink. Repair leaky plumbing, and prevent condensation on pipes. Wipe up spills of water or other liquids immediately.
- seal all the cracks and holes through which roaches enter, especially around baseboards.
- use bait stations (roach motels) to kill roaches, replacing them every 2–3 months. Boric acid or diatomaceous earth can also be used, especially in kitchen cabinets and under sinks and appliances.

While cleanliness is important, sometimes the problem is structural, and cockroaches persist despite vigorous cleaning. You need expert help from a pest exterminator if this is the case.

Apartment blocks are a particularly difficult issue. It is impossible to eliminate roaches from your apartment unless the whole block is treated, because roaches will simply enter from other apartments.

HEPA air filters are widely advertised, and may seem like the answer to this problem, but in fact they are of little value against cockroach allergen.

Unfortunately, even when cockroaches have been eradicated, a great deal of cockroach allergen often remains in the home, despite thorough cleaning. The reason for this is unclear, but it should not discourage you from trying to combat cockroach allergen, because even just reducing your exposure a little can have big benefits. In one American study that looked at asthmatic children who were allergic to cockroaches, the levels of the allergen at home determined how severe the asthma symptoms were. All the homes had cockroach allergen—not surprisingly, since this is what had caused the allergy in the first place. But children exposed to the highest levels of cockroach allergen at home were three times more likely to be hospitalized for asthma. They also missed more school due to asthma and had more sleepless, wheezy nights.

Cockroach allergens in food?

Flour is frequently contaminated with cockroach allergens. Cooking decreases the level of allergen but does not destroy it entirely. It is possible that contaminated flour could provoke a reaction when eaten by someone with cockroach allergy.

Other insects

Almost any insect that infests houses can cause allergic reactions in some susceptible individuals. Houseflies and carpet beetles have both caused allergies occasionally. Outdoor insects, including midges, mosquitoes, caddis flies, and mayflies, can cause allergies if they are especially abundant—as they are around the Great Lakes area in the breeding season, for example.

The Asian lady bug, introduced into the southeastern U.S. in the 1970s, frequently overwinters in North American houses, and can cause allergic symptoms in the nose and eyes. To keep the lady bugs out, you should caulk the outside of the house, to seal all gaps. Painting the house a very dark color is also suggested, because the insects seek out pale walls which resemble the light-colored cliffs where they overwinter in their natural habitat. Clean up well indoors to get rid of the existing allergen.

Mouse hazard

Until recently, no one had investigated the possible role of mice in causing allergies. Now researchers have shown that 18 percent of children in inner-city areas of the United States have an allergic reaction to mice, and that this can contribute to asthma. Exposure to cockroach allergen increases the risk of becoming sensitive to mice.

Tackling humidity indoors

In the modern drive for good insulation, one crucial thing has been forgotten—ventilation. Huge amounts of water vapor are generated in a house, and if it can't escape it creates humid conditions that are ideal for molds and dust mites. Apart from the steam generated by cooking and showering, you give off about 1 quart (1 liter) of water in sweat each night.

A household of four people pushes 74–148 quarts (70–140 liters) of water into the atmosphere around them every week. Combine this with modern draft-proofing and the result is air that is much too moist.

There are two distinct problems to be tackled:
- the overall level of moisture in the house
- localized areas of condensation, which are especially problematic with mold allergy because they create damp surfaces where molds can grow

The first step toward reducing moisture is to take out any humidifiers, repair any plumbing leaks, and rectify any structural problems, such as cracks in walls, a leaking roof, or rising dampness. Make sure there is no water seepage in the basement. Remember to look behind furniture for unnoticed damp patches.

Keep the kitchen door closed when cooking, turn off kettles as soon as they boil, and always use lids on saucepans to reduce steam. Think about having a range hood, for use when cooking. Alternatively, open a window while you cook and leave it open for a while afterward.

Try to dry clothes outside, or use a tumble dryer. Failing that, dry them in a well-ventilated utility room with the door into the house closed, so that the moisture goes out, not in.

Either fit a powerful exhaust fan in the bathroom, or just open the windows wide after baths and showers. (Baths are better, as they produce less steam.) Wipe down tiles and grouting with an old towel after showers, and leave towels and bathmats to dry elsewhere, not in the bathroom.

Note that all exhaust fans and tumble dryers must be *vented to the outside* (not, for example, to the attic).

Most important of all, ventilate the whole house whenever the air is dry outside. You should open several windows so that a draft blows right through. In addition, unblock any fresh-air vents, and reduce the amount of draft-proofing, to improve ventilation. If there are overshadowing trees or tall bushes around the house, cut them back to improve air flow.

Make sure that the vents in crawl spaces are not blocked and are working well. However, if the ductwork of your cooling system runs through the crawl spaces, it may be better to close the vents during the summer when humidity is high.

To eliminate condensation in colder rooms, heat all parts of the house to the same temperature. Loft insulation will help to keep ceilings warm and so prevent condensation upstairs. Keep closet doors open if they have any tendency to dampness, and/or warm the interior with a low-powered heater.

In the bathroom, strip off any vinyl wallpaper or alkyd/oil paints, as these are impervious to water. Replace with latex paint (preferably with a mildew inhibitor added) or with ordinary wallpaper. Both allow moisture to be absorbed into the wall and eventually to escape to the outside. Vinyl paper and oil-based paint keep condensation on the surface, encouraging mold growth there. For the same reason, tiles should be used just where needed, not all over the walls.

Don't have carpet in bathrooms or in basement areas.

Take out any metal window frames and replace with wood or vinyl frames, as cold window frames encourage condensation. If possible, fit double-glazed windows, which give a much warmer glass surface.

Wipe away any condensation that does occur around windows, or on windowsills, every day, and dry the cloths outside or in a utility room.

A device known as a hygrometer, which measures the relative humidity of the air, may be useful. Some garden centers and hardware stores sell them, as do a few suppliers of specialist allergy equipment (see p. 255). Aim for a relative humidity of less than 50 percent or (even better) less than 40 percent.

For new houses, or those that have just been completely renovated, ventilation is even more important. As much as 360 U.S. gallons (1,360 liters) of water are used in the construction of a house, mainly for plastering. Depending on the climate, this can take as much as a year to disperse. Using a dehumidifier may be worthwhile during this period, especially if there is a lot of rain, but do not speed the process up too much, as this can cause damage to the plaster, concrete, or lumber.

A special note about latex paint
People with an allergy to latex are reacting to rubber latex from the rubber tree. The world "latex" originally meant any emulsion of particles in liquid, and this is the meaning it has in the case of latex paint—so latex paints generally *don't* contain rubber latex. Only a few latex paints (mostly those used for ceilings) do contain rubber latex, and this is in a non-allergenic form.

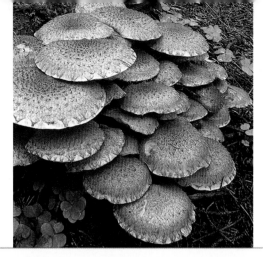

Molds
AND OTHER FUNGI

The air around us is full of bits and pieces that are mostly too small to be seen without a microscope—pollen grains, mold spores, fragments from plants, fibers from clothing, specks of ash from smoke, skin flakes, and diesel particles. Of these, mold spores are by far the most abundant.

Except in very dry climates, there are more mold spores in the air than anything else. In Britain—a relatively damp country where molds flourish—the record count is over 4,500 spores per cubic foot (160,000 spores per cubic meter) of air, compared to a record pollen count of only 80 grains per cubic foot (2,800 grains per cubic meter). Luckily, mold spores are not particularly allergenic, or even more people would be suffering as a result of inhaling such huge quantities of them.

Spores are produced by molds and other fungi, and they are to the fungus what seeds are to a plant—they can grow into new fungi. Doctors generally speak just of "mold allergy" because molds are the most common offenders, but larger fungi—mushrooms and toadstools—also produce allergenic spores. For example, a bracket fungus called *Ganoderma,* which infests dead trees and produces spores prolifically in mid-June, has been found to affect 16 percent of asthmatics in one part of New Zealand. Bracket fungi occur all over the world, but until recently no one had suspected them of causing allergic reactions, so the extent to which they cause allergies has not been investigated. The same is true of other large fungi.

Yeasts (single-celled fungi) are also found in the air, and it is possible—though this has not been investigated—that people with an allergy to yeast in food would also react to inhaled yeasts.

Indoors and out

Mold spores can be produced both indoors *and* out. There are different species of mold in different places and you may be lucky and react only to one or two uncommon species. But many molds grow in a very wide range of situations, both indoors and outdoors. There are also cross-reactions (see p. 14) between some of the molds, unfortunately, which means that people generally react to a great number of different molds. You will probably need to reduce mold growth inside your home as well as avoiding mold-rich places outside. Changes to your garden that eliminate havens for molds, such as leaf piles, may also be helpful.

Molds may be growing only in one part of a house—the basement perhaps—but can be carried all around the house on air currents.

The size of the allergen particles

Most mold spores are between 2 and 10 microns in size. A few species have spores that are smaller than 2 microns. (A micron is one thousandth of a millimeter.) Some people with mold allergy may be protected by an ordinary dust mask (see p. 109), but most will probably need a better-quality mask.

Avoiding outdoor molds

Molds live in the soil and grow on any decaying plant matter, such as dead leaves, dying plants, fallen trees, hay, and straw. Spore counts are highest in the fall. A thick covering of snow reduces the numbers of mold spores in the air dramatically. Once the snow melts in spring, molds flourish on the plants killed by the cold, so spore counts soon rise again.

The effect of the weather on spore release is very complex. Some molds like to release their spores when it is dry and windy, but others favor fog, mist, or dew. Rainfall washes a lot of spores out of the air, but it stimulates the release of some small spores.

A few pollen-information services also give a current mold-spore count, but making predictions of the spore count for the following day is nearly impossible.

Drastic avoidance measures, for those who are severely sensitive, include moving to a desert or semiarid area where there are far fewer mold spores in the air.

Listed below are the mold-rich situations and activities that could provoke your allergy symptoms. If they do, you should avoid them as much as possible, or wear a mask that will prevent the spores from being inhaled (see box on p. 120).

Places

- near fields of cereal crops in late summer, because of molds growing on the cereal leaves. Symptoms are likely at harvest time, when combine harvesters disperse the spores.
- in forests and old orchards, in gardens with compost piles or piles of dead leaves, and in greenhouses
- near springs and waterfalls, and in any damp, shady places

Times

- during late summer and autumn, when molds flourish outdoors
- following the first frost, which triggers spore release by fungi living in the soil

Activities

- disturbing compost piles, damp straw or hay, piles of grass clippings or heaps of fallen leaves, all of which are likely to be full of molds
- collecting up fallen leaves or fruit
- watering the garden because mold spores are released when water hits the dry soil
- mowing grass, if the clippings were not cleared up after the last mowing. Unless the weather is very dry, the clippings tend to go moldy.
- removing dead leaves or flowers from plants

A dangerous mold allergy

Anyone with asthma who also has allergy to the mold *Alternaria* should—with their doctor's agreement—increase their dose of preventer inhaler (for example, steroid or cromoglycate) during the spore-producing season. Research shows that severe near-fatal asthma attacks often occur during the *Alternaria* spore season among those allergic to this mold.

Spore release by *Alternaria* usually occurs in the summer or fall, but the timing varies from one part of the world to another, so check with your doctor or a local pollen/spore monitoring service. *Alternaria* can live outdoors in soil, and on seeds and plants. Indoors, it is a denizen of window frames, carpets, and textiles.

Indoor molds

These are the indoor conditions that can be difficult for mold-sensitive people. You should either avoid these, wear a mask, or tackle the problem at source—for example, by reducing dampness (see p. 119).

Places

- buildings that are damp, because moisture encourages mold growth. Never sleep in a room that has mold growing on the walls or windowpanes.
- old churches and church social halls
- houses with central evaporative cooling systems ("swamp coolers"); these tend to be very damp
- buildings that are near lakes, rivers, or the sea, because of the dampness of the air
- rooms with humidifiers
- bathrooms and shower rooms, unless well ventilated, owing to the steam and condensation
- rooms that are left unheated, and are therefore colder than the rest of the house, as these rooms tend to suffer from condensation
- buildings with dry rot. Not all mold-sensitive people react to the spores of these timber-rotting fungi, but some do
- buildings where old timbers are being removed, as this stirs up huge numbers of spores
- buildings where central heating has recently been installed, as the warmer temperatures in the building stimulates the existing molds to release their spores
- buildings with lots of indoor plants. There are molds you cannot see growing on the surface of the soil around a potted plant
- cellars and basements
- sun rooms, if not well maintained

- antique shops, farms, mills, vacation homes
- portable school classrooms.

Times

- during the winter, when there are usually more molds growing indoors due to condensation.

Activities

- Handling clothes, draperies, or other furnishings that smell mildewy: they may be dry now, but they will still be full of mold spores.
- Handling vegetables or fruit that have been stored a long time, or in damp conditions (for example, in plastic wrapping). Note that this can include mushrooms—they often have white molds growing on them, which can be quite inconspicuous.

If looking around your house for molds, bear in mind that they vary a great deal in color. Bread, vegetables, cheese, and other foods that are past their best grow green, gray, or white molds, often furry, and these are the ones most people are familiar with. But the black stuff on the walls of bathrooms and in the door seals of refrigerators is also mold. In some situations it takes a practiced eye to spot this type of mold—around window frames, for example, or in the patterns of bathroom-window glass, it can easily be mistaken for ordinary dirt. On shower curtains and cubicles you may find pinkish-red molds as well as these black kinds. Garden plants and crops can have bright orange molds (called "rusts") on their leaves, as well as the more familiar gray or black kinds.

Combating indoor molds

The crucial task here is to reduce dampness and condensation in the house—see p. 119 for the details—as this encourages mold growth on all kinds of surfaces, including walls, ceilings, windows, bathroom tiles, shower curtains, and even carpets. Once you have reduced the humidity, you can have a big cleanup and remove the spores that have been left by molds.

If your allergy symptoms are very bad, and you need some immediate relief, then you could get someone to clean away the mold growth and spores first, then tackle the humidity problem, *then* repeat the cleaning operation. Obviously, this is less efficient, but it may be the best approach if you are severely affected.

Note that the cleaning will, in itself, stir up a massive but unseen cloud of spores, so the allergy sufferer should not be at home during this work (see p. 109).

Cleaning away molds and stopping regrowth

There are two aspects to this task:

- an initial, major effort to clear the accumulation of mold growth and old mold spores—trillions of them are probably lying around your house—since these spores are the cause of the allergic reaction
- an ongoing effort to prevent the regrowth of molds in problem areas such as the bathroom

Get rid of any furniture that smells "mildewy;" it is packed with old mold spores. Fabric items that have this smell should be washed thoroughly. Old clothing, books, and newspapers may also be a source of mold spores.

Any carpets or other porous materials (for example, ceiling tiles and wall panels) that have ever been soaked by flood or storm waters should be disposed of now—and, unless everything can be dried within 24 hours, this should always be done if there is water penetration in the future. Research shows that such materials quickly become infested with molds. Check above the flood line, as water can seep up through the walls or paneling.

On refrigerators and freezers, clean out the rubber seals around the doors, going into all the crevices to get out the black mold that lives there. Also clean out the drip pans of fridges, freezers, and dehumidifiers. Keep showerheads and air-conditioning equipment (including the filters) very clean. This all needs to be done regularly from now on.

Clean off all the mold growing around windows, or on walls and ceilings, tiles or other surfaces. Undiluted mineral spirits or rubbing alcohol kills it very effectively, and it takes a long time to grow back again. You could, alternatively, wash the walls down with a mix of one part bleach to two parts water. (But note that chlorine fumes may be irritating to the airways of those with rhinitis or asthma.) Special anti-mold sprays are also available, but try them out cautiously, as they too may be irritants. Do not brush mold growth off with a dry cloth, as this simply disperses the spores. In the future, keep an eye out for new mold growth and remove it promptly.

Buy a new shower curtain and replace it regularly, or clean it thoroughly with an anti-mold spray.

Cut down on the number of houseplants, and find a new home for any that need constant moisture. With the remaining plants, take off dying leaves and flowers promptly, and remove the top layer of soil occasionally, replacing it with fresh soil or—even better—sand, or grit. Potpourri should also be evicted, as it can be full of mold spores.

Use vegetables and fruit promptly, and do not allow bread to go stale, or jellies, jams, and preserves to go moldy.

What to do if these measures fail:

Where there is an invincible humidity problem, a really powerful dehumidifier used during the day in bedrooms, and at night in the living room, will kill off most molds and defeat their efforts to regrow. Close all the doors and windows in the room where the dehumidifier is operating, and shut off air vents. Note that air-conditioning will also reduce the humidity of the air, but not as much.

Keeping mold spores out of the airways

Ordinary house dust can contain a lot of mold spores. The allergic individual should not dust, vacuum, sweep floors, or make beds until the anti-mold measures have begun to bite. Ideally the allergic person should go out while housework is done, and the house should be thoroughly aired before their return. If this is impossible, then wearing a good mask all the time is essential. A special vacuum cleaner that retains allergens, or vents them outside, may be helpful *in addition to* the mask.

Even though you have cut down on moisture and condensation and tackled mold growth, there could *still* be a lot of mold spores around, especially in an old house, one that has been very damp in the past, or one that is close to water. If symptoms persist, think about renting or buying a high-quality HEPA air filter (see p. 108) to take mold spores out of the air.

Do not use fans or fan heaters, as these churn up mold spores from the floor and other surfaces.

Beating athlete's foot

Allergenic fungi can grow on your body, as well as in your house (see pp. 16–17). If athlete's foot is playing a part in your allergies, it is vital to treat the infection thoroughly with drugs, because the fungus grows deep into the skin and can quickly stage a comeback if not completely destroyed. You should also be careful not to re-infect yourself:

• Always dry your feet very thoroughly, especially between the toes; soft paper towels do a better job than bath towels, and can be discarded, reducing the risk of reinfection.

• Wear cotton socks and shoes made of leather or canvas, which allow sweat to evaporate. Don't wear rubber boots or other footwear that make your feet sweat except when you really need to.

• Don't wear the same pair of shoes every day. When your feet get wet, change your socks and shoes promptly.

• Launder all towels and bath mats at high temperatures when you start the course of antifungal drugs, and again when you complete it.

• Never share towels, bath mats, socks, sandals, or shoes.

• Wear flip-flops at the swimming pool or sauna and in changing rooms; if any other member of the household has athlete's foot, take the same precautions in the bathroom at home—and make sure they seek treatment.

Occasionally, athlete's foot is a misdiagnosis for atopic eczema of the feet, a common problem among allergy-prone children (see box on p. 45). If the skin between the toes is not affected, it's unlikely to be athlete's foot and more likely to be eczema.

Cats, dogs,
AND OTHER PETS

If you or your child is allergic to your pet, you should really find it another home. But a survey in the United States showed that more than a third of people with cat allergy still keep their cat—so there is detailed advice below for those who want to keep the pet, as well as those who decide to part company.

Often people with severe allergies find that although they miss their pet badly at first, the vast improvement in their symptoms makes that difficult decision seem like a good one in the long run. Finding a home for an adult pet is often difficult, as most people want kittens or puppies, but try advertising locally, and explaining in your ad exactly why the pet needs a new home. Family and friends may be happy to help by offering your pet a home if you explain the problem. Ask around among your older neighbors, too—they may value having a mature pet that is calmer and already house-trained.

Cats

You can't *see* cat allergen—many people wrongly assume that it is cat fur that is allergenic, or flakes of skin. The main allergen is a protein found in the sweat and saliva of the cat, which wafts about in the air in microscopic specks. These lightweight allergen particles are carried throughout the house.

So small are these particles that they remain airborne for six hours or more, however still the air. If they do finally settle, they are easily made airborne again by the least little breeze. Simply walking around a room is enough to disturb them.

Parting with the cat

After your cat has vacated your home, there will be allergens everywhere—on and in the armchairs, sofas, and cushions, on shelves and lampshades, in the carpets and even stuck to the walls and draperies. They will also be *inside* the mattress if the cat once slept on the bed, and will shoot out every time you lie down.

Air the house very thoroughly to shift all the allergen that is just floating in the air. Wait a couple of weeks, and see how much your symptoms improve, before going further. If you still have troublesome symptoms that are worse at home, then you need to:

- Buy a high-suction vacuum cleaner that retains allergen particles (these are marketed for dust mites—make sure it is a good one) so that you can vacuum your furnishings without redistributing the allergen everywhere.
- Wash anything that can be washed: sheets, curtains, slipcovers, comforters and their covers, cushions and their covers, pillowcases, bedspreads, and so forth. Cat allergen is not affected by heat, so a cool wash is as good as a hot one—but you must wash all the allergen away, so use plenty of detergent and run the rinse cycle twice. No one knows if dry cleaning removes cat allergen.
- If the cat ever slept on your bed, consider buying new pillows and comforter. Covers designed for dust-mite avoidance (see p. 115) are an alternative option. They will keep some of the cat allergen from escaping into the air, but not the very smallest particles.
- Sofas and armchairs can be sprayed with 3 percent tannic acid or a polysaccharide (see box on p. 116) to deactivate the allergens. Vacuum very thoroughly to remove as much allergen as possible, then spray repeatedly for a few weeks or months. Test-spray a small area first to ensure color-fastness.

A clean getaway

The allergic individual should go out while this work is done and stay out for at least six hours afterward (see p. 109).

The size of the allergen particles

Cat allergen is the tiniest allergen—most of the particles are less than 2.5 microns and the smallest may be only 0.5 micron. (A micron is a thousandth of a millimeter.) You would need a really good dust mask or HEPA air filter (see pp. 108–9) for these particles. It probably won't remove the very smallest particles, but will certainly reduce the allergen load.

Even after the cat has gone and you have cleaned up meticulously, you may still sometimes have symptoms. Unfortunately, cat allergen is carried around on the clothes of cat-owners and gets into schools, movie theaters, buses, banks, and even the padded seats in hospital waiting rooms. However, only the most highly sensitized people are affected by these low levels of allergen.

Keeping the cat

Bear in mind that keeping the pet will result in significant continued exposure, however hard you try with the methods described.

- Improve the ventilation in your house, as this will reduce the amount of allergen in the air. If your house is tightly sealed against drafts, ventilation will actually make a huge difference. Air the house regularly. Always keep a window slightly open whenever the cat and/or the allergic person is indoors. You could use an HEPA filter to clean the air instead. HEPA filters work fairly well for the very small, lightweight particles of cat allergen, that can easily become airborne. Of course, an air filter cannot do anything to protect you from a cat sitting on your lap (though advertisements have sometimes implied that they can!).
- Provide the cat with a shelter outside where it can sleep some of the time, to reduce the amount of allergen in the house. Make it as warm and comfortable as possible, feed the cat there, and provide a little catnip to make it more attractive.
- If your cat is still allowed indoors, remove all soft furnishings and wall-to-wall carpeting. Buy leather- or vinyl-covered armchairs, which can be wiped clean of cat allergen.
- Keep the cat out of the bedroom entirely. If it has been in the habit of sleeping there, wash all the bedding and buy new pillows. The mattress and comforter should be replaced or covered with anti-mite covers (see p. 124).
- If you have an un-neutered tomcat, consider having him neutered; the amount of allergen produced declines when male cats are neutered.

The following measures are sometimes recommended, but in fact they don't work:

- treating the cat with acepromazine, an animal tranquilizer
- using a spray called Allerpet-C, which, so it is claimed, reduces the amount of allergen released. Scientific trials by a research group in Detroit have shown that it does not work.
- giving the cat a shower—that is, drenching it in water. After a cat has had such a shower, the washing water contains a lot of cat allergen, so everyone assumed that this meant less cat allergen in the air. New research shows that the amount of allergen in the air around a cat after showering is no less than before. However, actually immersing the cat for three minutes followed by rinsing in clean warm water does reduce the allergen level in the air considerably. Unfortunately, the cat probably renews its stocks of allergen very fast, as a washed dog does (see below) so you need to repeat the wash at least once a week to reduce the allergen level in the air.

Dogs

Most of the advice given above for cats also applies to dogs too because their allergens, too, are small and lightweight. Dogs produce less allergen than cats, and it seems to be less potent, but you would still need to clean up thoroughly after the dog has gone to another home.

If you decide to keep your dog, HEPA filters can be very useful, although you need also to take other measures, such as excluding the dog from bedrooms and keeping it outside for more (or most) of the time. Washing dogs thoroughly in a bath, using dog shampoo, reduces the amount of allergen in the air, but it builds up again to its former level within three days. You would need to wash the dog twice a week to achieve a useful reduction in allergen levels.

Other pets and domestic animals

Horses produce very powerful allergens, and people with allergies to horses are often so sensitive that even clothing that has been worn while riding and then brought indoors can elicit symptoms. Old furniture or mattresses stuffed with horsehair can sometimes cause problems, too.

In the case of small mammals, such as mice and guinea pigs, it is usually the urine that causes allergic reactions. Proteins in the urine become airborne and are carried around the house. You may be able to keep the pet if it is in a utility room or outbuilding, or caged and sheltered outside for the summer.

With pet insects, and with snakes, lizards, and other reptiles the allergens are found in tiny skin particles that float in the air.

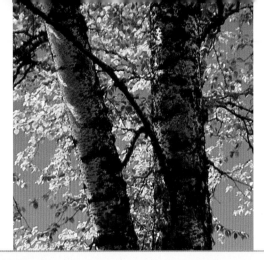

Pollen

Do you ever wake up in the middle of the night with an attack of hay fever or pollen asthma? And do you ever wonder how this can happen? The explanation is that warm air, rising up from ground level on a summer's day, takes pollen with it high into the Earth's atmosphere. When the air cools down after sunset, this pollen slowly descends again—an invisible "pollen shower."

It falls quite quickly in the countryside, reaching ground level between 8 and 10 p.m. but hot city pavements and buildings keep upward air currents going, and pollen stays aloft for longer. Most pollen lands on the city between about midnight and 2 a.m. That's why you wake up sneezing or wheezing—especially if you sleep with the windows open.

Understanding facts like these about pollen can help you to substantially reduce exposure. Pollen is by far the most difficult allergen to avoid, but don't believe the defeatists who tell you, "You can't do anything about pollen."

Pollen counts and forecasts

Pollen counts are based on the amounts of pollen collected at specific sites earlier in the day, or on the previous day.

Forecasts for the coming day are really just informed guess-work, based on the present pollen count, the time of year, the temperature and rainfall over the last few days, and the weather forecast for the next day. At best, pollen forecasts are only as good as the weather forecast.

Forecasts of pollen can be useful in deciding when to start taking antihistamines for hay fever or when to increase your asthma-preventer drugs. The starting times of the different pollen seasons are now predicted quite accurately.

Avoiding pollen outdoors

One thing that really can help here is turning on the air-conditioning in your car. In a non-air-conditioned car, closing the windows (and perhaps fitting a filter to the air intake) helps a lot.

The size of the allergen particles

The pollen grains that cause allergies are between 10 and 40 microns in size, with the majority between 20 and 35 microns. An ordinary dust mask takes out particles larger than 5 microns, so it will be adequate for most pollens. However, a few plants—including ragweed—produce tiny allergenic fragments, some no bigger than half a micron. These are about the same size as cat allergen and will therefore need much better masks. For these fragments, it is worth using an HEPA air filter and getting a high-quality vacuum cleaner.

A good exercising mask will keep out pollen grains and fragments during peak pollen times. Just wearing a scarf over the mouth and nose will also give some protection.

Another option is to smear a little Vaseline just inside each nostril and breathe through your nose only. Much of the pollen coming into your nose will stick to the Vaseline.

Timing is everything

Pollen release occurs at different times of day for different plants. Ragweed starts very early, releasing pollen between sunrise and 9 a.m., although damp conditions can delay release until as late as 2 p.m. Grasses release pollen from about 7:30 a.m. onward, but if the ground is damp, the release will be delayed until the moisture has evaporated. Unfortunately, a few species of grass wait until the afternoon, so there will be some pollen entering the air all day. If you get up at 6 a.m. for a walk or run, you can be safely home by 7:30. Alternatively, go out in the early evening, after grasses have finished releasing pollen, and before the evening "pollen shower." Birch is an afternoon pollen: release peaks between noon and 6 p.m. Unfortunately, there is no specific information at present about pollen-release patterns in other plants.

In general, all types of plants favor warm, sunny days for releasing pollen, and they all avoid rainy weather. Rain also washes residual pollen out of the air. On cloudy days there is a buildup of pollen in the flowers, so a massive release of pollen occurs on the next day of good weather.

Avoiding pollen indoors

Pollen grains have one huge point in their favor: compared to other allergenic particles, they are big and heavy. This means that they settle more quickly from the air. In a room with 10-foot (3-meter)-high ceilings, all the pollen will settle within four minutes, as long as the air is completely still. In other words, if you close all the doors and windows, block off any drafts, and sit fairly still, within four minutes you will be breathing pollen-free air.

This does not mean that all your symptoms will instantly vanish, because the "Late-Phase Reaction" (see p. 13) can go on for up to 24 hours. But you should feel better, and by not starting a new cycle of allergic reaction, you are improving the prospects for the next day. Escaping from pollen for a few hours every day should produce a general improvement in the long run, with your nose and airways becoming less inflamed.

Unfortunately, some plants produce allergenic fragments much smaller than the pollen grains. Ryegrass and ragweed both do this. These tiny particles take up to 6 hours to settle.

Some plants even produce "volatiles"—airborne chemicals that provoke symptoms. Birch trees release volatiles from their buds in early spring, weeks before the pollen itself is released, and they affect a great many people, including some who are *not* allergic to birch pollen. Volatiles can only be removed by masks or air filters that contain an activated carbon filter (see p. 109).

To cut down on the amount of pollen you inhale at home:
- Dry all your laundry indoors during the pollen season, to stop it from collecting pollen.
- Pets bring in pollen on their fur, so keep them outdoors during the pollen season, and avoid stroking them. Brushing them thoroughly before they come in is another option, but obviously the allergic individual should not do this.
- Close the windows, especially at times when your offending pollen is being released (see above), and in the evening or nighttime "pollen shower" (see p. 126).
- Change your clothes when you arrive home, since they will be coated with pollen, and wash or rinse your hair. Keep some clothes for indoor use only.
- Aim for still air (no drafts, no fans, and no vigorous movement) in the rooms where the allergic individual studies, sits, or sleeps. Air currents stir up pollen from the floor and furnishings. (No drafts means poor ventilation, of course, which is acceptable during the pollen season—but ventilate again afterward, to avoid encouraging molds and dust mites.)
- If tranquil air is an impossibility, consider getting a high-quality air filter, or air-conditioning. Alternatively, wet-dust and vacuum every day (using a vacuum cleaner that keeps allergen particles in—see pp. 116–17) to reduce the amount of pollen residue. People who are very sensitive may need to do this *as well as* having an air filter.
- Cover your armchair and bed with a sheet by day. In the evening, fold this up *very* gently and wash it. This removes the layer of pollen that accumulates during the day. If studying, cover your desk and books when you are not working.

Places to go, places to avoid

- For the grass-sensitive, mown grass is usually fine (it won't flower), although some people react to skin contact with grass (see p. 43). (However, pollen that has settled on the grass may be stirred up while the grass is actually being mown.) Unmown grass does flower and will cause symptoms. Wheat, barley, oats, and corn, although they are grasses, rarely cause problems. Rye and sugarcane do release pollen, and may affect some people.
- The levels of most pollens do not differ much between town and country. In fact, the upper floors of a high-rise building (with the air-conditioning off) may be one of the worst places, because of pollen rising on warm air currents.
- The seashore is often pollen-free thanks to onshore breezes. Mountain peaks and ridges are also good, but deep mountain valleys can be pollen traps.
- Places that often suffer from "inversions" (air trapped at ground level), can have very high levels of pollen.

Roses are not the problem

The pollens that cause allergic reactions almost all come from plants with inconspicuous greenish flowers. These plants are pollinated by the wind, which is why there is so much of their pollen wafting around in the air. Colorful and scented flowers are pollinated by insects and have big, sticky pollen grains that don't float about and rarely cause allergies. However, strong scents can irritate the nose of those who already have hay fever and make their symptoms worse.

Avoiding air pollution

Air pollution plays a variety of roles in allergic reactions. Some pollutants irritate the nose and airways (and sometimes the skin), making them more sensitive to allergens. These pollutants can worsen existing allergic symptoms and may promote the development of allergies in children, by making the airway membranes more permeable. Other chemical pollutants may affect the immune system directly, increasing any existing tendency to allergic reactions.

Indoor pollution

For many of us, the air in our houses is much more polluted than any outdoor air. Several of the indoor pollutants irritate the nose and airways, and some can trigger asthma attacks. A few of the pollutants found indoors can also make allergies and asthma more likely to develop in young children.

Background pollution

One of the worst irritants in indoor air is, of course, **tobacco smoke**. Other people's cigarette or pipe smoke can trigger asthma attacks in the short term, and makes asthmatics generally worse in the long run. Passive smoking may also affect the immune system, making allergies more likely to develop, though this is not proven. Do whatever you can to eliminate tobacco smoke from your home.

If you smoke yourself, there are many good reasons for giving up.
- If individuals from atopic families (see p. 8) smoke, they have a far greater chance of developing allergies and/or asthma when exposed to an allergen in the air.

Everyone is different

This section considers air pollution from the point of view of someone with hay fever or asthma. Those with chemical intolerance (see p. 84) may well be more severely affected by air pollution both indoors and out.

- For those who had asthma as children and have grown out of it, cigarette smoking doubles the chance of its coming back.
- Parents of asthmatic children who smoke indoors make their children's asthma worse. Teenagers can be just as badly affected by passive smoking as young children.
- Smoking during pregnancy significantly increases the risk of the baby developing allergies and asthma. (Smoking also leads to more premature births, stillbirths, and crib deaths.)

If possible, have an electric stove rather than a gas one — or install a powerful exhaust fan. Cooking with a gas stove generates a lot of **nitrogen dioxide**, a gas that you can't smell but which affects the airways. This same gas also comes from motor-vehicle traffic, but peak levels of nitrogen dioxide in kitchens with gas stoves are often ten times the average level on city streets, and frequently exceed standards for outdoor air set by the World Health Organization. Other sources of nitrogen dioxide include cigarettes, gas fireplaces, and kerosene heaters.

For *some* people with allergies, nitrogen dioxide enhances their response to the allergen. So if you inhale dust-mite allergen together with nitrogen dioxide, it may have more effect than the allergen alone. Breathing sulfur dioxide (see below) and nitrogen dioxide together boosts the reaction to allergen more powerfully than either gas alone.

Nitrogen dioxide might also make asthma attacks more likely, but the evidence on this is conflicting.

Smoke screen

Smoke particles from coal or wood do not seem to make allergies more likely to develop—in fact, quite the reverse. In rural areas of Germany, researchers have found that children with coal or wood stoves in their homes were less likely to have allergies or asthma. An Australian study made a similar finding. Bronchitis and pneumonia are more common in children living with wood and coal stoves, and these infections may stimulate the immune system in such a way that allergies are less likely to develop later. On the other hand, woodstove heating may worsen symptoms, if you already have asthma.

For young children, a high level of nitrogen dioxide at home may make the development of allergic reactions more likely. A recent Canadian study showed that children exposed to high levels of nitrogen dioxide in the home—usually from gas stoves—were *ten times* as likely to develop asthma as those breathing low levels of nitrogen dioxide. If a dog, cat, or other furry pet was kept, *and* there were high nitrogen dioxide levels, the risk of developing asthma shot up even higher, to 25 times that of children with low nitrogen dioxide and no pets. (Other studies have not produced the same dramatic results, but their methods of measuring nitrogen dioxide exposure were less precise.)

Try to eliminate materials that produce **formaldehyde** fumes, or seal the items with a good coat of paint. Formaldehyde is given off by pressed-wood products, including particleboard, hardwood plywood, and fiberboard. Injected cavity-wall insulation can also produce persistent formaldehyde fumes and is very difficult to get rid of—moving out is often the only option. A recent study from Australia showed that children exposed to formaldehyde especially in the bedroom, were more likely to develop allergic reactions: the higher the level of formaldehyde exposure, the more severe the allergic sensitization.

Those with asthma have more frequent symptoms if exposed to high formaldehyde levels. A recent study from Finland shows that easy-to-clean plastic wall-covering and flooring increases the risk of asthma in children.

A Canadian study found that children whose first home was less than 20–30 years old were 50 percent more likely to develop asthma than children living in older houses. One possible explanation for this lies with the materials used in the construction and fitting of new houses, especially the plastics, wood preservatives, and insulation materials. Solvents, and chemicals such as formaldehyde, are still being given off by these materials some years later. Another possible explanation may be better insulation and less ventilation, leading to higher humidity and indoor pollutant levels.

Air fresheners provoke asthma attacks in some people. For a few individuals they can cause general symptoms of ill-health that are similar to those described for mild chemical intolerance (see p. 84). Those affected generally don't realize that the air freshener is the source of the trouble. This malign effect is not entirely surprising, since air fresheners work by giving off a chemical that targets part of the brain—the part involved in processing sensory input from your nose. The chemical "freshens the air" by partially disabling your sense of smell. Better to open a window.

Cleaning products, furniture polish, and deodorant were never intended to go into the nose and airways, but that's what happens when they are sprayed from an **aerosol**, and they can trigger asthma attacks. Steer clear of aerosols as much as possible.

Pollution peaks

Read the instructions and ingredients lists on all products carefully. It is not just a question of what's in them, but also what gases they might give off when used. One asthmatic died within minutes when the de-rusting agent she was using on her dishwasher produced a large amount of **sulfur dioxide** gas: her airways tightened up so much that she couldn't even use an inhaler to save herself. "Sulfuric," "sulfate," or "sulfite" in the list of ingredients should ring warning bells if you have asthma: sulfur dioxide gas could be given off by this product.

Bleach, and other **chlorine**-based cleaning products, such as toilet cleaner and scouring powder, should be used sparingly and with plenty of ventilation. These products release chlorine gas, which in large amounts can irritate the airways of asthmatics. Never allow bleach or toilet cleaner to become mixed with any other product. Take care with any product containing hypochlorite, chloramine, ammonia, acids, or morpholine, and with the chemicals used for swimming-pool water. All these can trigger asthma attacks.

If doing repairs or do-it-yourself work around the house, take special care. Always ventilate the work area well, and wear a dust mask if sawing or drilling.

The smell of **paint** is due to solvents, and these can act as irritants to the nose and airways. When decorating, ventilate well, and use low-odor water-based paint. Some of the best low-odor paints, tested and shown to be safe for paint-sensitive asthmatics, are available only by mail order: see p. 255.

"Instant foam" kits sold for do-it-yourself insulation can provoke asthma in those who were not asthmatic previously. Two different substances are mixed to create the polyurethane foam, and during the mixing process, **isocyanate** is released—this is one of the most powerful asthmagens known (see box on p. 132). The level of isocyanate can breach the safety limit set for factories.

Avoid using fly spray or other **insecticides**: look for other methods of pest control. A study from Ethiopia showed that people using an insecticide in their houses were twice as likely to develop allergies. A study of Canadian farmers suggested that asthma might be linked to the use of carbamate insecticides. The sprays used for cockroaches can act as irritants for those with allergic rhinitis or chronic sinusitis.

If advised that your house needs spraying with insecticide, for powder-post beetles or other wood-boring pests, ask for more information before you go ahead. Is the spraying really necessary? What will happen if the house isn't sprayed? How quickly will it happen? Is there any other method of eradicating the pest? Spraying is often done when it is not really essential—houses remain standing in spite of heavy infestation. Unless you have an infestation that is threatening the structure of the house, you are probably better off *not* having the house sprayed. The heavy and ongoing exposure to insecticide that occurs in a sprayed house is something you and your family should avoid if at all possible. All the sprays used are toxic to some extent—don't believe those who tell you otherwise. A heavy exposure to pesticides can sometimes make allergic symptoms worse or precipitate chemical intolerance (see p. 85).

The garage, workshop, or toolshed can also be very polluted. Gasoline and kerosene can affect some people with rhinitis or asthma, and can bring on their symptoms. These fuels should always be kept in airtight containers. Paints sold for cars often contain isocyanates, among the most common causes of work-related asthma (see box on p. 132). If using such paint, wear a mask with an activated carbon filter (see box on p. 131) *and* make sure the area is well ventilated. And avoid prolonged or repeated exposure.

Outdoor pollution

Some of the pollutants in outdoor air can make allergic reactions worse and can trigger asthma attacks in people who are already asthmatic. A study of hospital admissions in London, Paris, Barcelona, and Helsinki found that high levels of pollution increased hospital admissions for asthma by about three percent.

The pollutants that matter to those with allergies are:
Ozone, which soars to high levels on sunny days, mainly in country areas that are near large cities. The reason for this is a chemical reaction that occurs when car exhaust fumes are exposed to sunlight, producing ozone, a highly reactive form of oxygen. Further chemical reactions, involving another ingredient of exhaust fumes, then break the ozone down again. Thanks to this second reaction, there is usually little ozone in city air. But in a relatively rural area 20 miles (32 kilometers) or so *upwind* of the city, the pollutants are too dispersed for the second reaction to occur, and the ozone from the urban traffic can accumulate.

Ozone levels in the air tend to peak in the late afternoon and early evening—but it takes between 4–24 hours for ozone to produce its effects on the airways. Indoors, ozone breaks down very quickly because of contact with other gases inside the house.

Ozone can increase the effects of allergens, such as pollen, on the nose and airways. In addition, ozone makes the airway muscles contract, even for people without asthma. Healthy people tend not to notice these effects, whereas some asthmatics may have more symptoms, and may need more drugs, on days when ozone levels are high.

Diesel particulates, which can become a problem in some downtown districts, and in areas close to main roads used by vans and trucks. Unlike ordinary gasoline, diesel fuel contains oil, so when it burns it produces tiny black particles. These consist of flakes of carbon (soot), coated with complex chemicals that are produced by the partial combustion of the oil. It is probably these surface chemicals, rather than the soot particles themselves, that have such bad effects on the nose and airways.

Some research suggests that diesel particulates might increase the risk of allergies developing—to pollen for example. Additionally, when levels of diesel particulates are high, asthmatics

But what about the ozone layer . . .?

Is ozone good for us or bad for us? People often get confused about this, because of all the discussion about "the destruction of the ozone layer." But that ozone layer (which screens us from harmful ultraviolet light) is a natural phenomenon, and it is far above the Earth, well away from our lungs. At ground level, in the air we breathe, ozone is unnatural and potentially damaging.

The size of the particles

Diesel particles are 1–10 microns in size, with most smaller than 2.5 microns. Tobacco smoke, coal smoke, fumes from oil-burning boilers, and the smoke from frying food all contain much smaller particles, down to a hundredth of a micron (.01 micron) in size. (A micron is one thousandth of a millimeter.)

In pollution reports, counts for particles in the air (mostly diesel particles these days, except in heavily industrialized areas) will often appear as "PM10," meaning "Particulate Matter less than 10 microns in diameter." This particle size is chosen because larger particles tend to settle in the nose and throat, and not reach the airways of the lungs. The term "Small Particles" is sometimes used to mean PM10.

To deal with air pollution, you need a really good mask with two filters: a dust filter that can take out very small particles and an **activated carbon filter** that absorbs irritant fumes and gases. Note that while activated carbon filters remove most pollutants, they do not take out nitrogen dioxide unless they have been specially treated.

tend to have more symptoms. If levels rise above 1.4 micrograms per cubic foot (50 micrograms per cubic meter), there is a sharp increase in asthma attacks—and a recent study in Birmingham, England, showed that such levels are regularly reached at roadsides.

Sulfur dioxide, which often reaches high levels in areas of heavy industry, particularly near coal-fired power plants and coking plants. This gas acts as an irritant to the airways and can trigger attacks in asthmatics, who are far more sensitive than healthy people to sulfur dioxide (see box on p. 207). However, at the sort of concentrations normally encountered, even in quite polluted air, sulfur dioxide does not have any effect on most asthmatics.

Nitrogen dioxide, which is produced by all types of vehicles, and by power plants and some factories. In towns and cities with heavy traffic, nitrogen dioxide can build up to high levels. Nitrogen dioxide is also found indoors (see p. 128)—often at far higher levels than outside.

In addition to these widespread pollutants, there are certain localized areas of air pollution, around industrial sites that are frequently said to cause health problems, including high rates of asthma. The kinds of industrial sites regularly mentioned include:

- oil refineries and oil-burning power plants
- cement works that use waste solvents for fuel
- dock areas where oil is loaded into tankers

There have been no detailed investigations into whether health problems are increased in these pockets of pollution, so it is impossible to say if there is a real link with asthma.

Avoiding outdoor air pollution

If you live in the kind of area that experiences high levels of ozone (see p. 130), plan your outdoor activities, especially jogging or sports, to avoid summer afternoons and early evenings.

If you are asthmatic, breathing through your nose may help as this can filter out some damaging pollutants before they reach the airways in your lungs. (If your nose is usually blocked, you could try the exercises on pp. 230–31).

Those who live very close to a highway with a lot of trucks going past would probably improve their own health, and reduce the chance of their children developing allergies and asthma, by installing air-conditioning, if they do not already have it, or high-quality HEPA air filters—or by moving to a cleaner area. But the benefits, in terms of decreased risk, are not enormous, and it is vital to take other preventive measures as well (see Chapter 8).

When driving, if you stop behind a truck or bus, keep your distance, close the window and turn off the fan. Diesel vehicles often emit a thick cloud of particles as they set off, and this can come straight into your car, setting off severe attacks for some asthmatics. Turning on the air-conditioning will reduce your exposure to diesel particulates while driving.

If you are buying a diesel-powered car, you can make a positive contribution to overall air quality by choosing one with a particle filter on the exhaust (now standard in German cars).

In the U.S., both the federal and state governments have strict regulations regarding vehicle-exhaust pollution. If you see a truck or bus pumping out black smoke, take the license number and report the violation to the appropriate authority (in many states, the state police).

When levels of ozone or sulfur dioxide are high, taking a supplement of vitamin C and eating plenty of foods that contain vitamin E and beta-carotene (see p. 207) can protect your airways.

Allergens and irritants at work

Some workplaces have very high concentrations of allergens in the air, especially if proper safety procedures are not being followed. Occupational allergies easily develop in these circumstances. The first signs may be symptoms in the nose, such as sneezing, blockage, or constant streaming (allergic rhinitis). You may also suffer from itchy or watery eyes (conjunctivitis), a cough, sweating, and a feverish feeling. Alternatively, direct contact with the allergen can produce a skin rash (dermatitis) or itchiness and swelling (contact urticaria—hives—and angioedema).

If you work somewhere with an allergy risk (see p. 133), be vigilant for such symptoms and see your doctor immediately. These symptoms can be the fore-runners of **occupational asthma**, which is a serious and potentially irreversible problem. Some allergens, such as latex, can even produce anaphylactic shock (a life-threatening allergic collapse). Prick-puncture tests (see p. 91) can show if you have developed an allergy to a substance encountered at work.

Acting promptly gives you the best possible chance of recovery and is vital if you have occupational asthma. Only if exposure to the allergen stops promptly do you have a good chance of shaking off the asthma. See a chest specialist as soon as possible, so that a definite diagnosis can be made. This is essential if you are going to make a claim for worker's compensation.

Far too many people with occupational asthma are just sent off with an inhaler when they first see their doctor. By delaying the moment when work is identified as the source of the problem, and the exposure to the allergen is stopped, drug treatment can turn occupational asthma into a disabling lifelong problem. Although drugs can be helpful in speeding your recovery *once expo-sure to the allergen has ended*, they should *not* be seen as a way of allowing you to go on working with the offending allergen or asthmagen.

If it seems plausible that your allergies or asthma are related to your work, your doctor might put you on temporary disability, so that you can have some time away from the workplace, to see if you recover.

The medical service at your workplace may be better at diagnosing occupational asthma than your own doctor, but be cautious. Some workplace medical offices offer genuinely confidential treatment, but in a few cases, information has been passed to the management, jeopardizing the jobs of workers

Other hazards

This section (pp. 132–4) deals mainly with *allergens* at work, that is, substances that provoke classical allergies.

In addition, there are skin irritants and antigens which can provoke **contact dermatitis** or **contact urticaria**: hairdressing involves several of these. Protective clothing and gloves are needed – but do not use latex gloves, especially the powdered variety, or you run the risk of developing latex allergy (see p. 133).

Some of the most dangerous workplace substances are chemicals that bring on asthma but are not allergens. These are usually called **low molecular weight asthmagens**. The most notorious of these are:

- platinum salts
- isocyanates (used in cement, in the manufacture of foam, plastics and varnishes, and for spray-painting auto-mobiles, aircraft and boats)
- colophony (used as a solder in electronics)
- glutaraldehyde (used in hospitals for sterilization procedures)
- persulphate (used in hairdressing)

Powerful respiratory equipment, supplying air from outside the area (see p. 134) is needed if you work with some of these substances, such as isocyanates for spray-painting.

with the early signs of occupational allergies and/or asthma. Most occupational health services *claim* to be independent, but they actually have to earn the trust of the workforce. Before you make any move, ask your colleagues for their views, especially those who have worked for your employer for many years.

Choosing a job

If you are looking for a job, and have any tendency to allergies, or come from an allergy-prone family, you should be very choosy about where you work. If at all possible, avoid workplaces such as the following, where there is heavy exposure to allergens:

• bakeries and flour mills, where the allergens concerned may be wheat proteins in the flour or enzymes added to the flour mix. These allergies can be very slow to develop—they may take years to begin.

• other food-processing plants, particularly those dealing with tea, soybeans, other beans, shellfish, and fish (especially if automated gutting machines are used without adequate ventilation).

• farms, docks, and cotton mills—or any other workplace generating dust from plant products. On farms, the dust from grain and hay may cause allergies, or mold spores (see p. 121) may be the culprit. Allergies to mites in hay, grain, and flour sometimes occur; eczema is the most common symptom.

• sawmills and carpenters' workshops, because of the wood dust, especially from hardwoods and from western red cedar (*Thuja plicata*).

• detergent and pharmaceutical factories handling enzymes— these are added to biological washing powders and are potential allergens.

• factories processing natural products, such as psyllium which is used as a laxative. Anyone who has been sensitized should avoid taking medicines containing the offending substance in future—a severe reaction could occur.

• hospitals and clinics, mainly due to latex used in gloves and equipment. Although nursing staff and surgeons are most susceptible, hospital administrative workers can occasionally be affected. Other workers who regularly wear latex gloves at work (for example, food handlers) are also at risk. The main problem is with powdered latex gloves, which release 15,000 times as much allergen into the air as unpowdered gloves. Unpowdered, low-allergen gloves greatly reduce the risk of latex allergy developing, and vinyl gloves are an even better choice.

• factories making or using rubber items. These places also may expose workers to the risk of latex allergy.

• laboratories and other workplaces where animals are kept. In the case of mice, rats, and other rodents, the allergen is found in the animals' urine, and becomes airborne as the urine dries. Insects and spiders (for example, those reared for biological pest control) are also allergenic, due to small airborne particles from their bodies.

Taking a risky job

If circumstances force you to take a job with an allergy risk, observe all the safety procedures that are in place, and where you have the option of turning on exhaust fans, wearing protective gear, or simply opening doors and windows, always do so.

Whatever you do, if you are in a risky job, don't smoke. At one salmon-processing plant, 40 percent of the smokers developed allergies, resulting in asthma, to the spray from the fish-gutting machine. Nonsmokers (who formed the overwhelming majority of the workers) were not affected at all. In U.S. cotton mills, workers who smoke are affected by levels of cotton dust in the air that are legally defined as "safe," while nonsmoking workers remain unaffected.

Passive smoking at work is also an important issue. An American study showed that nonsmokers were more likely to develop asthma if they worked alongside a smoker. Your employer has a duty to provide you with clean air. This includes ensuring that other employees do not impose their cigarette smoke on you.

Respiratory equipment

Where respiratory equipment is needed, your employer must provide this, and it must be the right equipment for the job. It should be inspected, tested, cleaned, and repaired after each use, and filters should be replaced regularly. These safety checks are your employer's responsibility, but make sure that they are being done, and always look the mask over before you put it on.

Two different types of respiratory equipment are in use:

- those that give you a supply of air from outside the work area, either from a compressed-air cylinder or via an air-hose (airline) supplied with outdoor air; these are called **breathing apparatus**
- those that use the surrounding air but filter it to remove allergens and asthmagens. These are called **respirators**. Ordinary respirators may pose problems for some asthmatics because they cannot breathe in strongly enough to draw sufficient air through the filter. Powered respirators can be the answer; they have a battery-powered unit to help with pulling in the air.

There are government regulations concerning the type of equipment required for each type of allergen and asthmagen. Large companies generally follow these regulations, but small businesses, such as local sawmills, carpenters' workshops, and car-repainting workshops, may not even know about them.

Any respiratory equipment that has a face mask must form a tight seal with your face. Facial hair will prevent this, and so will stubble, so shave carefully. Faces vary enormously in shape, and if your face mask does not fit, ask for a different type of mask or a different type of respiratory equipment. Persist until you get one that's right for you.

Carry out a "fit check" each and every time you wear the mask. For example, with respirators, you can check the fit by covering the air intake and breathing in sharply; if the mask fits properly, it should collapse onto your face, and remain stuck to your face for several seconds.

If you have difficulty breathing through the respiratory equipment, or if you can smell any of the substances you are working with, the replaceable filter cartridge or the equipment itself should be replaced.

Keep your mask on throughout the work period. If you find this impossible, talk to your employer or supervisor about getting a different kind of respiratory equipment—a powered device.

No form of respiratory equipment provides complete protection against allergens and asthmagens: there is always the chance of some small amount getting through. This is why respiratory equipment can't be used by those who have already developed occupational asthma but want to stay in their job.

Those who really cannot change jobs (for example, farmers) are sometimes able to use a powered respirator helmet, which allows them to go on working despite the allergen. But this is not an ideal solution from a purely health point of view. Farmers can also improve matters, where molds are the source of allergens, by keeping harvested crops dry and well ventilated.

Hand dermatitis

Housework is a major source of hand dermatitis—it is sometimes called "dishpan hands" or "homemaker's dermatitis." Bar staff, kitchen workers, nurses, and hairdressers are also very susceptible because of the constant exposure to soapy water and other irritants. Paint solvents and other synthetic chemicals can irritate the hands too. Indeed, almost any practical work can bring on hand dermatitis.

Hand dermatitis is very common and often very disabling. Sometimes it is due to atopic eczema, sometimes to contact dermatitis. Both may sometimes be playing a part—or the cause could be uncertain. A doctor can carry out patch tests for contact dermatitis (as well as ruling out other possibilities such as ringworm—a fungal infection—or psoriasis), but the cause of hand dermatitis frequently remains mysterious. However, the treatment of this problem is the same, whether atopic eczema or contact dermatitis is the cause, so exact diagnosis is not essential.

Caring for the hands is vital—they must be protected from irritants if healing is to occur. Instead of soap, use a non-soap cleanser (available at pharmacies). Ease up on handwashing; wear cotton gloves while at home, especially if doing vacuuming, dusting, and other housework. This keeps your hands clean so that they need less washing, as well as protecting the skin from many irritants. Most pharmacies stock inexpensive cotton gloves that are especially designed for protecting sensitive skin.

When you need to do wet work or gardening, put on waterproof gloves over the cotton gloves. Vinyl gloves are preferable to latex gloves, because of the risk of latex sensitivity. Make sure you have several pairs—there should be vinyl gloves available in the bathroom, the kitchen, and anywhere else where wet work occurs.

Disposable vinyl gloves (available from pharmacies) can be useful for delicate jobs such as peeling or chopping fruit and vegetables. In particular, protect the skin from tomatoes and the juice and peel of citrus fruits.

If the only gloves you can get are latex ones, make sure that they are *unpowdered* (the powdered ones are highly allergenic). Always wear cotton gloves underneath anyway, to reduce the risk of latex sensitivity to a minimum.

Once you have the problem under control and the dermatitis subsides, you can probably tolerate a lot more exposure because the skin is less permeable and therefore less sensitive. "For a while, I had three pairs of cotton gloves in use," says Lauren, who used to have severe hand dermatitis.

"One pair in the kitchen, for eating in, one pair in the bathroom, and one pair in my pocket, for use at all other times. I bought six pairs altogether—three in the wash, and three in use. That way, I managed to get through the whole day without washing my hands more than once. It was amazing how quickly my hands got better. Now I still use the cotton gloves a little, mainly for housework, but I don't need to be so obsessive about it. Gardening gloves and dishwashing gloves are always a must, of course."

You need to experiment a little to find a strategy that works for your particular lifestyle. Remember that friction—from tools such as hammers, screwdrivers, and wrenches—can irritate the skin almost as badly as chemicals. Dry, frosty air is another hazard, so wear gloves (preferably leather ones) in winter.

In addition to these protective measures, you also need treatment with steroid creams. Follow the doctor's instructions carefully—don't use either too much or too little. A non-perfumed moisturizer is also useful.

Should the rash not improve despite good treatment, there may be some internal cause rather than—*or in addition to*—an external one. This is especially likely if the rash is on the palms of the hands or along the sides of the fingers. Possibilities to consider include

- sensitivity to food—this can be checked with an elimination diet (see p. 194)
- sensitivity to nickel or another metal in food and water (see above). This is especially likely if there is a blistering rash that recurs regularly.
- an effect of cigarette smoking—this too can cause a recurrent blistering rash
- an effect of oral contraceptives or aspirin

Chapter 5

drugs and immunotherapy

"With my children, both of whom have allergies and asthma, I have always worried about the possible side effects of using Beclovent, Ventolin, and various antihistamines. But it seems to be a case of being "between the devil and the deep blue sea"—in other words, *not* using the drugs is far more risky than using them. I'm concerned about the effect of steroids on Michael's growth rate and bones, and about the effect of Ventolin on his heart. I've always wondered just how long these drugs have been around and if doctors could possibly know what the effects are on someone taking them for, say, 40 years. In the end, I've come to the conclusion that doctors simply don't have an answer to that question." Rachel, aged 37.

Rachel's concerns are probably shared by other parents of allergy sufferers—and by those who have allergies themselves. Their fear and suspicion of drugs are often fueled if doctors fail to mention side effects when prescribing.

The reason some doctors neglect to mention side effects is quite simple: being frank about potential minor side effects, such as headaches and nausea, greatly increases the number of patients who actually suffer from them. The power of the human imagination is such that a completely inert dummy pill can produce a wide range of minor side effects if these are expected. This is the flip side of the **placebo effect,** whereby a dummy pill can produce a distinct improvement if the doctor seems confident that it will help. So some doctors may keep quiet about side effects when they first prescribe a new drug—which does not mean that they are either complacent about or ignorant of them.

If you want to know about all the possible side effects of the drugs you are taking, that information is available here, along with information about how the drugs work and advice on using them to the best effect.

Before reading about the side effects of your drugs, bear in mind that **major side effects**—the ones that seriously damage health—are probably *not* going to happen to you. Only a few of the anti-allergy drug treatments—long courses of steroid tablets, for example, or high doses of theophylline—are *commonly* associated with major side effects. You probably have more chance of being struck by lightning than suffering some of the major side effects mentioned here. Even with the more hazardous treatments, you can tip the odds in your favor by being sensible—using your drugs correctly, taking the precautions suggested here, and keeping an eye out for warning signs.

Remember that the most common reactions are just **minor side effects**. In other words, they may be unpleasant or inconvenient, but they do not indicate that the drug is doing you any serious damage. These common side effects are noted during the safety trials that precede the release of a new drug and are studied closely to check that they are not a cause for concern. Careful testing is carried out on the patients involved in safety trials to exclude the possibility of any dangerous unseen side effects on the liver, heart, kidneys, and other vital organs. Carcinogenic effects are ruled out at an even earlier stage.

Unfortunately, these pre-release trials cannot possibly identify all major side effects. Everyone varies in their response to drugs. A drug might have a serious side effect that affects only one person in 10,000, and no safety trial can hope to identify such a rare response. Only when a drug is released and becomes widely used do such side effects come to light. Other unanticipated side effects can sometimes arise when people taking the new drug are much older than those in the safety trials or are from a different ethnic group with different susceptibilities. Combining the drug with certain other drugs can also be a potential source of trouble, although pharmaceutical experts can often predict such problems from their detailed knowledge of the chemistry of drugs and how they are broken down in the body. Side effects that take several years to develop—more than the timespan of most safety trials—will also fail to show up until after the drug has been released.

All this may sound very alarming, but in fact severe reactions to new drugs are not that common. And there are various safety nets in place—doctors keep a close eye on patients taking new drugs, and a special reporting system ensures that if unexpected side effects do show up, the information is quickly shared with others in the medical community.

In order to relate the information in this chapter to a particular medicine that you take, you need to know what drug category it belongs to. Does your inhaler contain a beta-2 reliever, a steroid, a cromoglycate-type drug (cromolyn) or an anti-cholinergic, for example? If you are not sure, ask your pharmacist.

Those are the **category names** for drugs: they denote families of drugs that are similar chemically and work in roughly the same way. Within each category, or family, there are a number of individual drugs. The individual drugs should, ideally, have a standard internationally agreed name—the **generic name**. Unfortunately, a few of the drugs used for allergies and asthma have more than one generic name—albuterol is called salbutamol outside the United States, and epinephrine is called adrenaline in Britain.

Finally there are the **brand names,** which are the ones most patients are familiar with. Unlike the generic names, brand names are always shown with a capital letter. Long-established drugs are usually made by several different pharmaceutical companies and are therefore marketed under several different brand names. A newer drug, which is still covered by a patent, will be sold under only one brand name.

The question of brand names is important in relation to advertising campaigns for prescription drugs. Such campaigns are a recent development in the United States, where more and more doctors are now faced with patients who have seen an advertisement for a prescription drug and want this instead of their existing drug. Frequently the advertised drug is little or no different from the patient's present drug. It may be exactly the same generic drug under a different brand name, or a drug that is very similar chemically and has much the same effects. These advertising campaigns are mostly pure hype—a pharmaceutical company has simply decided to spend money promoting a particular drug brand. It's obvious where that money will eventually come from: it will come from the price paid for the drug.

For those who wish to avoid drugs, or at least reduce their dosage, allergy shots (see pp. 164-9) are worth considering. They are not a treatment for the impatient, however—it may take a year or more before you see any benefits, and you need commitment and staying power to see the treatment through. Since they entail regular weekly appointments, they are also expensive, of course; but the outlay on allergy shots will probably be recouped in the long run, through a reduction in your expenditure on drugs.

Antihistamines

Antihistamines were first introduced in 1947 and are very widely used, so their safety—at least in the case of the older antihistamines—is beyond doubt. Most of the antihistamines have no major ill effects, and no one should feel concerned about taking them. At worst, they produce some annoying minor side effects, which often wear off in time.

These drugs are particularly valuable for **hay fever** and other allergies in the nose (**perennial allergic rhinitis**). They are also used for hives (**chronic urticaria**), sometimes in combination with another histamine-blocking drug—see p. 53.

Antihistamines are not much used for **asthma.** They have relatively little effect, probably because so many other messenger chemicals are involved in an asthma attack. However, doctors in Japan do use antihistamines for asthma, and it is possible that people of Asian origin react differently to them. Only one antihistamine, ketotifen, is widely used for asthma in the West, and this has other effects besides blocking histamine (see p. 159). A new role may soon develop for antihistamines in the treatment of asthma, combined with anti-leukotriene drugs (see p. 159).

If you suffer from **anaphylaxis,** you might be given antihistamines in a tablet or liquid form, for use in an emergency. Note that these are not enough in themselves to treat this dangerous condition—you *must* have an epinephrine injector (see p. 150).

In the past, some doctors prescribed antihistamines for **atopic eczema,** mainly for their sedative effect (see p. 139), which was thought to help children to sleep better and scratch less at night. This treatment has largely gone out of favor, because its value is in doubt. But a recent study has revealed that the non-sedating antihistamine known as cetirizine (Reactine in Canada; Zyrtec in the U.S.) may be useful for very young children with atopic eczema, not only in treating their skin but also in reducing the chance of their developing asthma (see p. 249).

Most people take their antihistamines in tablet or capsule form. Syrups and sugar-free elixirs containing these drugs are available for children.

Antihistamines can also be applied directly, in the form of nasal sprays or eyedrops. These are used mainly to treat hay fever and the conjunctivitis (inflammation of the eye) that often accompanies it. Levocabastine (Livostin) is particularly effective for the eyes.

Antihistamine creams are also sold, without prescription, for the treatment of insect bites—that is, the normal nonallergic reaction to such bites. These creams are not recommended for atopic eczema or other allergic conditions affecting the skin. Not only are they unlikely to help, but they may make matters worse because, with regular use, skin sensitization to the antihistamine can occur (see p. 54).

Some common brand names
Common brand names include:

non-sedating antihistamines—Allegra, Claritin; Mizollen, Zyrtec (U.S. only); Reactine (Canada only)

older (sedating) antihistamines—Atarax, Benadryl, Dimetane, Optimine, Periactin, Phenergan, Tavist

eyedrops—Emadine, Livostin

nasal sprays—Livostin; Astelin (U.S. only)

How antihistamines work

Of the messenger chemicals released when an allergic reaction occurs, the most important is **histamine**. This does its work by attaching to specialized **receptors** in certain parts of the body, and so triggering various reactions (see box on p. 12). The action of antihistamines is very simple: they bind to the same receptors as histamine, but they do not trigger any reaction. Histamine cannot bind to the receptor because the antihistamine is already there.

Unfortunately, the reverse is also true: if the histamine is already there, the antihistamine cannot elbow it off the receptor, which is why it is important to take the antihistamine *well before* the allergen is encountered. Taking antihistamines at the first sign of a sniffle or itch can also work, but the effects will not be nearly as good as taking them in anticipation of an exposure.

The best approach to treating hay fever, for example, is to start taking the antihistamines at least a week before the pollen season begins, and preferably two to three weeks before. You should then take them continuously until it is over. *This will make a huge difference to the degree of symptom control you achieve.*

Side effects of these drugs

The older types of antihistamines, such as diphenhydramine (Benadryl) are relatively nonspecific in their effects—they bind to several different kinds of receptors, not just those for histamine. As a result, they can have some unwanted effects, such as causing drowsiness and poor coordination. While these sedative effects are no cause for concern in themselves, they can, of course, be hazardous if you work with dangerous machinery or drive. Avoid both until you are sure how you react to the antihistamine. Note that the effects of alcohol may be increased.

Very occasionally some antihistamines have the opposite effect, causing stimulation rather than sedation; this is most likely to occur in children and old people. Lowering the dose may solve the problem.

The other possible side effects of the older antihistamines—all of which are minor ones—are headache, dry mouth, blurred vision, difficulty in passing urine, nervousness, shaky hands, upset stomach, and diarrhea. A few men suffer impotence while taking antihistamines, but this disappears when the drug is stopped.

The minor side effects of antihistamines, including drowsiness, often wear off after a while, although the benefits of the drug remain. So it is worthwhile persisting with an antihistamine, even if it causes some problems at first. Many people experience side effects from certain antihistamines but not from others, so try several different types to find one that suits you.

The problem of drowsiness has been reduced, in recent years, thanks to the development of new drugs that are far more specific for histamine receptors, the **non-sedating antihistamines**. (A few people do get drowsy even with these drugs. Again, the effects vary from one drug to another, so if the first one disagrees with you, you might try a different one.)

Hismanal and Seldane, two non-sedating antihistamines, have been withdrawn from use because they have been associated with abnormal heart rhythms in a minority of people. Mizolastine (Mizollen) a prescription non-sedating antihistamine (available in the U.S. but not in Canada) also has a potential for causing abnormal heart rhythms in a few individuals. This side effect can be made worse by:

- Exceeding the prescribed dose.
- Taking certain other medications while on Mizollen. Check with your doctor or pharmacist that other drugs taken are compatible with Mizollen.
- Drinking grapefruit juice while taking Mizollen—something found naturally in grapefruit may interact with the drug. If you have suffered abnormal heart rhythms in the past, make sure your doctor knows about this before prescribing Mizollen. Any side effects you experience while taking this drug must be discussed with your doctor.

In addition to these special precautions concerning Mizollen, *any* antihistamine should be used with caution by the elderly, and by people suffering from epilepsy, Parkinson's disease, glaucoma, prostate enlargement, kidney problems, urinary retention, a gastric ulcer, a thyroid disorder, porphyria, or liver disease. Always check with your doctor before taking antihistamines if you have any of these conditions.

It may be inadvisable to use antihistamines if you are taking sleeping pills, antidepressants or antianxiety drugs—again, see your doctor.

Stop taking antihistamines if you suffer any unusual kind of rash, or if your skin becomes more sensitive to sunlight.

If you are breast-feeding, check with your doctor, because many antihistamines pass into the milk, and they may make the baby sleepy.

Rescue treatment

Most antihistamines perform very badly if you take them once the allergic reaction has set in, but acrivastine (Semprex) can be good in these circumstances and is non-sedating. No prescription is required for this drug in the U.S. Semprex is not available in Canada.

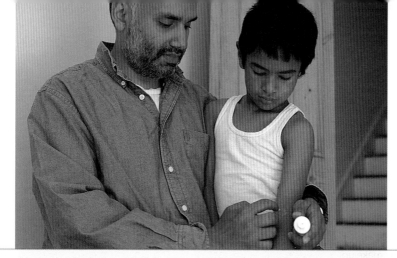

Steroids

Few drugs create quite so much alarm as **corticosteroids**. To some extent, this alarm is justified; if overused, they have dangerous side effects. But rejecting them entirely is a great mistake, because they are safe at the right dose and *immensely* useful for a variety of allergic symptoms. Armed with the information given here, you can use steroids as safely and effectively as possible.

Although their proper name is corticosteroids, these drugs are commonly—and rather inaccurately—called **steroids**. This name adds to their doubtful reputation by confusing them with the notorious anabolic steroids (see box on p. 142). However, the term "steroids" is used for corticosteroids in this book, simply because that is the name most people recognize.

Steroids do not deal with the allergic reaction itself, unlike antihistamines (p. 138) or cromoglycate (see p. 148). Instead, they tackle the consequences of the allergic reaction, **inflammation**.

What exactly is inflammation? The visible features of this phenomenon—for example, if it occurs in the skin, around a scratch or cut—are redness and slight swelling. There is also soreness, and some warmth. All these effects are produced by an influx of immune cells, intent on protecting the broken skin from infection. These immune cells generate messenger chemicals (see box on p. 10), which boost the inflammation, as well as attracting yet more immune cells to the area. When inflammation affects delicate membranes—as when you suffer a sore throat for example, there can be a great deal more swelling and discomfort.

The inflammation that follows allergic reactions is very similar to that provoked by infection, although the balance of immune cells and messenger chemicals is slightly different. Eosinophils (see p. 19) play a particularly important role in sustaining the inflammation produced by allergies.

This influx of eosinophils and other immune cells, which lights the fires of inflammation, occurs some hours after the allergic response itself. It is known as the **Late Phase Reaction** (see p. 13). Steroids work well for allergies because they curtail the Late Phase Reaction and have a calming effect on immune cells, especially eosinophils.

Steroid phobia

So many patients have a profound objection to taking steroids that doctors call it "steroid phobia." One of the hazards of giving information about potential side effects is that it may encourage "steroid phobia." That would be a tragedy, because steroids really are useful drugs that can do a lot of good and very little harm, if used correctly. The risks are very small when the steroids are used at low to medium doses and targeted directly at the inflammation. Even with high doses, the serious side effects can generally be avoided. Don't use this book's information to scare yourself—instead, use it to protect yourself while getting the most from steroid treatment.

Mimicking nature

All corticosteroids are chemically similar to **cortisol**, a substance produced naturally by the body. Cortisol—which is a hormone made in the **adrenal glands**, located near the kidneys—has a great number of different effects apart from damping down inflammation. It regulates the action of the kidneys, moves proteins out of the muscles and bones, and alters the pattern of fat distribution.

Like other hormones and chemical messengers that the body produces, cortisol achieves its effects by binding to **receptors** on target cells (immune cells, muscle cells, and the cells that make up the kidneys). These receptors vary a little, which gives researchers scope for making a synthetic version of the hormone, cunningly modified so that it binds well to one kind of receptor (the one on the immune cells, for example) but not so well to another (the one on the kidneys).

Hydrocortisone, the original steroid drug, is identical to cortisol, but the newer steroids have been modified chemically to have the maximum effect on inflammation and minimal effects on other body processes. While hydrocortisone can only be used for allergies at very low doses (as in nonprescription hydrocortisone cream), the modified steroids can be used at higher doses.

The side effects of steroid drugs are of two basic kinds:
- those due to suppression of inflammation (the desired effect of the drugs), because blocking inflammation partially reduces immunity to disease
- those due to the effects of steroids on other body processes—undesirable effects that have, as much as possible, been designed out of the modern drugs

These different side effects are discussed in more detail on p. 142. First, it is important to look at the crucial difference between taking steroids in tablet or liquid form and applying them directly to the affected area. Much unnecessary anxiety can be avoided by understanding this difference.

Targeting steroids

The risks of steroids fall dramatically if, instead of taking them in tablet form, you put them exactly where they are needed: that means sprays for the nose or drops for the eyes, inhalers to get the drug into the airways, or creams, lotions, and ointments applied to the skin.

The medical term for this is **topical application**, and it is infinitely preferable to taking steroid tablets. When a drug is swallowed, it does its job by being absorbed through the stomach lining into the bloodstream and then being carried around the body in the blood. This is called **systemic treatment** because it reaches the whole body system via the blood.

The areas that need the drug—the itchy skin or inflamed airways—get their dose, but so does every other part of the body. In order to get a useful amount to the afflicted parts, a fairly large total dose has to be taken, which inevitably affects the rest of the body, making the drug far more hazardous.

When a drug is targeted precisely, in sprays, drops, creams, or inhalers, the dose used can be much smaller. Some of the drug does get into the bloodstream, by penetrating the skin or the membranes of the nose or airways and entering the tiny blood vessels that lie just below. But the amount reaching the bloodstream is usually minuscule compared with the amount in the blood when you take steroid tablets. **Systemic side effects**—those due to the drug going around in the blood (see below)—are usually avoided, although there may be some local side effects, where the drug is applied.

Only with very powerful doses—as in the steroid inhalers used for severe asthma or high-potency creams for eczema—do topical steroids reach the bloodstream in sufficient amounts to cause systemic side effects. You have to be on these treatments for a long time, or be overdosing (a possible hazard with creams for eczema), to run the risk of systemic side effects.

Steroid tablets

Short courses of steroid tablets—which means three weeks or less—are pretty safe. They are usually sufficient to get the inflammation under control and can be taken three or four times a year without creating any problems.

Even if you have no choice but to take steroid tablets on a long-term basis, remember that the serious side effects can usually be avoided, or reversed if caught early (see p. 143).

Side effects of steroid tablets

Apart from changes that may (rarely) occur in the stomach lining, the side effects of steroid tablets are all **systemic side effects**.

In the early days of steroid use, a set of side effects resembling a disease known as **Cushing's syndrome** was frequently seen. The side effects included deposits of fat on the shoulders and abdomen and around the face, producing a "moon face," water retention resulting in puffiness, weakening of the bones, easy bruising, acne, and muscle wasting. All these changes are due to the unwanted effects of steroids on other body processes, not due to any effect on inflammation.

With the new and improved steroids (see left), plus a much more watchful approach by doctors, these severe side effects have become very rare, but they can still occur in people on high-dose steroid tablets. So long as they are noticed in good time (see p. 143), the problem can be reversed.

A few effects on other body processes remain, even with the new steroids:

- Raised blood pressure—this can occur even with short-term use of steroids.
- Children may stop growing, or grow more slowly. Usually they make up for this later.
- Quite commonly, there is increased hunger (though you don't actually need more food, and will put on weight if you eat more than usual). Insomnia and an agitated, edgy feeling during the day may occur. These are minor side effects and are no cause for concern.
- Side effects in the eye can occur: there is an increased risk of glaucoma and, with prolonged use, cataracts.
- Long-term use can also result in loss of calcium and phosphorous from the bones, leading to thinning and fragility (osteoporosis).
- Psychological changes may occur. Some people experience euphoria or greatly increased energy levels—with the opposite effects occuring when the course of steroids ends. At worst, steroids can trigger paranoia or severe depression and suicidal feelings. (These effects are more likely to occur in those with a history of mental illness. If you are concerned about this aspect, discuss the possible risks with your doctor before taking steroid tablets.)
- Some epileptics may suffer more frequent or more severe seizures while on steroid tablets.
- Very rarely, stomach ulcers develop, or other side effects in the digestive system.
- The skin may become thin, and the small blood vessels beneath it more fragile, leading to easy bruising and stretch marks (striae). This is also a potential problem with steroid creams, lotions, and ointments (see p. 146). Elderly patients are much more susceptible.
- Some diabetics need more insulin. In addition, anyone with the potential to develop diabetes is more likely to do so, but only if taking steroid tablets long-term. The diabetes usually goes when the steroids are stopped.
- A few men suffer impotence, but only with long-term use of tablets. This can be treated. Women may have irregular periods.
- Damage to the hip bones may rarely occur, usually with excessive doses of steroid tablets. This is called avascular necrosis and may require hip replacement.

In addition to these effects on other body processes, there are also some side effects that arise from the steroids' suppression of the inflammation. These can occur even with short courses. Again, however, these problems can almost always be prevented, or treated, or reversed if detected at an early stage.

- Skin wounds may be slow to heal and are more likely to become infected because of reduced immunity. This is not a serious problem—just keep all cuts and scratches clean.
- Infections by viruses and fungi (Candida, for example—see box on p. 83) may occur more readily.
- Some infections may be masked because fever is suppressed by the steroids. The disease may not be obvious until it has reached a more advanced stage than normal.
- Chicken pox and measles can be far more serious—even fatal—if steroid tablets are being taken *or have been taken for more than three weeks within the last three months*. This is something to be very careful about (see item 15 p. 143).
- Prolonged use can increase the risk of chest infections.
- Vaccination with live vaccines can cause problems.
- Older people who once suffered from tuberculosis (TB) may find that it comes back.
- High-dose steroids can lead to pregnancy if you are using an IUD (intrauterine device), because IUDs work by inducing a mild inflammation in the womb.

The most insidious effect of steroids—and remember again that this is a hazard only of *prolonged high-dose treatment*—is **adrenal suppression**. When steroid tablets are taken for more than three weeks, the adrenal glands' own ability to produce cortisol (see p. 141) starts to be slightly suppressed. The longer the course of steroids, the greater the effect. Stopping the steroids abruptly leaves the body without enough cortisol to protect itself, which, in the very worst cases, can lead to collapse. Less obviously, there may be greater vulnerability to the effects of accidents, serious illnesses, surgery, or childbirth—demanding events that would normally stimulate a rise in cortisol production to help the body cope with the stress.

If you take a short course of steroid tablets during this period, there is a greater risk of side effects than normal. Adrenal suppression can last for 6–12 months after treatment with steroids ends. It may be two years before the body can cope with surgery unaided and you will need low doses of steroids to get you through stress of this kind.

Will I look like a weight lifter?

Absolutely not. The steroids taken by unscrupulous athletes to pump up their muscles artificially are **anabolic steroids**. They are entirely different from the corticosteroids used to treat allergies.

Using steroid tablets safely

People taking steroid tablets for more than three weeks, or taking a lot of short courses, can protect themselves from serious side effects in the following ways:

1 Weigh yourself every day. If your weight suddenly starts to rise, despite eating normally, consult your doctor: this may be a sign of water retention.

2 If you develop hip pain, swollen ankles, muscle weakness, or acne, tell your doctor.

3 Get your blood pressure checked regularly by the doctor.

4 Get your eyes checked regularly by an ophthalmologist, who can detect any problems, such as glaucoma or cataracts, before there is irreversible damage.

5 In the case of children, make sure the child's growth is being monitored carefully by the doctor.

6 Stay as active as possible, with plenty of vigorous exercise, to protect against osteoporosis. Discuss with your doctor whether a calcium supplement would be advisable. Avoid getting too thin, as this is also a risk factor for osteoporosis. Reduce your salt intake, and don't drink too much alcohol. Ask your doctor to order a bone-density measurement periodically. Following menopause, women on steroid tablets should consider taking hormone replacement therapy (HRT), as this protects against osteoporosis.

7 Persistent unexplained back pain must be reported to your doctor; this can be a sign of osteoporosis. If you fracture your wrist in a fall (a Colles' fracture), make sure your doctor knows about this and prescribes urgent drug treatment for osteoporosis.

8 See your doctor if you are overtired, thirsty, or need to pass urine much more frequently—these are signs of diabetes.

9 Take your tablets after food to protect the stomach. See your doctor if you have persistent indigestion.

10 If you ever produce black, tarry stools, call your doctor immediately. This is a sign of bleeding from the stomach or elsewhere in the digestive tract.

11 With your doctor's permission, take all your daily steroids as a single dose in the morning. The long gap between one dose and the next stimulates the body to maintain its own steroid-making abilities and so reduces the risk of adrenal suppression. It can also protect against growth problems in children. Even greater protection comes from taking steroids on alternate days—one day on, one day off—although not everyone can keep their symptoms under control with this regime. Obviously, you must consult your doctor before you try. Your dose may need adjusting.

12 Adrenal suppression puts you at risk during any medical procedure. Tell your doctor, dentist, and anyone treating you in an emergency—*even if you stopped taking steroids up to two years earlier*. You should also carry a MedicAlert wallet card (see p. 255) at all times, in case you are unconscious.

13 Ask the doctor what you should do if you develop any kind of infection or suffer an accident. It is often necessary to increase the dose of steroid tablets.

14 Tell your doctor if you have ever had TB, as this can recur.

15 If you or your child have *not* had measles or chicken pox, avoid contact with anyone suffering from these diseases—or from shingles (herpes zoster), which is caused by the chicken pox virus. *See your doctor promptly if there is any contact with someone infected.* Emergency treatment to combat the virus must be started within 96 hours.

16 When being vaccinated, remind the doctor or nurse that you are taking steroid tablets.

17 Never stop taking steroid tablets abruptly if you have been taking them for more than 3 weeks, as some degree of adrenal suppression may already have begun. Your body needs time to recover its natural level of activity, so reduce the dose gradually. Get precise instructions from your doctor.

18 If you are asthmatic, at the end of any course of steroid tablets lasting more than 3 weeks, be extra careful about avoiding exposure to allergens and asthma triggers. You may be more vulnerable to severe asthma attacks for as much as a year after long-term steroid tablets are stopped or the dosage reduced.

Watch out for adrenal suppression

If you develop any of the following symptoms after stopping steroid tablets or syrup, or while reducing the dose, call your doctor as soon as possible:

- muscle weakness; muscle and joint pain
- feeling "under the weather"
- mental changes
- scaly or flaking skin
- breathlessness
- lack of appetite, or nausea and vomiting
- fever and weight loss
- painful, itchy lumps on the skin

Note that, very rarely, withdrawal of steroid tablets, or lowering the dose, can unmask a disease called Churg-Strauss syndrome (see p. 160).

Steroid nasal sprays

Most steroid nasal sprays contain very low doses of the drug and produce no significant side effects when used for short periods of time.

Steroid sprays for the nose are a very effective way of treating hay fever and perennial allergic rhinitis. They can be used after the symptoms have begun or in advance of encountering the allergen.

Steroid nasal sprays are also useful in reducing the size of nasal polyps (see p. 30) but only if they are inserted correctly. Gently blow your nose if needed. Insert the spray nozzle into your nostril and tilt your head slightly forward. Point the nozzle slightly to the side rather than straight up, and spray, while gently inhaling through the nose. Once the polyps have shrunk, keep them under control with regular use.

Always stick to the stated dose, as with any drugs—don't use the spray more often than you should. If you have a cold or other infection in the nose, stop using steroid sprays until it is better. Following a surgical operation on the nose, ask your doctor's advice before using steroid sprays.

Side effects

Minor short-term side effects may include dryness and irritation in the nose and throat and disturbances of smell and taste. Nosebleeds might occur and should be reported to your doctor. If you are a long-term user of steroid nose sprays, your doctor should check the membranes in your nose regularly, to be sure that they are not becoming thinned by the drug. Occasional eye checks may also be advisable with long-term use, as glaucoma can occur.

Allergic reactions to the steroid are possible, and they can cause bronchospasm (contraction of the airway muscles), though this is unusual. You should obviously stop using the spray and see your doctor if this occurs.

With very high doses of steroids in the nose, or prolonged treatment, some systemic side effects might occur. The main cause for concern is children's growth (see box on p. 145)—their height should be checked regularly.

Steroid eyedrops

Steroid eyedrops are sometimes given for severe inflammation of the eye during the hay fever season. However, the eye is vulnerable to infections if treated with steroid drops, and such treatment requires close medical supervision.

Side effects

Be extremely careful about infections—don't rub your eyes with your fingers, for example, or dry around your eyes with a towel unless it is absolutely clean. Follow your doctor's instructions very carefully, and go back immediately if your eyes become more uncomfortable, if redness increases, or if you have any other cause for concern.

With prolonged use, there is a risk of two serious side effects—glaucoma and cataracts. Consequently, steroid eyedrops are rarely used for more than a few weeks.

Using two forms of steroid

Allergy sufferers who need steroid nasal spray for hay fever or perennial rhinitis, as well as a steroid inhaler, often worry that they are getting too much steroid overall.

In fact there is no cause for concern, unless you are taking very high doses of inhaled steroid, in which case talk the matter over with your doctor. The amount in most nasal sprays is quite small, and relatively little gets into the bloodstream.

If you have allergies in the nose, this may well be making your asthma worse, and using steroid nasal sprays can be very helpful for the asthma symptoms (see p. 39).

Inhaled steroids and children's growth

If an asthmatic child inhales relatively high doses of steroids for many years, his or her growth can be suppressed somewhat. However, only a small number of children need these high doses, and with low to moderate doses most children's growth is unaffected. They may experience a short-term slowdown in growth, but their eventual height should be normal.

Unfortunately, there are a few children whose growth is stunted even by relatively low doses of inhaled steroids—and it is impossible to predict which children will respond in this way. However, if it is noticed in good time, and if the steroids can be withdrawn safely, the child's growth rate will almost certainly recover.

Your primary care doctor or pediatrician should be monitoring your child's growth. You can also measure this yourself and go back to the doctor if you are concerned. Keep the risks in perspective—uncontrolled severe asthma also stunts children's growth, as well as endangering the child in far more serious ways, so don't stop using the steroid inhaler.

Steroid inhalers

Inhaled steroids are a key part of the successful modern treatment of asthma (see p. 157).

Side effects

As with other topical treatments, inhaled steroids are a great deal safer than steroid tablets. However, some of the drug does get into the bloodstream, and with high-dose inhaled steroids taken for several years, the levels can be high enough to cause systemic side effects such as osteoporosis (see p. 142).

The dose is the crucial factor here. The leaflet that comes with your inhaler will tell you how much of the drug is delivered with each inhalation. To interpret the information about side effects correctly, you need to know your total daily consumption of inhaled steroid and whether this is a low, medium, or high dose:

- For budesonide or beclomethasone, two of the more common steroids, less than 400 mcg (micrograms) per day counts as a low dose for adults and children over the age of five. A moderate dose is 400–800 mcg per day, and more than 800 mcg a day is a high dose.
- For fluticasone (Flovent), less than 200 mcg a day is a low dose, 200–400 mcg is a moderate dose, and over 400 mcg is a high dose).
- All these figures should be halved for children under five (so a high dose of budesonide is more than 400 mcg per day, and a high dose of fluticasone more than 200 mcg a day).
- For other steroids, check with your pharmacist.

Anyone taking a low or moderate dose has very little to worry about as regards systemic side effects. Only those inhaling high-dose steroids for many years need feel concerned. The newer inhaled steroids, such as fluticasone, have a lower potential for growth suppression and other systemic side effects, while beclomethasone has the highest potential of the commonly used inhaled steroids.

If you may be at risk of systemic side effects, follow the protective measures described for steroid tablets on p. 143. Apart from growth suppression (see box above), the most likely effects are osteoporosis, adrenal suppression, and a recurrence of tuberculosis.

You can minimize the risk of systemic side effects from inhalers by swallowing as little as possible of the steroid. Always rinse out your mouth, gargle, *and spit out the water* after using your inhaler. Using your steroid inhaler morning and evening, just before brushing your teeth, will make it easier to remember to do this. (Using a spacer also reduces the amount of steroid that deposits in the mouth and throat, where it is not needed.)

Bear in mind that inhaling steroids regularly will help you avoid the need for steroid tablets. Asthmatics who are worried about side effects sometimes skip doses of their inhaled steroids, then find that their asthma is much worse and that they need a course of steroid tablets. Frequent courses of tablets increase the risk of serious side effects.

Minor local side effects of inhaled steroids include hoarseness and short-lived coughing due to direct irritation of the throat. These are no cause for concern.

If you are regularly inhaling steroids from a nebulizer, make sure the mask fits really well (see p. 163).

Because steroids reduce the immune defenses a little, one common side effect of inhaling them is a throat infection by *Candida* (see box on p. 83). Esophageal infections with *Candida* can also happen, but these are rare; the symptoms are heartburn and indigestion. Gargling with warm water after each inhalation will help prevent *Candida* infections. There are also antifungal drops or tablets if you are still having trouble. Keep inhaled steroids away from your lips if you suffer from cold sores (herpes infections) around the mouth. These can be made worse with steroids.

Fortunately, other infections are no more common when using inhaled steroids. This includes chest infections.

Steroid creams, lotions, and ointments

Steroid creams, lotions, and ointments are used for both atopic eczema and contact dermatitis. By delivering the drug to the place where it is needed, they reduce the dose required to an absolute minimum, and, if used correctly, are very safe. Dr. Ernst Epstein, a dermatologist at the University of California, observes, "All too often I encounter children who are miserable with uncontrolled atopic dermatitis because of their parents' unjustified fears of steroid side effects. It is cruel to the child and the family to forego topical medication."

It is very important to use a steroid cream of the right strength. For example, applying a nonprescription hydrocortisone cream to severe atopic eczema, or to poison ivy or poison oak rash, will be of no value. Similarly, only applying a prescribed cream occasionally, or only once a day when the doctor said three times a day, will mean that the rash never really succumbs to the treatment. Keeping old tubes of steroid cream in the bathroom cabinet, and using these instead of the newly prescribed cream, is another frequent mistake. If the earlier prescription was for a weaker steroid cream, which is not quite up to the job, you won't get the symptoms under control.

Inadequate treatment means that the rash goes on longer, so you probably apply *more* steroid in the long run—which exposes you to a *greater* risk of local side effects. It is far better to use a moderately strong steroid cream for a short period of time and get the inflammation fully under control.

Remember that steroid creams, lotions, and ointments are absorbed far more effectively immediately after a bath or shower, so this is a good time to apply them (see p. 48).

Don't stop using steroid creams too soon. The skin looks healthy and happy long before it is completely healed underneath. You must continue until the "hidden healing" has occurred. As a rough guide, the point when the skin looks good is just the halfway point; so the steroid creams should be continued for the same length of time again. If it took 3 weeks to get to the point where the skin looks fine, then you should go on applying the steroid creams for another three weeks after that.

In general, it is a good idea to phase steroid creams out slowly. Stopping abruptly may cause the rash to flare up—this is called a **rebound effect**.

Once you have atopic eczema under good control, you will still need some steroid cream at home for dealing with relapses. As soon as you notice any rough, itchy skin, apply the cream twice daily for 3 days, then once daily for another 3 days. This should be enough to curb the outbreak of eczema before it really gets going.

Side effects

To assess the risk of side effects from your steroid cream, lotion, or ointment, you need to know how strong it is. Four categories are recognized:

- mild
- moderately potent
- potent
- very potent

Ask your doctor or pharmacist which category corresponds to your cream, so that you can make sense of the information given below.

Unfortunately, if steroid creams are not used correctly, there can be some quite serious local side effects. Any steroid cream that is strong enough to work is also strong enough to produce side effects if overused, so this is a delicate balancing act. The main local side effects are thinning of the skin and striae (stretch marks). Teenagers and pregnant women are particularly susceptible to stretch marks if using steroid creams.

It is important to take care, because these side effects can be irreversible. The stretch marks, for example, may fade in time but never entirely disappear. Sustained overuse of steroid creams can produce permanent thinning of the skin. Thinning of the skin on the face may produce redness, with small blood vessels showing through. The fingertips may develop painful cracks.

Note that these side effects can come on very gradually. Some may be mistaken for symptoms of the disease itself.

Other local side effects may include an outbreak of pimples that look somewhat like acne. Increased hairiness or change in skin color are also possible. Fortunately these effects are reversible.

To avoid side effects, always follow the instructions for using steroid creams carefully, and don't apply too much or too often. If you have not been given clear instructions by your doctor on the quantity to use, go back and ask for more information. Ideally, you should actually be shown the correct amount of the cream to use each time. Remember to wash your fingers after applying steroid creams.

If potent or very potent steroid creams are slapped on with abandon, enough is absorbed into the bloodstream to produce **systemic side effects**, comparable to those that can occur with steroid tablets (see p. 142).

With very potent steroid creams, used for a long period of time, there is some risk of slight systemic side effects, even though the instructions for use are carefully followed. Young children are more susceptible. Bear in mind that covering the skin with bandages after applying the cream increases the amount absorbed into the bloodstream. The degree of adrenal suppression caused by using the cream (see p. 142) is probably going to remain unnoticed in everyday life, but a major illness, accident, childbirth, or a surgical procedure might reveal the problem—so tell medical staff what you have been using.

Different areas of the body respond differently to steroid creams. The skin of the face, and within skin folds, is more sensitive and generally requires a lower-strength cream, while the palms of the hands and the soles of the feet require a higher strength. The genitals and the area around the anus are particularly sensitive and these can become *permanently* damaged (and then a source of intense discomfort) by strong steroid creams; some dermatologists recommend using nothing stronger than 1 percent hydrocortisone.

Make sure you see your doctor regularly when using steroid creams continuously, especially if
- you are using very potent steroid cream
- you are applying a potent or moderately potent steroid cream over more than 20 percent of your body for more than a month
- you are applying potent steroid cream to a baby or young child

The vehicle—the cream, lotion, or ointment base in which the steroid is carried—is important because sensitivity reactions can occur to certain of its ingredients (see p. 44). Eczema sufferers can even become sensitized to the steroid itself, and this problem is difficult to diagnose because patch tests with steroids often give false negatives (see p. 91). If you are not getting better, ask the doctor if this could be the explanation. (If a rash *gets worse and starts to spread* when you begin using steroid creams, go back and see the doctor very promptly—you may have an infection called *tinea*, or ringworm, that flourishes all the more when steroid creams are applied.)

Some common brand names

Common brand names of steroids include:

nasal sprays—Flonase, Nasacort, Nasonex, Rhinocort, Vancenase

eyedrops—Inflamase, FML, Maxidex, Pred Forte

inhalers—Azmacort, Aerobid, Beclovent, Flovent, Pulmicort, Vanceril

tablets—Aristocort, Decadron, Medrol

creams, lotions, and ointments—Celestoderm, Cortate, Cyclocort, Diprolene, Diprosone, Halog, Kenalog, Lidex, Tridesilon, Topicort, Ultrarate, Valisone, Westcort

Other anti-allergy drugs

An allergic reaction is a lengthy, complex process, and the various anti-allergy drugs all work on different stages of that process. That is why it often makes sense to use several different drugs for the same allergic condition: they each tackle the problem in their own way.

Steroids (see p. 140) intervene at a very late stage, quelling the inflammation that follows on from an allergic reaction. Using a steroid is somewhat like calling the fire department to put out a fire, whereas using an antihistamine (see p. 138) is like having fireproof doors, to prevent the fire from spreading at an early stage.

Cromoglycate-type drugs (see below) intervene at an even earlier stage. They are like basic fire prevention—teaching children not to play with matches.

Anti-leukotriene drugs (see p. 149) work at roughly the same stage of the process as antihistamines but tackle a different aspect of the allergic reaction.

Cromoglycate-type drugs

These drugs are also referred to as mast-cell stabilizers or mast-cell blockers.

There are three drugs in this group, sodium cromoglycate (also known as cromolyn sodium or cromolyn), nedocromil sodium (Alocril, Tilade), and lodoxamide (Alomide). All operate at an early stage of the allergic reaction, stopping it before it actually starts. They stabilize the outer membrane of the mast cells (see box on p. 12), which then prevents the allergic response from occurring.

This is a far more satisfactory way of dealing with an allergic reaction than trying to tackle it after the reaction has occurred. But from a purely practical point of view, it has a drawback. In order to work at all, these drugs must reach the mast cells *in advance* of the allergen. They are of very little use if taken after the allergic reaction has begun.

For people who are taking cromoglycate-type drugs on a regular schedule, several times a day, it is very important to be conscientious about taking them on time.

If you are using these drugs on an "as-needed" basis, you should take them 30 minutes before an allergen is encountered, or 30 minutes before a bout of exercise if they are being prescribed for exercise-induced asthma. (Note that children sometimes respond differently, getting protection from these drugs immediately.)

The effect of these drugs takes time to build up. You should take them regularly for at least four weeks before deciding whether they are helping you or not.

One point in favor of cromoglycate-type drugs is that they are extremely safe, with few or no side effects in most people. Sadly, they do not work for everyone. A fairly high percentage of children

Some common brand names

Common brand names of cromoglycate-type drugs include:

inhalers—Intal, Tilade

eyedrops—Alocrile, Alomide, Opticrom

nose sprays—Nasalcrom (U.S. only); Cromolyn Nasal Solution (Canada only)

oral capsules—Gastrocrom (U.S. only); Nalcrom (Canada only) respond well to them, but the response rate is much lower for adults. Nevertheless, adult allergy sufferers, especially those who need steroids to control their symptoms, should always be given the opportunity to try out these drugs. When cromoglycate-type drugs do work, they are very effective and almost always trouble-free, so they are a good alternative to steroids.

Both sodium cromoglycate and nedocromil sodium are available in inhaler form for asthma (see p. 157). Sodium cromoglycate is also available as nose sprays for hay fever and other nasal allergies.

All three drugs are available as eyedrops. Recent evidence suggests that sodium cromoglycate eyedrops are less effective than the other two, particularly for the treatment of severe allergic conjunctivitis.

Sodium cromoglycate is available in capsule form for food allergy. Note that these capsules are of very limited value in food allergy, and are certainly not a substitute for food avoidance. They do reduce sensitivity a little and can sometimes be helpful for those with multiple food allergies (see p. 67).

Side effects of these drugs

There are no serious side effects at all for nedocromil sodium. Cromoglycate can, very rarely, cause joint pain and swelling. An allergic reaction to the drug itself is even more uncommon. Stop taking the drug and see your doctor promptly if either of these occur.

The only other side effects that have occasionally been reported are headache, nausea, and vomiting. None of these indicate any damaging effect by the drugs—they are all minor side effects.

Eyedrops containing these drugs may cause stinging and burning when inserted, but this is a minor side effect and usually wears off. Flushing and dizziness have sometimes been reported with lodoxamide eyedrops.

Nose sprays may also cause local irritation. This could be due to the drug itself, in which case it is a minor side effect. Alternatively, the irritation may be due to the preservative used or some other nondrug ingredient (see box on p. 33).

Occasionally cromoglycate nasal sprays cause bronchospasm—contraction of the airway muscles—but this tends to wear off quite quickly. Bronchospasm can also occur when cromoglycate-type drugs are inhaled (see p. 157).

Anti-leukotriene drugs

These drugs, which have a set of very specific effects (see p. 159), were originally designed to treat asthma. Their potential for treating other allergic diseases is currently being explored:

• Several studies show that they work well for **perennial allergic rhinitis**. In one trial involving people allergic to cats, taking an anti-leukotriene drug for a week reduced the symptoms brought on by cat allergen.

• They are especially useful for both rhinitis and asthma in patients suffering from the condition known as **aspirin-sensitive triad** (see box on p. 28). Research shows that they also reduce asthmatic reactions to very small test doses of aspirin, but they don't give protection against anaphylaxis brought on by normal doses.

• They have also been used successfully in cases of **chronic urticaria** and for some patients with **delayed-pressure urticaria.** It seems plausible that they would also be helpful for chronic urticaria linked to aspirin sensitivity.

• Preliminary trials suggest that zileuton (Zyflo) could be useful in **atopic eczema.** This anti-leukotriene drug helps to keep eosinophils (see p. 19) away, which may explain its beneficial effects. Eosinophils show up in the skin once eczema is well established and help keep the inflammation going. Zileuton is available in the U. S., but is not yet available in Canada.

For side effects of these drugs, see pp. 159–61.

More powerful anti-allergy drugs

Occasionally people with severe allergies, who are on constant high doses of steroid tablets or who fail to respond to steroids, need treatment with powerful anti-inflammatory drugs, such as methotrexate or cyclosporine. These drugs suppress the immune system and extremely careful monitoring for side effects is needed. Various new anti-allergy drugs may soon become available. One of these, omalizumab (Xolair) blocks allergic reactions by binding to IgE (see box on p. 12) and inactivating it.

Epinephrine

Anyone who has suffered anaphylactic shock (see p. 58) should be carrying a special syringe, called an auto-injector, loaded with epinephrine. The injector is very simple to operate and is designed for emergencies. Most allergy sufferers, even children, can give themselves the injection—or a parent or other adult can give it.

In the U.S., some asthmatics, and those with food allergy who suffer swelling of the throat, may be given epinephrine in inhaler form as well. This can be useful as an additional treatment, but it's definitely not a substitute for an injector. Inhaled epinephrine is not available in Canada.

Detailed instructions for using epinephrine in a crisis are given on pp. 98–9.

Wherever you go, take your injector with you. Always keep it close at hand: you need to be able to use it within minutes of the onset of the allergic reaction. You may be unable to speak (and therefore unable to ask someone else to fetch it) quite soon after the attack begins. The injector can be damaged by sunlight, excess heat, and freezing so don't leave it in a parked car.

If you are going camping or hiking somewhere remote, ask your doctor for a second injector or one that can deliver multiple injections. Also ask about the maximum number of injections that can be given, and never exceed this total.

It is vital that you be shown exactly how to use the auto-injector. In one Canadian study researchers discovered that only one out of four health professionals got the technique entirely correct when demonstrating how to use an auto-injector. In this study, pharmacists

Detailed instructions for using epinephrine in a crisis are given on pp. 98–9.

Some common brand names

Common brand names of epinephrine preparations include:

auto-injectors—EpiPen, EpiPen Jr

inhalers—Bronkaid, Vaponefrin, Primatene

were clearly the best bet as regards accurate instructions. Practice injectors are useful for training purposes, and they are available in most pharmacies.

When the epinephrine auto-injectors expire, they can be useful for practicing with, or for showing a new babysitter or teacher—practice on an orange or grapefruit.

Side effects of this drug

The important side effects of epinephrine involve the heart. Anyone with a heart condition should be given special advice by their doctor about using epinephrine. The same goes for people with diabetes, hyperthyroidism, or high blood pressure, and for anyone taking tricyclic antidepressants. Bear in mind that if you are taking beta-blockers for a heart condition, epinephrine may not have much effect. The crucial thing here is to talk to your doctor *in advance* of an emergency, if you have not already been given appropriate advice.

There are quite a few minor side effects from epinephrine, such as anxiety, trembling, nausea, sweating, dizziness, and cold hands and feet. These will soon wear off.

Drugs that can make you worse

Aspirin and its relatives have a very bad effect on some people with rhinitis and/or asthma (see box on p.151). Unfortunately, recent research shows that acetaminophen is not safe either. It makes asthma more likely to develop in those who do not yet have the disease, and increases the severity of asthma symptoms for those who do. Unlike aspirin, acetaminophen affects everyone, because it lowers the levels of a natural antioxidant, called glutathione, which the body makes to protect the lungs from oxidants. The greatest effects are seen in people who take acetaminophen regularly (once a week or more), but even an occasional dose makes some difference.

All the other drugs that can make you worse are prescription drugs, and your doctor should be alert to the dangers. But doctors are overworked and sometimes forget, so it is sensible to know about the risks for yourself. If you have any doubt about the drugs you are taking, ask a pharmacist.

Beta-blockers are a major hazard for people with allergies. They can make the airways contract and can bring on a serious asthma attack. They also make anaphylaxis more likely in someone who already has allergic reactions (see p. 59), and they increase the risk of a severe reaction to allergy

shots (see p. 166) or skin tests (see p. 91). Beta-blockers are prescribed for high blood pressure, angina, other heart problems, migraine, and thyroid disease. There are alternative drugs in all cases. Asthma sometimes develops in people who have been taking beta-blockers for years. Although the beta-blockers are not responsible for this, once asthma has begun, they will make symptoms worse. Eyedrops for glaucoma may also contain beta-blockers, and can have a bad effect on asthmatics.

ACE inhibitors, used for heart conditions, may cause a cough and swelling that could result in airway narrowing. They may also increase the risk of a severe reaction to immunotherapy.

Female hormones affect asthmatics, so taking the **contraceptive pill** or **hormone replacement therapy** (HRT) may make asthma worse. Progesterone-only contraceptive pills tend to cause fewer problems.

The drug **isoniazid** (INH), prescribed for tuberculosis, makes the body far more susceptible to histamine in foods (see p. 200.)

An allergic reaction to a specific drug (for example, penicillin) can also occur in some people, resulting in urticaria, or even anaphylactic shock.

Aspirin sensitivity

Aspirin sensitivity is not an allergic reaction. What causes this problem is a metabolic abnormality—a malfunction in one aspect of the body's chemistry. The details of this are very complicated: you may simply want to read about how to cope with the problem.

The exact nature of aspirin sensitivity is still far from clear, but it seems to involve a relatively poor production of **prostaglandins**, combined with a plentiful production of **leukotrienes**. Both these substances are **messenger chemicals** which, broadly speaking, promote inflammation. But the details of their pro-inflammatory activities differ. It seems that, ideally, the body should have a harmonious balance between the two, and an imbalance produces problems.

Both prostaglandins and leukotrienes are manufactured from certain fats that are found in the diet. These fats are the raw materials and worked on initially by two different **enzymes**—one that leads to the production of prostaglandins and another that leads to the production of leukotrienes.

If one of these enzymes is defective, it may mean that the other is oversupplied with raw materials, resulting in a serious imbalance between prostaglandins and leukotrienes. In people with aspirin sensitivity, or at risk of developing aspirin sensitivity, the enzyme that produces prostaglandins seems to be defective.

Even in the absence of aspirin, this imbalance between prostaglandins and leukotrienes causes problems. It leads to symptoms such as chronic urticaria (see p. 52) or rhinitis, nasal polyps, and asthma (a cluster of symptoms that is commonly called **aspirin-sensitive triad**—see box on p. 28).

Taking aspirin can make the imbalance between prostaglandins and leukotrienes even worse in a person with this underlying abnormality. Aspirin exerts its painkilling effects by disabling the main prostaglandin-making enzyme—the enzyme that is already defective.

When someone with aspirin sensitivity takes aspirin, they may suffer worsening asthma, a severe asthma attack, or—the worst-case scenario—collapse. This is a potentially fatal reaction similar to anaphylaxis (see p. 101).

The greatest puzzle about aspirin sensitivity is why it often takes so long to develop in someone who already has the symptoms of aspirin-sensitive triad—indicating the basic metabolic abnormality. It may be as much as 20 years from when someone has their first symptoms (for example, nasal polyps) to when they begin reacting badly to aspirin.

If you have triad symptoms already, but no aspirin sensitivity yet, what should you do? Unfortunately, there are no safe tests for aspirin sensitivity at present—taking a small dose of aspirin and seeing what happens is very hazardous. It is probably best to assume that you are going to become sensitive to aspirin at some stage and avoid all aspirin and aspirin-like drugs. Caution is the best plan here, because aspirin sensitivity can come on very suddenly and be life-threatening the first time it occurs. Note that some aspirin-sensitive triad sufferers have polyps and rhinitis but no asthma until they actually develop aspirin sensitivity—a dose of aspirin suddenly brings on their first asthma attack plus other symptoms of aspirin sensitivity.

Avoiding aspirin itself is not difficult, but aspirin-like drugs pose more of a problem. Every year there are a number of deaths from these drugs. Some of these cases occur because a busy doctor momentarily forgets that a patient should not take these drugs. The drugs that must be avoided are all known as **nonsteroidal anti-inflammatory drugs** (NSAIDs) or **COX-1** and **COX-2 inhibitors**. However you will not see either of these names on the packet. These drugs are very widely used for pain relief (for example, in backache and headache remedies such as Advil), for the treatment of arthritis, and for several other inflammatory diseases.

There are dozens of nonsteroidal anti-inflammatory drugs available, and many are sold under several different brand names. The list grows every year, as new drugs or new brands are launched. The only way to avoid these drugs is to be very cautious:

• When buying any cold- or flu-remedies, painkillers, medicines (including those you apply directly to the skin) for sprains or sports injuries, headache tablets, or migraine tablets, always buy them at a pharmacy, rather than a supermarket, and check with the pharmacist that they do not contain aspirin or aspirin-like drugs.

• Be cautious also about remedies for an upset stomach. A few (for example, Alka-Seltzer and Pepto Bismol) have aspirin-like ingredients.

• Don't take any drugs unless you are 100 percent sure of what they contain. Remember that the ingredients of a familiar brand name can sometimes change—read the label every time.

• When a doctor prescribes any new drug, always mention that you are sensitive to aspirin or that you have nasal polyps. Alternatively, check with the pharmacist when the prescription is filled.

• Aspirin-free painkillers almost always contain acetaminophen, a drug that can cause a severe reaction (similar to the collapse induced by aspirin itself) in about 5% of people with aspirin sensitivity. If you are taking acetaminophen for the first time, start with half a tablet. Be sure that, for the next two to three hours, you have a way of getting to hospital quickly should you start to feel ill. (Note that acetaminophen has an entirely separate effect, increasing the severity of asthma, and it is best not to take it too often—see box on p. 150)

Avoiding all aspirin-like drugs will prevent you from having anaphylaxis or severe attacks of asthma. Unfortunately, symptoms such as asthma and nasal polyps will not go away, however careful you are about avoiding aspirin.

It is well worth trying the new anti-leukotriene drugs (see p. 149), especially if you have aspirin-induced asthma. They seem to help by curtailing the activities of leukotrienes and so redressing the balance between leukotrienes and prostaglandins.

Drugs for asthma

The drug treatment of asthma is far more complex than for any other allergic disease. Drugs prescribed for asthma fall into two basic categories: those that open up the airways by relaxing the airway muscles, called **relievers**, and those that treat the inflammation in the lining of the airways, called **preventers**. The former offer a "quick fix"—like taking an aspirin when you have a headache. Just as the actual cause of the headache is not treated by an aspirin, so the actual cause of the asthma attack is not addressed by relievers. Preventers, on the other hand, tackle the basic problem—the inflammation that triggers the contraction of the airway muscles (see p. 36).

In the past 10 years, there has been a quiet revolution in asthma treatment, with far more people being given preventer inhalers, usually low-dose steroids. The aim is to get the airways in better condition, with the inflammation thoroughly damped down, so that the airway muscles don't go into spasm. The ultimate objective is to make people less reliant on reliever inhalers, because the potential hazards of overusing them are now realized.

The details of modern asthma management and the different approaches used are described on p. 160, following the discussion of the main types of drug used for asthma treatment.

Beta-2 relievers (beta-agonists)

Our airways open up when we produce epinephrine (better known to many people as adrenaline). Generating epinephrine is the body's natural response to feeling angry or frightened. The epinephrine widens the airways so that we can run faster or fight more vigorously.

Epinephrine, given as a drug, was among the earliest treatments for asthma. However, it also stimulates the heart to beat faster and raises the blood pressure. While it is useful for emergency treatment (see p. 150), the side effects make it too hazardous for routine use.

The beta-2 relievers work by mimicking epinephrine—they bind to the same receptors in the airways, the beta-2 receptors. Binding to these receptors stimulates the airway muscles to relax, so that the airways open up.

In other respects, the beta-2 relievers are *not* like epinephrine. Clever chemical manipulation has made them sufficiently different from epinephrine to have little effect on the heart and other organs when taken at normal doses.

Beta-2 relievers are best taken by inhalation. Although tablets and syrup are available, these are far more likely to bring on side effects, because the dose needed, in order to ensure that enough reaches the airways, is so much bigger. Inhaled beta-2 relievers target the drug on the airways so the dose can be smaller. They also have the advantage of taking effect soon after being inhaled and of giving full relief within 10–15 minutes.

There are two different kinds of beta-2 relievers:

- the traditional **short-acting beta-2 relievers**, whose effects last for 3–6 hours (usually about 4). The modern consensus is that these should be used only when needed, not taken routinely.
- the newer **long-acting beta-2 relievers**, which last up to 12 hours. These drugs are prescribed for more severe forms of asthma (see p. 154) and are generally used routinely, twice a day.

A key question for asthma sufferers is: How often can short-acting beta-2 relievers be used? Ideas about this have changed considerably over the last 20 years, and no doctor would now want to have patients using a Ventolin inhaler five, six, or more times a day—something that was quite common in the past. This level of need for beta-2 relievers indicates that the asthma is poorly controlled and requires treatment with a preventer, to quell the inflammation in the airways.

Detailed policy on beta-2 relievers still varies from one part of the world to another. Canadian guidelines state that if a short-acting beta-2 reliever is needed more than three times a week for symptom relief, a preventer should also be prescribed. U.S. guidelines recommend that a preventer be added if reliever medications are needed more than twice a week for symptom relief. In both cases, the use of a beta-2 reliever once a day, before exercise, is allowed in addition to this.

How safe are these drugs in the long term?

The cause of the big rethink on beta-2 relievers was an epidemic of asthma-related deaths in New Zealand between 1976 and 1988. The death rate from severe asthma attacks was 2–4 times its previous level for a while, and more than a thousand New Zealanders died in the epidemic.

There has been a huge controversy over what exactly caused these deaths. Most researchers now agree that the main cause was a new brand of inhaler which delivered a double dose of the drug fenoterol, a short-acting beta-2 reliever with a very powerful effect on the airways and quite high levels of side effects involving the heart. The same brand of inhaler may have been linked to increased death rates in Canada and Germany.

Research suggests that the problem was greatest in New Zealand because sales of the new inhaler were highest there and because many patients got their inhalers through repeat prescriptions. As a result, people whose asthma was deteriorating badly were not seen by a doctor and were using large amounts of beta-2 reliever, rather than taking preventer drugs. This is now believed to be a major cause of asthma deaths. There are three separate factors involved:

- The beta-2 reliever covers up the effects of the severe inflammation of the airways. People feel reasonably well, because the reliever is opening up their airways, and don't realize just how bad their asthma really is. The untreated inflammation in the airways can eventually lead to a serious, and potentially fatal, asthma attack.
- The short-acting beta-2 reliever, used regularly, makes the airways more sensitive to exercise and to allergens such as dust mite and pollen. This means that an asthmatic who is already allergic to these allergens reacts to them at much lower levels in the air.
- The airways become less and less responsive to the beta-2 reliever itself, so that when a serious attack occurs, requiring hospital treatment, huge doses of beta-2 reliever are needed to open up the airways. These massive doses carry a risk of serious side effects involving the heart.

The details of the New Zealand epidemic still evoke controversy. Was fenoterol itself, which is stronger than other beta-2 relievers, the cause of the deaths? Or was it just that the inhaler delivered a double dose—would any short-acting beta-2 reliever be dangerous at twice the normal dose? Or was it overuse of all beta-2 relievers and lack of preventer drugs?

Some common brand names

Common brand names include:

short-acting beta-2 relievers in inhalers—Ventolin; Maxair, Proventil (U.S. only); Berotec, Bricanyl (Canada only)

short-acting beta-2 relievers in tablets—Bricanyl, Novo-Salmol (Canada only)

short-acting beta-2 relievers in syrup—Ventolin

long-acting beta-2 relievers in inhalers—Serevent; Foradil, Oxeze (Canada only)

Until this is resolved, safety-conscious asthmatics may want to assume that any of these possibilities could be correct. An ultracautious approach would include:

- Avoiding fenoterol if possible. (Fenoterol is not available in the U.S. In Canada it is sold under the brand name Berotec.)
- Not routinely taking two puffs of a single-dose inhaler (check with your doctor if you have been told to take two puffs).
- Using any short-acting beta-2 reliever only "as needed"—which should be two doses or less per week according to U.S. guidelines, and three doses or less per week according to Canadian guidelines (not counting once-a-day doses before exercise). Note that with this level of use, there is absolutely no risk from these drugs; it is only regular overuse that is damaging and dangerous.
- Using a peak flow meter and ensuring that you are assessed regularly by your doctor.
- Always taking your preventer medication as prescribed.

Since about 1990, the death rate from asthma has been falling, particularly in countries with a policy of reducing use of beta-2 relievers, and increasing inhaled steroids. The death rate in New Zealand is now the lowest it has been for 50 years, and at the same level as in other Western countries.

Unnecessary alarm

While investigating the causes of the New Zealand epidemic, medical researchers discovered that patients inhaling a short-acting beta-2 reliever four times a day had more irritable airways after just two weeks. Their airways were also less responsive to the drug, even after this brief period of use.

Some researchers began to ask if the asthma epidemic itself—the increasing number of cases of asthma—*could actually be due to these drugs*. Maybe children with mild wheezing, which might have cleared up if left untreated (and which would have gone untreated in the past), were becoming full-blown asthmatics *because* they were now using beta-2 inhalers?

Many doctors and researchers became very concerned about these questions, and a leading medical journal *The Lancet* published an article with the provocative title *"Worldwide worsening wheezing—is the cure the cause?"* That was in 1992. Since then, much more research has been done, and it is clear that this particular fear about beta-2 relievers was unfounded.

Unfortunately, there are a few books and other publications around that are spreading unnecessary alarm about these drugs by reporting the debate as it was in 1992. They have taken up that question "*Is the cure the cause?*", assumed that the answer is "yes," and ignored all the subsequent research, which shows the opposite.

Beta-2 relievers in severe asthma

A few patients with severe asthma remain breathless and wheezy, even though they are inhaling moderate doses of a steroid preventer every day. Increasing the dose of inhaled steroids does not make a huge difference to their symptoms, and it substantially raises the risk of steroid side effects.

Taking a **long-acting beta-2 reliever** frequently works wonders for such patients. These relatively new drugs relax the airway muscles and go on working for 12 hours or more.

There has obviously been concern about long-acting beta-2 relievers having the same kind of insidious side effects as their short-acting counterparts (see p. 153), and so increasing the likelihood of deaths from asthma. However, studies of people taking these drugs suggest that the risks are minimal.

Other studies show that the chemical differences of the long-acting drugs, as well as prolonging their effects, also give them a more complex set of actions in the body. For example, they improve the effect of steroids in calming inflammation and may even have some small anti-inflammatory effect of their own.

Doctors believe that, for patients with troublesome asthma, the benefits of long-acting beta-2 relievers greatly outweigh the risks. But they should be used only in combination with inhaled steroids. Inhalers that contain both a steroid and a long-acting beta-2 reliever have been introduced in Canada (Advair is an example); they are not currently available in the U.S. Various other options, such as allergen avoidance and the new anti-leukotriene drugs (see p. 159), should probably be investigated as well.

If you are taking long-acting beta-2 relievers, use them regularly, once every 12 hours—the good effect gradually builds up with consistent use.

Generally speaking, you should not take additional doses in between. Long-acting beta-2 relievers are not intended for use if you have a sudden asthma attack—your doctor will prescribe a short-acting beta-2 reliever for this. This limitation on the use of long-acting beta-2 relievers is certainly appropriate for salmeterol (which was the first of the long-acting beta-2 relievers to be developed) because it is very slow to take effect on the airways. However, one of the newer long-acting beta-2 relievers, called formoterol (available in Canada, but not yet in the U.S.), begins to work just as quickly as a short-acting beta-2 reliever. Formoterol could, in theory, be used on an "as-required" basis to combat asthma attacks. You may want to discuss this possibility with your doctor.

Finally, don't stop taking your preventer drug (inhaled steroid or cromoglycate), even if you feel a lot better. Long-acting beta-2 relievers are *not* a substitute for preventers.

Some patients with very severe asthma need to take regular doses of short-acting beta-2 relievers *as well as* long-acting beta-2 relievers. You should obviously follow the advice of your asthma specialist closely if you are on this kind of drug regime, and not change anything without medical approval. However, it might be worth discussing other options, such as anti-leukotriene drugs. In addition, take every opportunity to reduce your asthma symptoms in other ways—by reducing allergen exposure, avoiding asthma triggers (see p. 39), and other self-help measures (see p. 41).

Immediate side effects of beta-2 relievers

Minor immediate side effects of these drugs include headache, nervousness, trembling, restlessness, flushing, dry mouth, anxiety, and muscle cramps. Children may become more excitable. These side effects—all of which are due to the resemblance of beta-2 relievers to epinephrine—usually wear off quite quickly. Some long-acting beta-2 relievers may cause nausea and vomiting.

A pounding heart is usually a relatively minor side effect, but it can be more serious, and should be reported to your doctor.

A few asthmatics find that their airways narrow when these drugs are inhaled, rather than opening. This is called **paradoxical bronchoconstriction**. If this happens, stop using the inhaler and see your doctor as soon as you can.

Even more rarely, asthmatics can develop allergic reactions to the drugs or suffer hallucinations or seizures. Obviously you should stop using the inhaler immediately if you experience side effects of this kind and should see your doctor.

There can be an interaction between beta-2 relievers and other drugs or medical conditions. Should you need a diuretic, tell the doctor or pharmacist that you are also taking a beta-2 reliever, and ask which types of diuretic are safe. If you have high blood pressure, a heart problem, or a thyroid condition, make sure the doctor remembers this when prescribing beta-2 relievers.

Asthma alert

If you ever find that your short-acting beta-2 reliever has no effect within 10 minutes, or is needed more than once every four hours, this indicates a serious asthma attack, and you need urgent medical help (see p. 100).

During a severe asthma attack, while getting to the hospital or waiting for a doctor to arrive, up to 30 puffs of a short-acting beta-2 reliever should be taken as an emergency treatment, to get the airways open. *There is a risk of death if you don't use the reliever fully in this situation.* (This emergency dose is safe for almost everyone, but there may be risks if you have a heart condition—get detailed advice from your doctor in advance.)

Ephedrine

Ephedrine and orciprenaline belong to the previous generation of reliever drugs. They are chemically very similar to epinephrine and therefore cause a lot of side effects, especially involving the heart.

These drugs are no longer recommended and will likely be phased out completely. Some older asthmatics may still be using them, just because they have been on them for years and no one has reviewed their treatment.

If you are taking such drugs, ask your doctor about switching to a newer form of reliever—it will be more effective as well as having fewer side effects.

Anticholinergics

These drugs, also known as anti-muscarinics, are relievers. However, they work in a completely different way from the beta-2 relievers. They block the action of the **parasympathetic nervous system**, a set of nerves which is the biological equivalent of autopilot—working without the intervention of conscious thought. The parasympathetic nervous system has many effects on the body, including keeping the airway muscles nicely toned (see box on p. 235). By blocking the parasympathetic, anticholinergics help the airway muscles to relax.

The only anticholinergic used for asthma treatment in North America is sold under the brand name Atrovent. It is taken by inhalation, generally requires 1 to 2 hours to reach its maximum effect and lasts for 8 hours.

For most asthmatics, especially those with a strong allergic component to their asthma, anticholinergics are generally less effective than beta-2 relievers. But they are useful to children under one year, who may not respond to beta-2 relievers. They

also have a role where asthma is combined with chronic bronchitis—here the anticholinergics can sometimes be more effective than beta-2 relievers—and they are particularly useful for asthma with a lot of mucus, because blocking the parasympathetic tends to reduce mucus production. For severe asthmatics, anticholinergics may be combined with beta-2 relievers.

Anticholinergics should be taken only when needed, not regularly several times a day. If used regularly, they can make the airways more sensitive, just as short-acting beta-2 relievers can (see p. 153).

Side effects

Minor and immediate side effects of anticholinergics may include a dry mouth, blurred vision, constipation, and irritation of the mouth and throat. A few people suffer nausea or difficulty in passing urine.

Serious side effects are rare. Any increase in the stickiness of the sputum coughed up may be a cause for concern, especially in children. If there is an increase in wheezing or coughing, stop taking the drug.

If you already have glaucoma or prostate problems, you should be monitored carefully by your doctor, as these conditions can get worse with anticholinergic drugs.

When anticholinergics are used in a nebulizer, it is vital that the mask fits well (see p. 163).

Anticholinergics for the nose

Another use for anticholinergics is in nasal sprays, for the treatment of vasomotor rhinitis, a nonallergic condition that is frequently mistaken for allergic rhinitis (see p. 29). In this disorder, the constant flow of mucus is caused by a malfunction of the parasympathetic nervous system, which is why anticholinergics work well.

Steroid inhalers

Most asthmatics nowadays are given a steroid inhaler at some point, as part of their asthma treatment (see p. 160). It will probably be a low-dose inhaler, and the risks of side effects from this are very small. Even at higher doses, inhaled steroids are relatively safe. Many people are unnecessarily afraid of inhaled steroids and refuse to use them until their asthma becomes really incapacitating. It is important not to delay using an inhaled steroid for too long, as this could cause permanent damage to the airways: inflammation eventually thickens the airway wall, leaving it less flexible and therefore less capable of widening.

For side effects of inhaled steroids, see p. 145; and for common brand names, see p. 147.

Steroid tablets

These are usually a treatment of last resort. But if your asthma is badly out of control, they can, quite literally, be a lifesaver. On the other hand, if there are any other means by which you can tackle your asthma, so that you do not need steroid tablets again in the future—avoiding allergens and irritants, for example, or using other preventer treatments—those means should be taken.

For side effects of steroid tablets, see pp. 141–3; and for common brand names, see p. 147.

Cromoglycate-type drugs

For asthma, these drugs are taken by inhalation only. They work by blocking the allergic reaction (see p. 148), and are therefore a type of preventer drug.

Cromoglycate-type drugs are usually inhaled four times a day, although your doctor may recommend more frequent inhalations to begin with. Once your asthma is well controlled, you may be able to reduce the dosing regime to three times a day, or possibly twice a day: ask your doctor's advice about this.

Should you decide to stop taking these drugs at some point, talk to your doctor first. It is generally best to reduce the dose gradually, over a period of 7–10 days. Some asthmatics need to introduce (or reintroduce) steroids at this time, to maintain control of the airway inflammation.

Side effects of these drugs

When inhaled, cromoglycate-type drugs can produce short-lived irritation in the throat, which may lead to coughing. This sometimes develops into temporary bronchospasm, causing you to wheeze, but this is really only a minor side effect—it does not indicate that the drug is making your asthma worse.

Asthmatics are sometimes advised to use a short-acting beta-2 reliever (such as Ventolin) before their cromoglycate inhaler, to overcome this problem. However, this would involve using the beta-2 reliever four times a day, which is no longer considered a good idea (see pp. 153–4). Talk to your doctor again if you have been given this advice.

A better way around the problem of throat irritation may be to switch to an aerosol inhaler, because the irritation is much less than with dry-powder inhalers. Using a spacer along with the aerosol inhaler (see p. 162) will help even more.

Serious side effects of these drugs are very rare (see p. 149). For common brand names, see p. 148.

Theophylline

Theophylline-type drugs are also known as **xanthines** or methyl-xanthines. These drugs are chemically similar to caffeine. They cannot be inhaled, so are taken as tablets or syrup. They start working about 30 minutes after being taken and their effects last for 6–8 hours. Slow-release preparations take 90 minutes to start working, but they last 12–24 hours and are therefore useful for nocturnal asthma.

In North America, doctors generally regard these theophylline-type drugs as reliever drugs (see p. 152), but rather risky ones whose use is justified only for people with severe asthma. They are given, as an additional treatment, to asthmatics who are not responding well to the usual drug program (see p. 160). Unfortunately, fairly high doses are needed for theophylline-type drugs to act as relievers, reversing bronchospasm. There is a very narrow margin between such a dose and one that causes major (and sometimes dangerous) side effects.

Such side effects usually occur while the doctor is still trying to work out the correct dose—this varies from one person to another, so prescribing theophylline-type drugs is no easy matter. Once you are established on a safe dose (and provided your general health and your intake of alcohol, nicotine, and medicinal drugs does not vary—see p. 158), you can usually continue taking theophylline without serious side effects.

In the United States, theophylline-type drugs, at much lower doses, may sometimes be given to people with mild asthma. At these low doses they do not act as relievers, but they have a slight anti-inflammatory effect and therefore act as preventers. The risk of toxicity is much less. Taking low doses of theophylline allows people with mild asthma to reduce their use of beta-2 relievers. However, inhaled steroids are usually more effective in this role, and are the preferred treatment.

Side effects of these drugs

Typical side effects of theophylline-type drugs include nausea, vomiting, stomach pains, diarrhea (sometimes with blood), headache, anxiety, restlessness, insomnia, dizziness, pounding heart, or irregular heartbeat.

Any side effect of these drugs should be taken seriously and reported to your doctor as soon as possible. If you cannot get an appointment quickly, it may be best to stop taking the drug before seeing the doctor, so long as you have other drugs to control your asthma. Call your doctor for advice.

It is remarkably easy to overdose when taking these drugs at higher doses (see p. 157). Such overdoses can be fatal. The symptoms include repeated vomiting, shaking, feeling unusually hot, needing to urinate frequently, severe thirst, maniacal behavior, and irregular heartbeat (palpitations). Delirium and convulsions may occur shortly afterward, so get hospital treatment *urgently* if you have any of these symptoms.

Unfortunately, a serious overdose can sometimes occur in people who have taken theophylline-type drugs without trouble for many years. There may be no advance warning that anything is wrong—no mild side effects preceding the serious ones. To protect yourself against this, you need regular blood tests from your doctor.

One fundamental problem with theophylline-type drugs is that many different factors—including diet, illnesses other than asthma, and taking other drugs—can alter the way your body deals with the drug. If your liver is breaking the drug down more slowly than usual, the amount in your blood will rapidly increase and can reach toxic levels.

These are steps that can help prevent an overdose with theophylline-type drugs:

- If you start taking a new drug of any kind, or stop taking a drug (especially the contraceptive pill), or if you change your intake of nicotine or alcohol, ask your doctor—*preferably in advance*—if your dose of theophylline-type drug needs changing.
- Many drugs interact with theophylline-type drugs, including the new anti-leukotriene drugs. You should always be cautious with any drug, but take particular care with two antibiotics—ciprofloxacin (Cipro) and erythromycin (various brand names)—and with cimetidine (various brand names), used to treat stomach ulcers and heartburn.
- If you have flu vaccinations, or develop certain illnesses, especially viral infections, heart disease, or liver disease, watch for the typical side effects of theophylline-type drugs (see above) and consult your doctor immediately if any occur. These conditions all change the effects of theophylline-type drugs.

- Don't eat meals that are very high in fats or oils at the same time as taking theophylline. A lot of fatty food causes too much of the drug to be released at once from the slow-release preparations and increases the risk of side effects. Avoid sudden, major changes in your diet.
- See your doctor regularly for checkups. Simply getting older changes your reaction to these drugs; your dose may need to change over the years.
- If you are at all forgetful about tablets, keep a careful record of when you have taken your theophylline-type drugs. Be very careful never to take a second dose by mistake.
- Talk to your doctor if you are not taking a slow-release form of theophylline (see box below for brand names). There are usually fewer side effects from these than from the regular forms of the drug.
- Wear a MedicAlert bracelet (see box on p. 95) saying that you are taking theophylline-type drugs. If you have a severe asthma attack and are taken to the hospital, it is important that medical staff know this, so that they do not give you more drugs of this type.
- Neither you nor your pharmacist should switch to another manufacturers' slow-release form of theophylline without first discussing the change with your doctor.

While pregnant or breast-feeding, it may be advisable to stop taking theophylline-type drugs; discuss this with your doctor. Although the drugs do not affect most unborn or newborn babies, there are occasional reports of toxicity. Less seriously, theophylline-type drugs get into breast milk and may make babies irritable and restless. This problem can be solved by always taking the drug just after a feeding—this reduces the amount in the milk.

The theophylline-type drugs might produce behavioral problems and learning difficulties in young children although this is unproven. Research shows that there are no problems for children over six.

Some common brand names

Common brand names of theophylline-type drugs include:

slow-release preparations—Phyllocontin, Quibron T/SR, Slo-Bid, Theochron SR, Theo-Dur, Uniphyl

ordinary preparations—Choledyl, Theolair

Ketotifen

Ketotifen (Zaditen) for asthma treatment is currently available in Canada, but not in the U.S. It is an antihistamine (see p. 138), although it has other effects in addition to those of ordinary antihistamines. Most significantly, it stabilizes mast cells in a similar way to cromoglycate. One advantage of ketotifen for many people is that it is taken by mouth (in tablet or syrup form). When it was first introduced, doctors hoped that it would be of particular help in asthma, but it has not lived up to expectations. However, some asthmatics do find it effective. It is worth trying because, if it works, it could permit you to reduce your dose of steroids.

Ketotifen requires up to six weeks to take effect, so continue taking your previous drugs at the same dose for at least six weeks, or you will risk losing control of your asthma.

Side effects of this drug

Minor side effects from ketotifen include nausea, behavior change, headache, increased appetite and weight gain, drowsiness, dry mouth, and slight dizziness. Do not drive until you are sure that ketotifen does not make you drowsy. Alcohol may pack a more powerful punch than usual, so drink very moderately at first. If drowsiness is a problem, take the drug in the late evening. The sleepy feeling may wear off after a few weeks of taking the drug.

There are no serious side effects from ketotifen, except if taken with drugs for diabetes.

Anti-leukotriene drugs

Leukotrienes are among the messenger chemicals produced by mast cells during an allergic reaction (see box on p. 12). They help to perpetuate the inflammatory process begun by histamine, and they amplify the reaction by attracting more immune cells into the area.

The anti-leukotriene drugs fall into two distinct groups:
- those that bind to the receptors for leukotrienes, called leukotriene-receptor-antagonists. Currently, there are two drugs in this group, montelukast (Singulair) and zafirlukast (Accolate). A third drug, pranlukast, is in the pipeline and currently going through its safety trials.
- those that block the production of the leukotrienes altogether, called 5-lipoxygenase inhibitors. There is only one drug in this group at present, zileuton (Zyflo). It is available in the U.S., but not in Canada.

As regards tackling inflammation, the anti-leukotriene drugs work in a completely different way from either steroids or cromoglycate. This makes them useful as an add-on treatment, supplementing the effects of existing anti-allergy drugs. They can also be used alone, for the treatment of mild asthma.

For asthmatics, anti-leukotriene drugs may be particularly good in combination with antihistamines—whereas antihistamines alone are singularly unsuccessful in asthma (see p. 138). Recent research suggests that taking antihistamines together with anti-leukotriene drugs is an effective way to control airway inflammation. However, there have been no large-scale trials of this treatment option yet, and it may be a while before it comes into general use.

In the airways of people with asthma, leukotrienes can directly trigger bronchospasm (contraction of the airway muscles), as well as fostering inflammation and increasing mucus production. This multiple action of leukotrienes makes anti-leukotriene drugs very valuable for asthmatics because they act as both relievers (reversing bronchospasm) and preventers (tackling inflammation).

All the anti-leukotriene drugs are taken in tablet form. If you are trying an anti-leukotriene drug for the first time, don't expect any noticeable effects to occur for about three days. Once you are taking the drug regularly, each dose requires 2–4 hours to have its full effect, but goes on working for 12–24 hours in total.

Although anti-leukotriene drugs have a reliever effect, they cannot give you *immediate* relief from bronchospasm. Asthmatics must therefore also carry a short-acting beta-2 reliever (see pp. 152–3), in case of an asthma attack.

For those who dislike inhalers, the fact that these drugs are taken in tablet form makes them an attractive option.

Side effects of these drugs

The side effects noted in safety trials of these drugs were all minor ones:
- zafirlukast—headache, infection, nausea, diarrhea, pain
- montelukast—headache, diarrhea, abdominal pain, cough, and flulike symptoms
- zileuton—upset stomach

According to the data gathered so far, more serious side effects are unlikely. However, as with all new drugs, **you should report any unusual symptoms to your doctor**, just in case these represent a rare or long-term side effect of the drug (see p. 137).

Very occasionally montelukast causes anaphylaxis, or other allergic reactions, such as itchiness, hives (urticaria), or swelling (angioedema).

Zileuton can cause liver damage, but again this is very rare. Your liver function should be closely monitored by the doctor with regular blood tests, and the drug withdrawn at the first sign of trouble. You should not be given zileuton if you have liver disease.

The most worrying development noticed to date is the appearance, in a very few people taking zafirlukast or montelukast, of a disorder called Churg-Strauss syndrome. The symptoms may include a blotchy purplish rash (due to vasculitis—see second box on p. 73), a flulike illness, worsening asthma, and numbness or tingling in the limbs. The heart, lungs, and nerves are all affected, because eosinophils (see p. 19) are present in large numbers and cause damaging inflammation.

A study of the cases reported so far suggests that this syndrome may not be due to the anti-leukotriene drugs themselves but to other causes, most commonly a reduction in the dose of steroid tablets. Other patients who are not taking anti-leukotriene drugs, but are reducing or stopping steroid tablets, may also (again, very rarely) develop Churg-Strauss syndrome. Doctors now suspect that all these patients were already suffering from an underlying eosinophilic disease, which first showed itself simply as asthma and was quelled by the steroid treatment prescribed for the asthma. The disease was thoroughly masked as long as the patient was using steroids, but when steroids were withdrawn, the underlying disease flared up, producing a wide range of symptoms. In most cases, reintroducing steroids brings these symptoms under control again.

Putting it all together

What is the ideal combination of asthma drugs? That is something that your doctor can only work out slowly, because it varies from one individual to another.

The conventional approach to asthma treatment is to start patients on a short-acting beta-2 reliever and then, if the symptoms are not controlled, to add other drugs. This approach is called "stepping up." The standard steps, or stages, are as follows:

1 Use a short-acting beta-2 reliever only.

2 Add cromoglycate or low-dose inhaled steroids.

3 Add a long-acting beta-2 reliever to the low-dose inhaled steroids, or go to moderate or high dose inhaled steroids.

4 If adequate control is still not achieved with moderate to high doses of inhaled steroids, add any of the following: long-acting beta-2 reliever, anti-leukotriene drugs, or theophylline. More rarely, a combination of these drugs is used.

5 If there is still no success in controlling symptoms, add regular steroid tablets.

Short courses of steroid tablets may be used at any stage, for the control of sudden, severe attacks.

Over the last ten years, there has been a change of strategy, and very few people are now kept on Stage 1. Inhaled steroids are now given to most asthmatics, even those with relatively mild asthma. Research from Sweden, where widespread use of inhaled steroids first became general policy, shows considerable benefits to this approach.

If you have gone beyond Stage 2, "stepping up" is usually followed by "stepping down." In other words, when the symptoms have been well controlled for 3–6 months, doses of some drugs are reduced, or certain drugs stopped altogether. If the asthma flares up again, the dose is increased or the drug reinstated. If there are no problems, and symptoms remain stable for a month or two, another reduction is tried.

An entirely different approach to asthma management is now being tried with some patients—starting off with moderate to high doses of inhaled steroids (equivalent to Stage 3) and then "stepping down." The idea is to get the inflammation under control promptly and fully at the outset. This often seems to be the best strategy.

A few asthmatics don't get much benefit from steroids. If your dose of steroid needs to be raised repeatedly, or you still need to use your reliever daily in spite of taking steroids, you may have **steroid-resistant asthma**. There are other drugs that can help, including anti-leukotriene drugs and the more powerful anti-allergy drugs (see p. 149.)

Alcohol, caffeine, and asthma

Some asthmatics experience bronchodilation (opening up of the airways) when they drink alcohol, while others experience bronchospasm (tightening of the airways). For those whose airways open up, there is probably no harm in sometimes having a drink to relieve your asthma symptoms. Clearly, it would be wrong to make a daily habit of this.

If your airways tighten up with alcohol, it may not be the alcohol itself. Alcoholic drinks contain a variety of other ingredients, either derived from the original ingredients or generated during the fermentation process. Called "congeners," these vary from one type of alcoholic drink to another, and they are often the culprits in asthma. So you may well find that while one kind of alcoholic drink has a bad effect, another type of drink is fine.

Caffeine has a far more uniform effect—it opens up the airways for most asthmatics. However, the amount needed to relieve an asthma attack will also produce unpleasant side effects, such as a pounding heart or shaky hands. There are also long-term problems with such high doses of caffeine, including insomnia, headaches, nervousness, and "restless legs." It is much better to use your reliever inhaler to control an attack; the drug in the inhaler has been chemically tailored to give the maximum therapeutic benefit with the minimum of side effects. Anyone who consumes tea or coffee excessively can suffer too much stimulant effect, resulting in palpitations or diarrhea. Occasionally there are more serious ill-effects (see p. 235), and it is not always obvious that caffeine is the cause.

Using inhalers

The value of using an inhaler, rather than taking tablets or syrup, is explained on p. 141 for steroids. The same principle applies to all drugs.

The oldest type of inhaler is the "puffer" or aerosol inhaler, which delivers the drug as a fine moist spray. Its proper name is "pressurized metered-dose inhaler" or MDI. In addition, there are now many devices that deliver drugs in dry-powder form.

If you or your child finds aerosol inhalers difficult, you may do better with a dry-powder inhaler. Your doctor should have several different inhalers available for you to try out, to see which one suits you best.

When you are given an inhaler, you must be shown how to use it by a doctor or nurse. Many asthma patients have a "poor inhaler technique," and as a result get too little of the drug. This often leads to their asthma getting out of control. The advice given here for using inhalers is no substitute for proper training and should be used only to supplement what your doctor, pharmacist, or nurse has told you.

When using an aerosol inhaler or MDI, remember to shake the inhaler well, or you will not get the right dose. Your in-breath must coincide exactly with pressing the canister down; this is the part that many people find difficult. You must breathe in slowly and deeply, otherwise you do not get much of the drug into your airways.

Many asthmatics stop inhaling the moment the spray from the aerosol inhaler hits the back of the throat. The spray contains a **propellant**, which makes it very cold, and there is a natural reflex response to this cold liquid which stops inhalation. This response may be impossible to control. If so, you need a dry-powder inhaler (see right), or a spacer (see p. 162) to use with your aerosol inhaler.

Breath-operated aerosol inhalers, such as the Maxair Autohaler (available in the U.S. but not in Canada), can be useful for those who find ordinary aerosol inhalers hard to use. With these devices,

Arthritis and inhalers

People who suffer from arthritis in their hands often find inhalers difficult to use. There are several aids now available to help with this problem—ask your doctor.

you do not have to push the canister down because your in-breath triggers the release of the drug. Take care not to block the air-intake holes with your hands, and don't stop breathing when you hear the inhaler click. (If there is no click, start again and breathe in more forcefully this time.)

One hazard with aerosol inhalers is that, when almost empty, they produce no drug—just the propellant. Although they still "puff" normally, they are not effective. It may be hard to tell when your inhaler is running low, but you can find out by removing the metal canister and placing it in a bowl of water. It sinks if it's full, and floats horizontally if it's nearly empty. An inhaler that floats vertically, nozzle downward, is half full. This is not very accurate, however, and it is best to keep track of the doses or days of use.

Many asthmatics find dry-powder inhalers, such as the Spinhaler, Rotahaler, Diskhaler, Diskus, and Turbuhaler, the easiest to use. Because they have no aerosol device, they cause no propellant-associated problems.

On the other hand, nothing pushes the drug into your mouth and lungs with a dry-powder inhaler; you have to do all the work yourself. This means that you have to breathe in quite hard and fast. During a severe asthma attack you may not be able to breathe in hard enough to get a good dose of the drug. Some asthmatics have an aerosol inhaler as well, often combined with a spacer (see p. 162), for use during severe attacks.

For the parents of asthmatics, who want to keep an eye on how much of a drug is being used, most of the dry-powder inhalers allow you to do so.

Do hold your breath

Whichever type of inhaler you use, it is important to give the drugs a chance to do their work. Breathe in slowly and deeply with an MDI. Breathe in hard, fast and deeply with a dry powder inhaler. After inhaling, and when your lungs are full, you should hold your breath for at least 10 seconds.

Side effects from nondrug ingredients

There are other ingredients in inhalers besides the drug, and they occasionally cause side effects.

Aerosol inhalers are the worst offenders. They can contain up to five non-drug ingredients, such as propellants and surfactants. Some asthmatics are sensitive to one of these and respond with coughing or bronchospasm when they inhale it.

If inhaled in large amounts, the propellants in aerosol inhalers can give a mild "high," and asthmatic teenagers and their friends may—*very rarely*—begin abusing inhaled beta-2 relievers. Parents should be alert to the possibility of such problems, but should not worry unduly.

Dry-powder inhalers do not need propellants or surfactants, so they are suitable for anyone who develops a sensitivity to these. However they may contain lactose, or milk sugar, in addition to the drug. Sufficient lactose is deposited in the mouth and swallowed to provoke symptoms, such as diarrhea and gas, in people who suffer from severe lactose intolerance (see box on p. 79). Trace amounts of milk proteins in the lactose may be a problem for people with severe milk allergy.

CFCs and inhalers

Aerosol inhalers have long contained CFCs, which, at ground level, are very inert gases and usually safe to inhale. Unfortunately, they cause serious damage when they reach the ozone layer, high above the earth, so they are being phased out in asthma inhalers, as they are in all aerosols. Other propellants, called hydrofluoroalkanes (HFAs), are being introduced to take their place. The spray from an HFA inhaler may taste and feel different, but it should do exactly the same job as a CFC inhaler; the drug it contains remains the same. Research suggests that these new propellants are very safe, but tell your doctor if your reaction to your inhaler seems to change suddenly.

These new propellants deliver medication more efficiently into the lungs, so that usually only half the previous dose is required. Unlike CFC-type inhalers, they will deliver a constant dose until empty. In addition, they are not affected as much by below-freezing temperatures.

Inhale—then brush your teeth

Asthmatic children are more prone to dental decay than other children, and inhalers are suspected of causing the problem. No one knows, as yet, exactly which ingredient of the inhalers is the culprit—it could be a drug, or a non-drug additive such as a propellant. Alternatively, the fact that the spray from some inhalers is slightly acidic could explain this side effect. As a preventive measure, brush the teeth after using the inhaler, or simply rinse out the mouth with water.

Using spacers

A spacer is a large, empty chamber that can be fitted to an aerosol inhaler (a puffer or MDI) to make it more effective and easier to use. The aerosol spray enters at one end of the spacer, and the asthmatic breathes it in from the other end.

When using a spacer, you can breathe normally; you don't have to take all the drug in at once or hold your breath after you've inhaled. But you should try to breathe as slowly and deeply as possible and hold your breath for up to 10 seconds if you can.

Note that spacers are for use with aerosol inhalers only: they are no good with a dry-powder inhaler. Spacers allow the aerosol propellant (see p. 161) to evaporate, leaving tiny airborne droplets of the drug to be inhaled. Once the propellant has evaporated, these droplets are no longer cold, so the reflex response that stops you from inhaling is avoided.

During an asthma attack, spacers are immensely valuable, because they allow you to get some of the drug into your airways even though you are unable to take a deep breath. There is a collapsible spacer, called the E-Z Spacer, which folds up into a plastic case small enough to be slipped into a pocket. In a severe asthma attack, having such a spacer could save your life.

In an emergency, if no spacer is available, you can improvise one (see p. 100).

Babies and small children, who cannot yet coordinate the in-breath with pushing the aerosol canister down, need spacers for everyday use. There are spacers designed for young children with masks that fit over the nose and mouth.

When using a spacer, shake the inhaler and then spray it into the spacer once only. Inhale slowly and deeply within five seconds. During a severe asthma attack, you can add another dose from the inhaler every 10 seconds, until the attack begins to subside, but keep a count of how many puffs you use (see p. 100).

To treat a young child, shake the inhaler well, and fit it to the spacer. Put the mouthpiece into the child's mouth, or put the mask on. Tell the child to breathe in and out steadily with the mouth open, and listen for the clicking of the valve on the spacer—this shows that it is opening and closing. (Or look for the valve opening and closing—in Canada, the

Priming a spacer

Prime a new spacer, or one that has been washed, by firing the inhaler into it five times. The drug will coat the spacer, due to an electrostatic charge on the plastic. You won't be able to see the drug as it forms a very thin coating.

When you come to use the spacer, no more of the drug will stick to the spacer walls, because they are already coated, so the full dose will be available for you or your child to inhale.

Priming new spacers is particularly important when the asthmatic is a young child, because there may be some delay between firing the inhaler and the child taking a full breath. The longer the delay, the more chance the drug has to stick to the unprimed spacer walls.

Some brands of spacer (for example, the AeroChamber) are made from a type of plastic that does not need to be primed, but must be washed before first use.

valve is made of soft plastic and does not produce a click.) When the child's breathing is regular, puff a single dose into the spacer. The child should breathe in and out 5–8 times before you take the spacer away.

A spacer can be used on a baby while he is asleep, which may make life easier for you both. If you need to use the spacer while a baby or toddler is awake, stroke the mask against the child's cheek first. Keep smiling and talking, so that the situation doesn't seem so frightening. If the baby does start to cry, keep the mask in place; the crying will bring on a deep in-breath, which is just what is needed.

For an older child, decorating the spacer with colored stickers can make it appear less daunting. Try to make using the spacer seem like a game. If this fails, don't get into a battle with the child—leave it a while and try again later.

Nebulizers

A nebulizer delivers a high dose of asthma drug in an easily inhaled form. It is generally used for severe asthma only, or in an emergency to relieve asthma attacks.

A nebulizer can be attached to an oxygen cylinder, which enriches the air-drug mixture with oxygen. This is useful in severe asthma.

The only people who need to have a nebulizer at home for emergencies are those with brittle asthma, whose condition can deteriorate very suddenly and sharply.

For routine use, only a very small minority of asthmatics require a nebulizer. They include

- those with such severe asthma that they depend on large doses of drugs to control their symptoms
- very small children or elderly people with severe asthma, who have difficulty using inhalers. For them, a nebulizer may be the easiest way to take their drugs.

The fact that the hospital's nebulizer is so effective in an emergency gives it a special mystique for many people, who assume that nebulizers are a magical cure for asthma. Nebulizers are widely advertised in specialist publications for asthmatics, and while they are expensive, they can appear to be the answer to a prayer. Many asthmatics, or their parents, mistakenly believe that owning a nebulizer will be the answer to all their problems. In fact the nebulizer works so well only because it delivers a much higher dose of the reliever drug—a dose that also carries a higher risk of side effects. This high-dose treatment should not be used on a regular basis unless it is absolutely essential. No one should buy a nebulizer without first discussing the matter with their doctor.

Asthmatics who own a nebulizer should have detailed written instructions from a doctor about when and how to use it, and how much of the drug to put in. One hazard of owning a nebulizer is that it may give you a false sense of security during emergencies, and delay you from getting expert medical help when you need it. If the nebulizer is for emergency use, you should be told the exact signs that indicate a need to use it and—no less important—the signs that show the attack is out of control and needs hospital treatment.

Take care, when using a nebulizer, not to allow the mist to escape and settle on the face or eyes. Regular exposure to steroid mist can cause cataracts and thinning of the skin on the face. Anticholinergics (see p. 156) can cause glaucoma if they come into contact with the eye. The mask must fit very tightly. As an additional precaution, place a scarf around the upper edge of the mask to close any gaps. Wash the face after using the nebulizer with steroids.

Keep off the cough syrup

Coughing can be a useful reaction in an asthma attack, as it evicts mucus from the lungs. But in some asthmatics the cough does not produce mucus and seems to be no more than a reflex reaction to the airway inflammation. This type of cough can be debilitating, but it is *not* a good idea to treat it with cough syrup which has no benefit and may mask the seriousness of the asthma. The best course is to tackle the airway inflammation with preventer drugs such as steroids. Simple **expectorants** that loosen mucus may be tried, but are rarely helpful—ask your pharmacist about these.

Allergy shots

"My allergist talked to me about allergy shots several times," says Al, "but I thought I was OK on the inhalers, and I really hate needles. Then—it must have been about six years ago—there was a real bad ragweed season. One day it was so hot, and suddenly I just couldn't breathe at all. That was scary. I wound up in hospital on oxygen and a nebulizer, and I thought, 'OK, that's it, I'll give the shots a try.' Now—well, I just wish I'd done it when I was younger. My asthma is a whole lot less trouble."

Not everyone responds this well to allergy shots, but for those allergy sufferers who do benefit, they are an excellent treatment. One of their attractions is that they tackle allergies right at their source, by teaching the immune system to react differently to the allergen. Another advantage over treatment by drugs is that with allergy shots there are no concerns about insidious long-term side effects. The side effects are all short-term and entirely obvious (see p. 166).

More correctly known as allergen immunotherapy or simply immunotherapy, this form of treatment was devised by an English physician, Dr. Leonard Noon, who reported his successes with hay fever patients in 1911. Other names for this treatment that you may come across are specific immunotherapy (SIT), incremental immunotherapy (IIT), hyposensitization, and desensitization.

The uses of allergy shots

Allergy shots are used mainly for airborne allergens such as pollen, dust mite, cockroach, and mold spores. Allergies to animals can also be treated with allergy shots, but the treatment cannot work miracles—if you keep your cat, you are inhaling such a high dose of cat allergen every day that there is a limit to the impact the shots can make on your immune system. In general, it makes sense to avoid an allergen if you can, rather than have allergy shots against it and continue exposing yourself to it.

People with simple allergic reactions affecting the nose and eyes (allergic rhinitis and conjunctivitis) respond well to allergy shots. In patients with hay fever, for example, the success rate is about 80–90 percent. When nasal allergies are complicated by chronic sinusitis or nasal polyps, the success rate is a little lower.

Some studies of the long-term effects of allergy shots suggests that if they are given to children with hay fever or perennial rhinitis, those children are less likely to develop asthma or new allergies.

How about using allergy shots in the treatment of established asthma? Unfortunately, asthma is a more complex disease than hay fever, and allergies are only one factor among many (see p. 38) involved in causing asthma. Consequently, the benefits of allergy shots for asthma are less certain. Shots may be a great help for an asthmatic such as Al, who has a strong allergic reaction to a single airborne allergen, but they are frequently less useful to other asthmatics. It is difficult to say in advance exactly who will do well with allergy shots, but research shows that the following asthmatics are unlikely to benefit:

- those with severe long-term asthma
- those with aspirin sensitivity
- those with chronic sinusitis
- those who are sensitive to several year-round allergens, including dust mite

The value of allergy shots to children with asthma is a subject of great debate among doctors. One recent study of asthmatic children, by a team at Johns Hopkins University, discovered that allergy shots don't add any substantial further benefits when the asthma is being well treated by means of allergen avoidance and asthma drugs. However, this influential trial has been criticized for not including shots for cockroach, a major allergen among asthmatic children in urban areas. Inclusion of this important allergen might have made the immunotherapy far more effective.

In making a decision about allergy shots for childhood asthma, the possible long-term advantages are worth considering. Some studies suggest that if asthmatic children with allergies are given a full 5-year course of immunotherapy, they tend to have fewer asthma symptoms and need less medication as young adults.

Chronic urticaria (hives) is occasionally caused by airborne allergens, in which case allergy shots may help, but shots are not recommended for atopic eczema. However, when people with eczema also suffer from asthma or rhinitis, they often want to try allergy shots for their nose or airway symptoms. Some find that their eczema lessens in response to the immunotherapy treatment, but more often the skin gets worse and the shots have to be stopped. One of the alternative forms of desensitization (see p. 211) may be more helpful for atopic eczema.

Insect-sting allergy is a prime candidate for allergy shots, but food allergy is not (see pp. 168–9).

How allergy shots work

Allergy shots are small injections, just under the skin. The injected liquid contains an extract of the offending allergen—for example, ragweed pollen or dust mite. The injections are given at regular intervals, usually once a week, although other schedules are possible (see p. 167).

At the outset, a very dilute version of the allergen extract is used, way below the threshold that will generally cause an allergic reaction. For people who, on the basis of their skin tests, seem highly sensitive, the doctor will begin with an extract that is even more dilute.

For the next injection, a slightly higher concentration of the allergen extract is used, and the concentration is increased with each successive injection. The idea is to habituate the immune system to the offending allergen by very gradually raising the dose. Eventually, when the dose reaches a level that is known to give beneficial effects, no further increases are made.

Unpleasant reactions to allergy shots do occur (see p. 166), and if an allergy sufferer reacts badly on several successive occasions, the dose may be leveled off before the ideal maximum dose is reached. However, a good allergist will persist for some time in trying to increase the dose, because stopping at a lower level may cause the therapy to be ineffective (see p. 166).

The first stage of immunotherapy, when the concentration of the allergen extract is being increased week by week, is known as the **buildup stage**. The second stage, when the dose is being kept at the same level, is called **maintenance therapy**, and the dose used is the **maintenance dose**.

There will not necessarily be any obvious improvement when the buildup stage is complete. The benefits of the treatment should begin to appear within 6 months of reaching the maintenance dose, but some people have to wait a year, or even two, before they improve.

For people with troublesome pollen allergies in mostly one season (for example, tree, grass, or ragweed pollen), a more convenient schedule of 3–12 weekly injections may be given each year, before (pre-seasonal) and sometimes during (co-seasonal) the specific allergy season. The allergy extract is usually modified to allow larger doses to be given with less risk of local reactions. This may not be as effective as year-round (perennial) immunotherapy, but for some allergy sufferers the time saved is worth the trade-off.

As the immunotherapy begins to take effect, your symptoms should decline, and you will probably need fewer drugs. What lies behind these changes? In other words, how is the immune system affected? There is no simple answer to this question because no two allergy sufferers react to allergy shots in quite the same way. Research has revealed a surprising number of different changes that may occur. Frequently there is a shift in the kind of antibodies that the body produces against the offending allergen. Levels of IgG antibodies (which help to block the allergic reaction) go up, while levels of the allergy antibody, IgE, tend to stabilize and eventually go down. The numbers of mast cells (see box on p. 12) may also decline, and they can become less responsive to the allergen. The balance of power between Th1 cells and Th2 cells may also shift, with the pro-allergy Th2 cells (see p. 11) becoming less influential.

Multiple allergies

Allergy shots tend to work well for people with a single allergic sensitization—allergic only to dust mites, for example—but there is some debate over how useful allergy shots are for people with multiple allergies.

Allergists generally deal with multiple allergies by combining all the relevant allergens for each patient, and using this mixed extract for the allergy shots. During the buildup phase, the ceiling on the maximum dose is set by one allergen, the one that is the least tolerated. It is difficult to hit on the right maximum dose for each individual allergen when working in this way, so the results of immunotherapy are unlikely to be as good as when treating a single allergic sensitization.

However, giving immunotherapy for just one or two key allergens, when a patient has multiple allergies, is not the answer either. Many immunotherapy failures are probably due to undertreatment of this kind.

If you have multiple allergies, ask your allergist about the prospects for success before you begin allergy shots.

What can go wrong

The secret of safe immunotherapy is to go at exactly the right speed for the immune system of the individual being treated. A good allergist looks for feedback from the immune system— signs that show how well it is coping with the steadily increasing dose of allergen—and uses this to pace the immunotherapy schedule.

Going too fast—getting ahead of the immune system's ability to cope—is hazardous. A severe allergic reaction, called anaphylaxis (see p. 58) can occur, and this is potentially life-threatening. So long as epinephrine and resuscitation equipment are available, even such an extreme crisis can be dealt with safely, but deaths have occurred, usually when patients have suffered anaphylaxis after leaving the doctor's office. Between 1985 and 1989, 17 deaths resulting from immunotherapy were reported in the United States alone.

Serious reactions to allergy shots usually occur
- during the initial buildup phase; maintenance therapy is much safer
- during the pollen season, for those with pollen allergy
- when a new vial of allergen extract is first being used, due to variations in concentration (see below)
- when there is a dosing error

Those people most vulnerable to severe reactions are
- people with asthma, especially severe or unstable asthma
- those who have experienced systemic allergic reactions in the past
- anyone who is extremely allergic, as revealed by skin tests
- anyone taking beta-blockers (see box on p. 150)

With care, fatalities can be avoided, and the advice given on pp. 167–8 will help you to protect yourself.

When the shots don't work

Life-threatening reactions to the shots affect only a tiny minority of people. The other thing that can go wrong—and this is far more common—is that the allergy shots simply have no effect.

One likely reason for this failure is that the maintenance dose is not high enough. In other words, the allergist should have continued raising the concentration of the allergen extract but stopped too soon. Often doctors settle for a low maintenance dose because they are being cautious—the lower the dose at the leveling-off point, the smaller the risk of a serious reaction. Safety is clearly important, but a long course of shots that has no effect is a terrific waste. You would be better off with an allergist who uses a moderate or high-maintenance dose, and who has excellent safety procedures in place to prevent bad reactions or to deal with them when they occur. Discuss success rates at your initial meeting with the allergist. Ask how the maintenance dose that he or she aims to use compares to the maintenance doses generally recommended for the allergen concerned.

Standardizing allergens

Another possible reason for the failure of allergy shots—more common in the past than now—was that the allergen extract simply did not contain enough of the relevant allergen. In an attempt to address this problem and improve safety, much research effort has been invested in standardizing allergen extracts, so that they always contain exactly the same amount of the allergen.

This is a difficult process, because the starting material—cat dander, for example, or dust mite droppings—is a natural material and therefore variable. Some samples contain far more of a particular allergenic ingredient than others.

One way around this problem is to develop accurate methods of measuring the amount of the allergens in the extract. Another approach is to abandon the whole business of making extracts, and produce allergens artificially in a laboratory. This is done by inserting the gene for the allergen—the gene for the Der p1 allergen of dust mite, for example—into bacteria. The bacteria then act as production units, manufacturing large amounts of the allergen every day. With this high-tech approach, the exact content of the allergen preparations can be controlled.

These high-tech allergen preparations are extremely pure, and therefore very effective—so long as you are sensitized to the particular allergen that is included.

Unfortunately, most natural allergic materials contain two, three, or even more separate allergens. In dust mite droppings, for example, while Der p1 is the main allergen—the one that affects most people—there is also an allergen called Der p2. A few people are more sensitive to Der p2 than to Der p1.

Artificially-produced allergen preparations usually include the main allergen only. If you belong to the minority of people who are more severely allergic to one of the other allergens, such preparations will probably not work for you, or will not work well. If immunotherapy fails, a good allergist will consider this possibility and will try other options, such as treatment with an old-fashioned extract containing all the allergens.

Some of these treatment failures could be avoided if more thorough and precise skin testing took place before allergy shots began. Skin tests with individual allergens, such as Der p1 and Der p2, rather than with an allergen extract containing a mix of allergens, would help considerably. As the new high-tech allergens become more widely used, this more sophisticated approach to testing will probably become commonplace.

The timing of allergy shots

There are various different approaches to the timing of allergy shots. The basic method, which is favored by most North American allergists, starts with injections once a week. This approach has a good safety record.

After the maintenance dose has been reached, injections are given once every 2–4 weeks. If you have pollen allergies, the frequency of the maintenance injections may be increased during the pollen season, although the dose may be lowered to reduce the risk of reactions.

It is the regularity of the injections that gradually creates, and then sustains, immune tolerance; so make sure to keep all your appointments. You will jeopardize your chance of success by not doing so. During the buildup phase, leaving a gap of more than a week between injections also increases the risk of severe reaction.

Once you have had two years with no symptoms, your allergist may suggest stopping immunotherapy. It usually takes 4–5 years of regular therapy, from the time of your first shot, to get to this point. You should find that the benefits persist for many years, perhaps indefinitely, even without any further shots. If symptoms do recur eventually, another course of immunotherapy should put you back on track.

Trying to speed up the process of immunotherapy greatly increases the risk of a severe reaction (anaphylaxis). However, there are situations in which fast results are needed, and in such cases rush immunotherapy, also called accelerated immunotherapy, may be used.

During the buildup stage of rush immunotherapy, injections are given every day, or even several times a day. All the usual safety procedures (see below) are observed with particular care, to reduce the chance of a severe reaction. In semi-rush immunotherapy, the buildup injections are given twice a week.

Minimizing the risks

There is much you can do to minimize the risk of suffering a severe reaction to allergy shots. (Most of the precautions listed below are already taken by conscientious allergists.)

• Before you agree to a course of allergy shots, ask the allergist about his or her success rate, how often severe reactions occur with the technique being used, and if epinephrine and resuscitation equipment are on hand. (If the answer to this last question is "No," go elsewhere.) Be wary of anyone who seems casual about the risks involved. Take note of the attitude of the nursing staff, since they usually give the shots. You need to know that you are in safe hands—the staff must be extremely careful about checking the dose of allergen and verifying that the allergy extract is yours before giving the shot. They should also be well trained in emergency treatment for anaphylaxis.

• If you are taking beta-blockers (see box on p. 150) or if you have a heart condition, discuss the safety issues with your doctor at the outset. Beta-blockers (given for heart conditions or migraine) make immunotherapy much more dangerous. ACE inhibitors (given for high blood pressure, heart failure, and some complications of diabetes) also increase the risks. If these drugs cannot be avoided or discontinued during immunotherapy, great caution is necessary.

• At each visit, inform the doctor if you have an infection of any kind, as this can alter your reaction. You should also tell the doctor about any new medicines you are taking, including eyedrops for glaucoma—some of these products may contain beta-blockers (see box on p. 150).

• Report any reactions that occurred after your previous shot, such as redness, itching, or swelling around the injection site, or (more seriously) symptoms elsewhere on the body, such as hives, itchy skin, sneezing, a runny nose, red or itchy eyes, tightness in the throat or chest, coughing, or wheezing. Always make a note of such symptoms, so that you don't forget to mention them at the next visit. This is crucially important, for such reactions can indicate that the immune system is being hurried along too fast.

• If you are asthmatic, never have a shot when you are experiencing asthma symptoms. If you have a peak flow meter, always check your peak flow immediately before the appointment, even if you feel fine. If your peak flow is less than 70 percent of your best reading, don't have the shot. Check your peak flow again before you leave the doctor's office, and if it has declined sharply, tell the doctor.

• Never leave the doctor's office until at least 30 minutes after the shot was given. Although many allergists ask you to wait for only 20 minutes, research shows that severe reactions often occur after that point, and a 30-minute wait increases the safety margin substantially. Unfortunately, 30–50 percent of reactions take place *after* 30 minutes. If you have a history of severe allergic reactions, waiting for an hour is not excessive—take a book or, in the case of a child, anything else that will make the time pass happily.

• If waiting 30 minutes is impossible, talk to your allergist about carrying an epinephrine auto-injector, for use in the event of a severe reaction after you have left the office. Some allergists believe that everyone undergoing immunotherapy should carry epinephrine on the day a shot has been given. *Note that using the epinephrine injection is just the first step in treating anaphylaxis* (see p. 98). If you have to give yourself an epinephrine shot, you must then go back to your allergist or to a hospital emergency room.

• Severe reactions can begin some hours after the allergy shot, so stay within reach of a phone for about 24 hours.

• Avoid strenuous exercise for two hours after a shot. The increased blood flow during exercise can cause more rapid release of the injected allergen extract into the bloodstream, increasing the risk of a reaction.

• If you have pollen allergies, be extra cautious during the pollen season, especially if you are asthmatic.

Giving yourself allergy shots at home

Some allergists will allow certain patients—those at least risk of a severe reaction—to give themselves allergy shots at home. The hazards of anaphylaxis (see p. 166) are such that many doctors feel this is unwise, particularly during the buildup phase of immunotherapy. Neither the American Academy of Allergy nor the Canadian Society of Allergy recommend home shots.

You should discuss the safety issues very fully with your allergist before deciding on home treatment.

If you do decide on home treatment, despite the risks, or if you are already giving yourself shots, you should study all the safety measures given above and implement those that are appropriate. You should have an epinephrine injector available for emergencies *and* someone on hand to help you if you need to get to hospital quickly. Be particularly cautious if you are asthmatic.

Allergy shots for insect-sting allergy

Allergy shots provide highly effective protection for those with insect-sting allergy and should be given to anyone who has had a severe systemic reaction (see p. 60). They are also recommended for adults who have had a cutaneous systemic reaction (see p. 60), on the basis that they may well progress to a severe systemic reaction with the next sting.

Studies of people who have suffered severe systemic reactions and are then treated with allergy shots show that 97 percent have no systemic reaction to insect stings while on the shots. For the 3 percent who are not fully protected, the severity of the reaction is much reduced and far less likely to be life threatening. In other words, this is an excellent treatment that can save lives.

Not everyone with insect-sting allergy sees the insect that caused the reaction. Skin tests may not give the answer either, because there are often positive reactions to several different venoms. Some of these may be false positives (see p. 91), so it is impossible for the allergist to say which one(s) are actually relevant. Most allergists will recommend immunotherapy for all of them, using a mixture of venom extracts.

Where the guilty insect was seen and identified, but other venoms also give positive skin tests, a more difficult decision has to be made. Some allergists carry out immunotherapy for all the venoms that gave a positive skin test, on a "better safe than sorry" basis. Since there are cross-reactions between venoms (see box on p. 113), there is some sense in this. Other allergists give immunotherapy just for the insect that did the deed.

Will immunotherapy against one insect protect you against a related insect? In the case of two closely related insects, such as wasps and hornets, which have many allergens in common, it might do so—but there is no guarantee. The problem is that, besides the shared allergens, each venom also has its own unique ingredients. With the tests now available, it's impossible to say if you are reacting mainly to shared allergens or to unique ones. So immunotherapy against wasp venom *may* give you protection against hornet venom, but it will not necessarily do so—and vice versa. In the case of bumblebee allergy (seen almost exclusively in people, such as horticulturists, whose work involves handling bumblebees), a more definite answer is possible—honeybee immunotherapy does *not* work. Immunotherapy with bumblebee venom does work but, unfortunately, this is not currently available in North America.

Injections are normally given weekly during the buildup phase. If protection is needed urgently—for example, to deal with work-related sting allergy—rush immunotherapy may be used. Once you have reached the maximum dose, you will need a maintenance injection every 4 weeks. After a year, this maintenance dose can be given every 6–8 weeks.

After 3–5 years of immunotherapy, you will probably be skin-tested again, and if your results are negative, the immunotherapy will be stopped. Research shows that even if your skin test is still positive when immunotherapy ends, there's an 80–90 percent chance that you will *not* have a systemic reaction to future stings.

More long-term studies indicate that, for up to 15 years after immunotherapy ends, there is a 10 percent risk of a systemic reaction. (Note that the 10 percent risk applies whether skin tests were positive or negative at the time of stopping.) However, these reactions are generally mild.

It is recommended that people with insect sting allergy continue to carry their epinephrine treatment kits after immunotherapy is discontinued. Venom immunotherapy for life may be considered for the following groups, who are at higher risk:
- anyone who has had a previous near-fatal sting allergy
- anyone who had a systemic reaction to immunotherapy
- anyone who has a honeybee allergy

Some people prefer to continue with immunotherapy simply for their own peace of mind. In fact, research shows that a near-fatal systemic reaction has long-lasting psychological impact and that many people continue to feel anxious despite completing immunotherapy *and* reacting negatively to skin tests.

At one time, challenge stings with live insects were given to check whether immunotherapy had actually worked. Few North American doctors do this now, but it is still common practice in other countries, such as Germany. Your allergist may be prepared to do a challenge test if you ask. The fact that the psychological consequences of insect-sting allergy are so persistent suggests that challenge tests with live insects may have a particular value.

Unfortunately, even challenge tests do not give an absolute guarantee. For unknown reasons, an insect-venom allergic person may not react to every sting, and some sting challenges may be negative the first time but produce a systemic reaction the next. This is observed in the real world where the risk of repeat allergic reaction when stung by the same type of insect is only 30–60 percent (not 100 percent) for untreated people. However, a challenge test will give you some indication of the effectiveness of the allergy shots. If a challenge test is used, epinephrine and resuscitation equipment must, of course, be on hand.

Allergy shots for food allergy?

The hope that allergy shots might help people with severe food allergy has not as yet been realized. With respect to food allergy, doctors are aiming simply to protect against the effects of accidentally eating a tiny amount of the food—no one is expecting that a child with nut allergy will be able to eat peanut butter cookies along with the rest of the family.

Even this rather limited aim still seems like a distant dream. The process of giving the shots is nerve-racking because of the constant risk of a severe reaction. This risk prevents the dose of allergen from being increased very much, so the beneficial effects are small. While there may be some reduction in sensitivity, it is not enough—or not reliable enough—to be of any practical value.

Research is now focused on developing modified forms of the food allergens (**allergoids**) that could induce tolerance without any risk of a bad reaction. Peanuts are currently at the center of this research, and modified peanut allergen could become available in the next few years. Even if it works, it is unlikely to allow patients to eat peanuts without restriction.

Mild allergic reactions to food are a different matter. One report indicated that some patients receiving allergy shots for hay fever noticed an improvement in their fruit and vegetable allergies if they had Oral Allergy Syndrome (see box on p. 63).

The future of immunotherapy

Allergoids (see above) could be useful with any type of allergy. The allergen is carefully altered so that IgE antibodies no longer recognize it (eliminating the risk of a bad reaction to the shot itself), yet it can still interact with T-helper (Th) cells. An allergoid made from cat allergen can teach cat-specific Th cells not to give the "go ahead" signal for a reaction to real cat allergen. The safety of allergoids allows a very fast schedule of allergy shots. Some experimental vaccines may even work with a single shot.

A far more radical approach is to shift the immune system away from allergy altogether, by altering the balance of Th1 cells and Th2 cells (see p. 11). Inspired by discoveries about hygiene (see p. 21) researchers have made a vaccine from soil bacteria and used it to treat adult asthmatics. At least one third showed far less reaction to inhaled allergen after receiving the vaccine.

diets for allergy and intolerance

This chapter covers two main types of diets: avoidance diets and diagnostic diets. Both are intended for people with sensitivity to food.

An **avoidance diet** is for people who already know what food or foods affect them and simply need to avoid those foods. A **diagnostic diet** is for those whose symptoms suggest that they might be suffering from food sensitivity of some kind and who cannot be diagnosed by indirect methods such as skin tests because true food allergy is not involved. A diagnostic diet is intended primarily to show whether or not food is causing the symptoms.

The diagnostic diets themselves fall into two basic categories. First, there are diets that, by a process of elimination, identify a particular food (or foods) as a cause of symptoms. Called **elimination diets**, these are used to diagnose idiopathic food intolerance (see p. 74) and certain other sensitivity reactions to particular foods. An elimination diet is *purely* diagnostic—simply a means to establish which foods are at fault. To this end, all commonly eaten foods are avoided at the outset, and each food is then tested individually. Once an elimination diet has been completed, the information gained from it is used to establish a suitable avoidance diet. For example, if milk, wheat, and oranges caused symptoms during the testing phase of the elimination diet, those foods are all avoided in future.

Second, there are **specific diagnostic diets**, which are a great deal simpler to carry out than elimination diets. A specific diagnostic diet aims to reduce the intake of a particular substance found in certain foods. The substances concerned—histamine or nickel, for example—are known to cause particular symptoms in susceptible people.

A specific diagnostic diet simply cuts out all the foods that contain large amounts of the substance under suspicion. If this diet alleviates the symptoms, and does so consistently, it is plausible that the substance concerned is indeed the culprit. However, the diet should be stopped and then started again, preferably several times, to check the response. Once the sensitivity is confirmed, the subsequent avoidance diet that follows is basically the same as the diet used for diagnosis.

Note that there is no agreed terminology for these different kinds of diet, and the definitions given above will not necessarily be used in other publications. You may even come across "elimination diet" being used to mean "avoidance diet," which is particularly confusing. If you are consulting other sources of information, check the context to see what meaning is intended.

There is one exception in this chapter—the diet to protect against asthma, described on pp. 206-7. It is neither an avoidance diet nor a diagnostic diet, but a health-promoting diet of the kind commonly advocated to combat other widespread conditions, such as cancer and heart disease. In fact, it has a remarkable number of similarities to diets that reduce the risk of these other diseases.

The anti-asthma diet is immensely healthy, whereas many avoidance diets carry a risk of malnourishment. An allergic individual—especially a child—following any kind of restrictive diet should be assessed for the possible risks. That is why it is important to talk to your doctor before starting any dietary treatment or investigation. A referral to a dietitian or nutritionist may be necessary.

When malnutrition does occur as a result of self-treatment, there are often very complex factors at work. One potential hazard with dietary treatment is that psychological problems can easily become entwined with obsessions about food. Eating can be a potent form of self-expression, or a way of exerting control over oneself and others. Many doctors have seen patients who are mistakenly convinced that food sensitivity is at the root of their health problems, or those of their children. In some cases, no amount of objective evidence to the contrary will deflect people from such beliefs.

A few people with mistaken beliefs of this kind impose very restrictive diets on themselves—or sometimes on the whole family. The food rules that they establish may be a way of limiting contact with the outside world, avoiding other problems and issues by making diet the central focus, or simply making demands on other people's time and attention.

The current fad for identifying "food allergy" using very dubious diagnostic tests (see p. 93) will probably send many more psychologically vulnerable people down this route.

Another unhelpful trend in the dietary field is the wholesale (and usually ineffective) use of vitamins, minerals, and other supplements for a great variety of diseases, including allergy and other forms of sensitivity. It is important to realize that none of the sensitivity diseases described in this book have nutritional deficiency as their primary cause, so supplements are not a major part of treatment in most cases. For the majority of people with some kind of sensitivity disease, a supplement will make only a small difference, if any. However, it is true that, with *some* sensitivity problems, certain supplements may be helpful to certain individuals. The use of Vitamin C in asthma (see p. 000) is one example of this, and there are some other instances mentioned in Chapter 2.

Generally speaking, it is better to get the vitamins, minerals, and other nutrients you need (such as antioxidants) from food, not from tablets. Studies of adult-onset asthma have shown that only natural vitamin E protects against the disease; supplements have no effect.

Many plant and animal extracts (or foods enhanced with these extracts—so-called functional foods), are now being promoted vigorously as health-enhancing products. Regulators are concerned that the distinction between nutritional value and medicinal effects is becoming increasingly blurred, and are trying to establish clear guidelines and laws.

Some of the claims made for "functional foods" are based on good scientific evidence and conform to existing regulations. However there are also claims that are not based on any reliable evidence. Efforts are currently being made to clamp down on manufacturers making these false claims, but in the meantime consumers should be on their guard against some of these products. Useful information on them can often be found on the Internet (see p. 255).

Allergy-prone consumers should also be alert for foods or supplements containing herbal extracts that might actually trigger sensitivity reactions, such as echinacea and ginkgo (see p. 221). Those with aspirin sensitivity and asthma should be cautious about foods or supplements containing high levels of omega-3 oils (see box on p. 221).

Reading food labels

What exactly is in ready-made food? People with food sensitivity, especially those with severe food allergy or celiac disease, need a straight answer to this question, but frequently they don't get one. Research among food-allergy sufferers has found that, in the course of a year, half of them inadvertently eat the food they are trying to avoid, owing to a lack of information about ingredients. Restaurants and cafeterias are responsible for many of these accidents, and most of the resulting fatalities (see p. 111), but packaged food also plays a part.

Unfortunately, many potentially allergenic food ingredients, such as milk and eggs, are found in packaged food without appearing on the label in everyday language. The information is usually there somewhere, however—you just need to know what words to look out for.

Decoding food labels

The problems with the wording used on food labels fall into two general categories:

- Some of the ingredients are described using technical terms. These are usually specific constituents of the original foodstuff, for example lactalbumin, one of the proteins found in milk.
- Some manufactured ingredients can be made from different starting materials. So an item such as "edible starch" could be made from either wheat or corn, while "hydrolyzed protein" could be made from soy, corn, or yeast, sometimes with wheat added.

One day, no doubt, manufacturers will realize what a burden this type of obscure labeling imposes on their allergic customers and start using plain language. In the meantime, food-allergy sufferers just have to learn all the terms that may be used for their culprit food.

Labels used in health-food stores and delicatessens are another matter altogether. Here the problem is with exotic-sounding items such as kamut that are actually a potentially allergenic food (wheat).

These are the words that you need to look out for, plus some of the unlabeled items that could, unexpectedly, contain your problem food:

Corn

Items always made from corn: cornmeal, cornstarch, dextrose, polenta

Items sometimes made from corn: baking powder, cereal starch, edible starch, food starch, glucose syrup, hydrolyzed plant protein, hydrolyzed protein, hydrolyzed vegetable protein, malt, malt flavoring, modified food starch, modified starch, starch, textured vegetable protein, vegetable gum, vegetable protein, vegetable starch

Note that the adhesive used on envelopes and stamps is sometimes made from corn and that many medicines contain cornstarch.

Eggs

Items always made from eggs: ovalbumin

Items sometimes made from eggs: lecithin (this is rare in foods—lecithin is usually derived from soy; only in pharmaceuticals is lecithin likely to be derived from egg), lysozyme

Fish

Be very cautious when traveling. The use of fish meal as an ingredient of spicy sauces is common in Southeast Asia and in some parts of Africa. The strength of the spices may make the fish undetectable.

Milk

Items always made from milk: casein, caseinate, lactalbumin, whey

If you see the term "dairy-free" on standard packaged foods, you can safely assume that the contents are free from goat's and sheep's milk as well as cow's milk. But be more wary with home-made or locally produced foods labeled "dairy-free"—some people think that "dairy" refers only to cow's milk.

Parev (parve, pareve) is a term used for kosher (sanctioned by Jewish law) food that contains neither milk nor meat. However, contamination with traces of milk is possible.

Lactose is a sugar produced from milk, and while it is not allergenic itself, it may contain a trace of allergenic milk proteins. The amounts involved are tiny, and will only affect the most sensitive individuals.

The label "non-milk fat" sometimes misleads people if they just glance quickly at labels. The fact that a product contains non-milk fat does not, of course, mean that it is entirely milk-free—remember to look for all the synonyms of milk (see above).

Nuts

Items always made from nuts: frangipane, marzipan, praline

Standard packaged food will almost always include the nuts by name, but if you are buying other food (for example, from a stand selling home-made food), watch out for the above names.

Be very cautious about nut oils (see p. 110). Almond essence may be produced chemically, in which case it is safe, but some is made from real almonds and could therefore be allergenic.

Peanuts

Items always made from peanuts: arachis oil, peanut oil, satay sauce

Alternative names for peanuts: arachide, beer nuts, cacahueta, cacahuete, earth nuts, goober nuts, goober peas, groundnuts, mandelona nuts, monkey nuts, new nuts, Nu-Nuts,

You are likely to encounter these names only on imported food, or

when traveling. Always be very careful with food from India or Southeast Asia, where the use of peanuts is very common (for example, in sauces) and often not at all obvious.

Items sometimes made from peanuts: hydrolyzed plant protein, hydrolyzed protein, hydrolyzed vegetable protein (The usual source is soy, wheat, or yeast, but some is derived from peanuts.)

If your child is highly allergic to peanuts, read the label on all vegetarian foods and on *everything* sweet, even jelly beans, ice cream and milk shakes. Also watch out for home-made play-dough, and some animal food (for example, mixes for birds or gerbils, or the pellets used at petting farms), if your child reacts to skin contact with peanuts.

Avoid chocolate from Poland, which often contains peanuts that are not declared on the label.

Sesame

Items always made from sesame or containing some sesame: gomashio, halva, hummus (houmus), tahini

Standard packaged food will almost always use the term "sesame" on the label, but if you are buying other food (for example, from a health-food store or a stand selling home-made food) watch out for the above names. Check carefully for sesame in any Chinese packaged food (for example, stir-fry oils) and in the drink Aqua Libra. Sesame oil is allergenic (see p. 110). Watch out for contamination by traces of sesame in bakeries and delicatessens where goods are sold unwrapped.

Shellfish

Items sometimes containing shellfish: curry paste, fish sauce and other sauces/pastes used in Southeast Asian cooking

Standard packaged food should mention shellfish specifically, but you may need to read the label carefully. Be cautious about bottles of imported sauce, and home-made or take-out food.

Soy

Items always or usually made from soy: miso, soy protein, soy protein isolate, soy sauce, textured vegetable protein, tofu, vegetable protein

Items sometimes made from soy: hydrolyzed plant protein, hydrolyzed protein, hydrolyzed vegetable protein, lecithin, vegetable gum, vegetable starch

Changes in ingredients

Unfortunately, the ingredients of a product can change without any obvious warning on the label, or any change in the packaging. You should always check the label in detail, every time—even on foods that you have eaten before without any trouble.

Wheat

Items always made from wheat: bran, flour, graham flour, hard flour, strong flour, whole-wheat flour (there are nonwheat brans and flours, of course, but the word "bran" or "flour" without any qualification usually means wheat)

Regional names for particular types of wheat: bulgur or bulgar wheat, chilton, couscous, dinkel, durum, einkorn, farro, fu, kamut, semolina, spelt, triticale (a hybrid of wheat and rye), triticum

Items sometimes made from wheat or containing a little wheat: baking powder, cereal binder, cereal filler, cereal protein, cereal starch, edible starch, food starch, hydrolyzed plant protein, hydrolyzed protein, hydrolyzed vegetable protein, modified food starch, modified starch, starch, textured vegetable protein, vegetable protein, vegetable starch

Assume that bread, crackers, crispbread, pastry, pasta, and noodles are made from wheat, unless definitely labeled otherwise (and read the label in detail, too, because a little wheat is often added to items such as rye bread and crackers).

Note that buckwheat is not wheat at all—it is not even a cereal. Nor does it commonly affect celiacs, as is sometimes claimed, though a few celiacs may develop an intolerance reaction to it, through eating it very regularly.

For more information on avoiding gluten, see p. 177.

Yeast

Items usually made from yeast: leavening

Items sometimes made from yeast: hydrolyzed plant protein, hydrolyzed vegetable protein

Labeling loopholes

Manufacturers do not have to include on the label
- any ingredients used in an earlier manufacturing process; for example, yeast used to make bread for breadcrumbs, or bread used to inoculate blue cheeses with mold—this can leave minute traces of gluten in the cheese.
- residues left by substances used during processing, such as wheat flour used to dust processing lines or prevent dried fruits from sticking together. Manufacturers do not need to declare these residues (sometimes called "incidental additives") on the label because the substance serves no function in the final product and is present in amounts that are considered insignificant. The vast majority of people with celiac disease or food allergy will tolerate such microscopic traces, but the most sensitive individuals may not. Some celiacs are affected even by food additives manufactured from cereals (see p. 177).
- incidental ingredients used in flavorings. Flavorings are covered by the terms *spice*, *natural flavor*, and *artificial flavor*. The incidental ingredients they might contain include wheat, milk, corn, or potato. All would be present only in trace amounts—not enough to be a problem for most people, but they could affect extremely sensitive individuals. Spice can also include garlic oil, a rare cause of allergies. Pressure is being exerted on U.S. and Canadian government agencies at present to make these labels more accurate and informative.

Take care when traveling abroad, because labeling laws vary from one part of the world to another. You can access information on this via the Internet (see p. 255).

"May contain" labels

Labels reading "Contains peanut ingredients" or "May contain nut traces" are springing up like weeds on packaged food. Similar labels relating to sesame, milk, and eggs are also starting to appear.

Allergy sufferers, suddenly unable to eat brands of breakfast cereal, candy, and other foods that they formerly enjoyed, feel very frustrated about this development. Many suspect that these labels are often just a defensive tactic—warning off consumers with food sensitivity when the chance of the food's containing the allergen is actually very small. The danger is that some allergy sufferers may stop taking the labels seriously. Teenagers, in particular, are increasingly dismissive of "May contain" labels, and this is a huge worry for parents.

Could the need for "May contain" labels be eliminated altogether with more careful factory procedures? The problem here is that, with nuts, perfect cleaning of production machinery is extremely difficult. Most machines have nooks and crannies in which a nut from one production process can become lodged, only to free itself later during the making of a non-nut product. It is quite possible that someone could encounter a whole nut, or substantial pieces of nut, in a non-nut product. That is why no one with nut allergy, even if it is relatively mild, should disregard "May contain nut traces" labels.

Some makers of confectionery and cookies have now set up dedicated nut-free production lines, with stringent precautions to avoid any possibility of contamination. This allows them to market products that are guaranteed nut-free. If you cannot purchase these locally, you may be able to order them by mail or over the Internet (see p. 255).

Note that packaged foods that have been produced on nut-free production lines in the past can be switched to different production lines that necessitate a "May contain nut traces" label.

In some cases, a product is manufactured in two separate places, one of which is nut-free, while the other is not. Consequently, the same product may sometimes be sold with a "May contain" label and sometimes without. Don't disregard these labels, however illogical they might seem.

Packaging errors

As most people with food allergy are now aware, ready-made foods sometimes go out in the wrong packaging. Alarming cases that have occurred in recent years include hazelnut yogurts labeled "Toffee yogurt," and vegetable casseroles containing nuts sold in packages intended for Vegetable Lasagne (no nuts).

Manufacturers are increasingly aware of the hazards, and when mistakes are discovered, medical information web sites and organizations such as the Food Allergy Network (FAN) in the U.S., the Anaphylaxis Network of Canada, and the Canadian Food Inspection Agency are quickly informed, so that they can alert allergy sufferers.

Belonging to such an organization, and/or checking web sites regularly (you don't have to join in order to use the web site), is definitely recommended for anyone with food allergy. (See p. 255) for the contact details.) However, you should bear in mind that no information service can protect you completely from this hazard. The odds against it are high, but one day you might just be the unlucky person who first discovers a packaging error by suffering an allergic reaction to packaged food. To protect your-

When is a nut not a nut?

Those with nut allergies often worry about eating nutmeg and coconut. In fact, allergic reactions to these are rare. People with nut allergy are no more likely to react to nutmeg or coconut than anyone else.

Tiger nuts or chufa nuts are not nuts at all, but the roots of a sedge plant—they are most unlikely to cross-react with true nuts.

Peanuts, botanically speaking, are not true nuts at all. They are legumes. There can be cross-reactions with soy and/or lupin (proceed very carefully with this novel food ingredient) but reactions with other legumes are rare. Cross-reactions with tree nuts such as almonds and Brazils, are quite common however (see p. 15). Many people with peanut allergy can in fact eat tree nuts, but they should be aware that a cross-reaction could develop at some stage.

Because cross-reactions between tree nuts are so common, doctors tend to speak simply of "nut allergy." However, it is possible to be allergic to one type of tree nut, without being allergic to others.

self as much as possible, take these precautions:

• Always check that the food in the package looks like the photograph on the package.

• Double-check, when you serve the food, by noting the conspicuous ingredients of the meal (carrots, for example) and ensuring that they are indeed on the list of ingredients—any discrepancy should make you suspicious.

• Note the smell and appearance of any ready-made food, before you taste it. Do this even for very simple things such as flavored yogurts.

• Take only a very tiny mouthful at first, and if you have any tingling of the lips or mouth, stop eating immediately (this is helpful for true food allergy only, not for celiac disease).

• Be especially cautious about vegetarian food if you are allergic to nuts or soy.

Latex in food

People with latex allergy may react to very small traces of it in food. This sometimes occurs with packaged food or restaurant food that has been prepared by workers wearing latex gloves. On one occasion, a highly allergic individual reacted to a water glass that had been handled by someone wearing latex gloves. The amounts of latex involved are minuscule, and only affect those with severe latex allergy. However, there is a strong case for workers handling food to wear non-latex gloves, especially with the rise in cases of latex allergy.

There are also reports of people with latex allergy reacting (usually very mildly) to cold-seal adhesives in food wrappers, such as those used for ice cream. The reaction only occurs if the wrapper actually touches the lips or mouth.

Gluten-free and wheat-free diets

Eve's apricot and apple dessert

When it comes to making bread and cakes, wheat has some remarkable cooking properties that nothing else can match. Its characteristic proteins, called **gluten**, form very strong elastic threads. These make a stringy dough that can be stretched and stretched as the bread rises. As a result, the bubbles of gas given off by the yeast or baking powder are all embraced by the dough, giving an open, airy consistency to the finished product.

Have no illusions—without wheat flour you cannot make a crisp baguette or featherlight blueberry muffins. If you are able to eat rye, then rye flour makes a pretty good substitute, because it also contains gluten, though not as much as wheat flour does. But a gluten-free diet excludes rye, too (see p. 177), and then baking definitely becomes a challenge.

Even on a gluten-free diet, however, you can still make several perfectly edible, even delicious, types of bread and cake. The secret, especially with bread, is to accept that the texture is going to be different from wheat-based bread but to add enough interesting flavors to give the finished product its own special character. The gluten-free bread you make at home will taste vastly better than the pale and unappetizing commercial substitutes—and at a fraction of the price.

Wheat-free and gluten-free bread tends not to keep as well as regular bread, so make a batch of small loaves and freeze some of them. You can slice them before freezing and then extract and defrost a few slices at a time, as needed. Bread that is not frozen should be kept in a plastic bag in the refrigerator. Even when kept in this way, the bread gets rather dry and tough after a few days and will benefit from being toasted. Try spreading it with butter, margarine, or solidified olive oil (see p. 183) *before* putting it under the broiler—this revives bread far better than ordinary toasting.

Pastry making without wheat is also a challenge (see p. 180), but cakes and other sweet items are much less of a problem. As long as you accept the limitations of nonwheat flours, cakes can be made perfectly well using gluten-free flours. With the right culinary tricks, you can even make a light, fluffy sponge cake (see pp. 180–81).

If you have an allergy or intolerance to other foods besides wheat, the recipes here can be adapted accordingly. For example, commercial egg replacers (see p. 186) can be used in place of eggs, and milk substitutes (see p. 183) can replace cow's milk.

Wheat-free diets

This section is for people with an allergy or intolerance reaction to wheat. Those with celiac disease should read the section on gluten-free diets.

In devising a successful diet for yourself, you need to take account of two factors:

1 How sensitive are you? If you have a true allergy (see p. 62) to wheat, you may be very sensitive and need to avoid even the tiniest amount of wheat. But if you are just intolerant of wheat (see pp. 74–6), you probably won't react to such small amounts, so you don't need to be so careful.

2 Are you sensitive only to wheat, or do you also react to related cereals, namely rye, barley, and oats? Some people have to avoid these as well, because of cross-reactions (see p. 14).

Those who are highly sensitive to wheat and have cross-reactions to related cereals need to follow the same kind of diet as the most sensitive celiacs (see Gluten-free diets). Ready-made gluten-free foods (such as bread and biscuits) can be useful, and they should be safe for you, unless you are ultrasensitive.

People who don't have any cross-reactions to related cereals can tolerate the following:

- rye bread and rye crackers, as long as they are 100 percent rye—always double-check. If you buy rye bread from a local bakery, and it is unlabeled, make sure the staff understand that you must always have 100 percent rye bread. Ask them to tell you if they ever change the recipe—and jog their memories about this from time to time.
- beer—as long as it is brewed using barley. Most beer is, but watch out for German Weissbier, which is made from wheat.
- oatcakes, as long as they don't contain wheat flour or bran. Check the label carefully.

Gluten-free diets

A gluten-free diet is more restrictive than a wheat-free diet, since gluten is also found in rye, barley, triticale, and spelt. All these must be carefully avoided.

At one time, this list would have included oats as well, but new research suggests that the proteins found in oats, called **avenin**, are sufficiently unlike gluten to be safe for many celiacs. If you have celiac disease, you *must* have medical approval before eating oats. Only people who are healthy and doing well on a gluten-free diet should try oats, and they should not eat more than one small serving (less than 1¾ ounces/50 grams) per day. It is vital that the oats be grown, harvested, transported, milled, and packaged separately from all wheat to avoid contamination.

Various flours are used to make gluten-free breads, including flours derived from rice, potatoes, soybeans, and buckwheat (not a true wheat). These special flours are sold in health-food stores, and can also be bought mail-order. In some cities you can find chickpea flour and gram flour in Indian grocery stores. There are also special gluten-free bread mixes available in both health-food stores and pharmacies, but these almost always contain soy, and it is best to avoid eating too much soy (see p. 71).

Celiacs who are extremely sensitive to gluten and have to avoid all traces of it should be very careful about ready-made food. These are just some of the unexpected sources of gluten:

- Thickeners and stabilizers sometimes contain traces of gluten. These additives are widely used in ready-made foods.
- A number of food additives (including caramel, citric acid, dextrin, mono- and di-glycerides, gum base, malt, malt flavoring, maltodextrin, maltose, monosodium glutamate, and vegetable gum) are manufactured from wheat, barley, or oats. Although the amount of gluten/avenin they contain is extremely small, it can affect a few celiacs.
- Barley enzymes, used to make rice milk, some brands of soy milk, soy sauce, and miso, can leave minute traces of gluten in the finished product. Blue cheese can also contain minute traces of gluten (see p. 174).
- Whisky and gin—both grain-based spirits—can contain gluten. So can distilled white vinegar. (These will affect only the most sensitive celiacs, whereas beer must be avoided by all celiacs, since it is made from barley.)
- Flavorings and spices in packaged food can include tiny quantities of wheat flour (see p. 174).
- Wheat flour may be used as an aid to food preparation, leaving tiny residues in the food (see p. 174).
- Nonwheat flour may be delivered to the manufacturing plants, or transferred from one area to another, through hoppers or vacuum tubes that have previously been used for wheat flour. Very low levels of contamination can occur in these ways, sufficient to affect those celiacs who are extremely sensitive. This is one problem with gluten-free foods (see below), unless they are made in dedicated gluten-free manufacturing plants.
- "Gluten-free" products bought outside North America may not be suitable for the most sensitive celiacs. The international standard is "not more than 200 parts per million"—this is less stringent than the standards used in the U.S. and Canada. Only Sweden has U.S.-style standards. (However, it is not true, as one major U.S. celiac support group claims, that European gluten-free products can contain up to 3 percent gluten. Levels are much lower than this and are safe for most celiacs.) The United States, Australia, and several European countries allow the use of purified wheat starch in gluten-free baked products, which may contain minute traces of gluten. Canada does not allow this.

There is a great deal of useful detailed information about gluten in food on the Internet, but there is also some very misleading information on one particular web site.

Wheat-free baking powder

Some brands of baking powder contain a little wheat flour. You can make your own wheat-free version by mixing 2 oz (60 g) baking soda with 4½ oz (130 g) cream of tartar and 2 oz (60 g) of a nonwheat flour. Sift together thoroughly.

The following recipes give the nearest cup equivalent to the metric measurements.

Brown bread

This mixture of buckwheat and potato flour makes a light-textured bread that is also good toasted.

PREPARATION TIME: 15 minutes, plus about 1 hour rising time

COOKING TIME: about 35 minutes

MAKES: 1 large loaf

2½ cups (250 g) buckwheat flour
2 cups (250 g) potato flour
1 teaspoon salt
1 package quick-rising active dry yeast
2 tablespoons (25 g) butter
1 tablespoon molasses
1 extra-large egg, beaten

Stir together the flours, salt, and yeast in a large bowl. Using your fingertips, rub in the butter. Add the molasses and egg, and mix to a soft dough with 1 cup (225 ml) tepid water. Transfer to a large buttered bread pan, wrap in a plastic bag and leave in a warm place for about 1 hour, or until the mixture has risen to the top of the pan. Meanwhile, preheat the oven to 425°F/220°C.

Bake until risen and firm to the touch, about 35 minutes. Remove from the pan and tap the bottom—it should sound hollow. If not, return to the oven for 5 minutes more. Let cool in the pan 10–15 minutes, then turn out onto a rack to cool completely.

Variation: Many different kinds of flavorings can be added to this bread. Try seeds such as poppy seeds, mustard seeds, caraway seeds, and onion seeds (Indian stores usually stock these with their spices). Sunflower seeds and sesame seeds—either plain or lightly toasted—are also good. A combination of black olives, sun-dried tomatoes, and a pinch of mixed herbs makes a Mediterranean-style bread.

Seeded rice bread

This delicious "nutty" textured loaf is yeast-free as well as wheat-free. It is good as toast.

PREPARATION TIME: 30 minutes

COOKING TIME: 40 minutes

MAKES: 1 small loaf

¾ cup (150 g) long-grain brown rice, well rinsed
¾ cup (100 g) rice flour
1¼ cups (100 g) rolled oats, ground to a fine meal in a food processor
1 teaspoon wheat-free baking powder
1 teaspoon salt
⅓ cup (50 g) sunflower seeds
3 tablespoons flax seed
1 large, slightly underripe pear, peeled, cored, and coarsely grated
2 extra-large eggs, beaten
2 tablespoons vegetable oil
4 tablespoons buttermilk, plain yogurt, milk, or milk substitute

Cook the rice in plenty of boiling water for 15–20 minutes until tender. Drain thoroughly and let cool slightly.

Preheat the oven to 400°F/200°C.

Combine all the ingredients in a large bowl. Then transfer the dough to a small, well-greased bread pan and bake until slightly risen, golden, and firm to the touch, about 40 minutes. Let cool slightly in the pan, then turn out onto a cooling rack. Leave to cool completely. Serve cut into thick slices.

Banana loaf

This semisweet bread is yeast-free as well as gluten-free. It is good for packed lunches—and it makes good toast.

PREPARATION TIME: 10 minutes

COOKING TIME: about 1 hour

MAKES: 1 large loaf

4 medium-ripe or underripe bananas
2½ cups (300 g) brown rice flour

7 tablespoons (100 g) butter, softened
2 tablespoons wheat-free baking powder
2 extra-large eggs
1 cup (225 ml) milk or soy milk

Preheat the oven to 350°F/180°C. Butter a large bread pan and line the bottom with parchment paper. Peel and cut up the bananas and place in a food processor with the remaining ingredients. Blend until thoroughly mixed, then transfer the mixture to the prepared pan. Bake until risen and firm to the touch, about 1 hour. Let cool slightly in the pan, then turn out onto a rack and leave to cool completely.

Rich herb bread

A tasty and nutritious bread made with herbs and olive oil.

PREPARATION TIME: 20 minutes

COOKING TIME: 30–40 minutes

MAKES: 1 small loaf

1 cup (110 g) chickpea or gram flour
1 teaspoon honey
2 tablespoons olive oil
1 teaspoon salt
1 unripe pear, peeled and grated
¾ cup plus 2 tablespoons (200 ml) boiling water
2 large eggs
½ onion, finely chopped
fresh herbs (thyme, tarragon, or marjoram)

Preheat the oven to 350°F/180°C. In a large bowl, stir together the flour, honey, olive oil, salt, and grated pear. Then pour the boiling water over the mixture and stir in. Separate the eggs into two bowls. Beat the yolks thoroughly and stir into the cooled flour mixture, along with the onion and herbs. The mixture should now be the consistency of heavy cream. If too thick, add a little more water.

Beat the egg whites until soft peaks form, then carefully fold into the flour mixture. Pour into a small well-greased bread pan and bake 30–40 minutes until firm to the touch.

Crispy millet skillet cakes

Tasty and filling, these are popular with children. They make no pretense of being bread, but are an excellent substitute for breakfast toast or a lunchtime sandwich. They are free from yeast, milk, and eggs, as well as wheat. They can be frozen and then fried without thawing for a quick meal.

PREPARATION TIME: overnight soaking, plus 30 minutes
COOKING TIME: about 40 minutes
MAKES: about 20 small skillet cakes

1 heaping cup (225 g) millet
1 teaspoon salt
½ cup (150 g) peanut butter (or cashew, pecan, or other nut butter)
1 teaspoon sesame seeds, toasted until golden
vegetable oil for frying

Rinse the millet and soak overnight. Rinse again to remove the starch, drain, and add 2 cups (600 ml) water plus the salt. Boil gently over low heat for 20 minutes, or until the water is absorbed.

While still hot, add the nut butter and sesame seeds. Mix together well, using a potato masher to break up the millet.

While the mixture is still warm, roll into small balls between the palms of your hands, then flatten. Fry the cakes in oil in a skillet over low heat about 20 minutes, or until the outside is golden and crunchy. Serve with fruit or a salad.

Cumin and coconut griddle cakes

This savory variation on pancakes makes a good substitute for bread. The griddle cakes are delicious served warm from the pan. When cold, they can be reheated in a moderate oven (350°F/180°C) for 5 minutes if required. They can be frozen.

Seeded rice bread

PREPARATION TIME: 25 minutes
MAKES: about 27 griddle cakes

¾ cup plus 2 tablespoons (100 g) chick-pea or gram flour
¾ cup (100 g) rice flour
1 teaspoon wheat-free baking powder
1 tablespoon ground cumin
⅛ teaspoon salt
1 extra-large egg
1¼ cups (300 ml) coconut milk
vegetable oil for frying
To serve:
choose from skinned and chopped fresh tomato mixed with a little freshly chopped cilantro, or fried mushrooms with chopped scallions and parsley moistened with a little crème fraîche.

Mix the dry ingredients together in a bowl, then beat in the egg and coconut milk to give a thick batter. Set a large nonstick griddle over medium heat. Generously oil the surface of the pan, then drop well-spaced tablespoons of the mixture into the pan.

Cook until the edges of the cakes start to form bubbles and the base of each is golden, then carefully turn and cook on the other side until golden. Keep warm, covered with a clean dish towel, while you make the rest.

Pressed prune and walnut bread

Serve warm, spread with butter or with one of the suggested savory mixtures.

Variation: For sweet griddle cakes, omit the cumin and add 2½ tablespoons (30 g) granulated sugar and either a sweet spice such as cinnamon, or the finely grated zest of a lemon or orange.

Pressed prune and walnut bread

Based on a traditional Spanish recipe, this is delicious served with cheese, or as a snack on its own.

PREPARATION TIME: 10 minutes, plus overnight cooling
COOKING TIME: 1 hour
MAKES: 1 9-inch (23-cm) loaf

2¼ pounds (1 kg) ready-to-eat pitted prunes
1 cup (200 g) walnut or pecan halves
1 cup (50 g) brown rice flour
2 extra-large eggs, beaten

Preheat the oven to 325°F/170°C. Combine the ingredients in a bowl. Press into a greased round 9-inch (23-cm) cake pan, cover with greased foil, and bake 1 hour. Place a heavy weight on top and leave to cool overnight before unmolding. Cut into thick slices using a serrated knife.

Walnut macaroons

Lemon surprise pudding

Millet "tabbouleh"

Tabbouleh is a salad from the Middle East that is traditionally made with cracked wheat. Millet makes a very good wheat-free alternative. This dish can be useful for packed lunches.

PREPARATION TIME: about 7 minutes
COOKING TIME: about 25 minutes
MAKES: 4–6 servings

scant 1 cup (175 g) millet
7 tablespoons olive oil
salt and pepper
3 tablespoons lemon juice
3 tablespoons each freshly chopped mint
    and flat-leaf parsley
2 scallions, finely chopped

Put the millet in a saucepan with 1 table-spoon of the oil and cook over medium heat, stirring, for 2–3 minutes until lightly toasted. Stir in 1½ cups (350 ml) boiling water and simmer uncovered until the water is absorbed and the millet seeds are just cooked, about 20 minutes. Transfer to a bowl, stir in the rest of the oil and season generously. Stir in the lemon juice, forking it through the mixture. Leave to cool, then stir in the herbs and scallion.

Variations: Add finely chopped tomato, cucumber, bell pepper, or dried apricots.

Wheat-free tart shell

Make an unfilled tart shell as suggested below. Alternatively, you can chill the pastry dough, then grate it roughly over a savory or sweet pie filling.

PREPARATION TIME: 15 minutes, plus
    30 minutes freezing
COOKING TIME: about 20 minutes
MAKES: 1 8-inch (20-cm) tart shell

1 cup (125 g) fine cornmeal
½ cup (50 g) chickpea or gram flour
¼ cup (25 g) arrowroot
⅓ cup (25 g) ground almonds
6 tablespoons (75 g) butter or vegetable
    shortening
white of 1 large egg, lightly beaten

Stir the dry ingredients together in a bowl. Using your fingertips, rub the butter and dry ingredients together until the mixture resembles coarse meal. Stir in the egg white and mix to a soft dough. Press the pastry dough evenly into an 8-inch (20-cm) fluted tart pan and leave in the freezer for a minimum of 30 minutes. In the meantime, preheat the oven to 400°F/200°C. Bake the tart shell for about 20 minutes, until lightly golden.

Variation: For sweet pastry, add 2 table-spoons granulated sugar.

Rich cheese crackers

These crisp, mouthwatering crackers are good to serve with drinks.

PREPARATION TIME: 20 minutes
COOKING TIME: about 25 minutes
MAKES: 20 crackers

½ cup (55 g) soy flour
⅓ cup (40 g) potato flour
6½ tablespoons (40 g) rice flour
½ cup/1 stick (115 g) butter, softened
1 cup (115 g) grated Cheddar cheese
1 extra-large egg, separated
2 tablespoons celery or poppy seeds

Mix the flours together in a bowl, then work in the butter, cheese, and egg yolk to give a firm dough. Roll into 20 balls. Lightly whisk the egg white and turn the balls in it until lightly coated, then dip in the seeds to lightly coat.

Space the balls well apart on baking sheets and press down firmly to flatten. Bake in a preheated oven at 400°F/200°C for about 25 minutes until golden. Cool slightly, then transfer to a wire rack and leave until completely cold and crisp.

Sponge cake

The secret of this sponge cake's lightness is in the beating. A trail of the batter, falling from the beaters onto the surface, should remain visible there for at least 30 seconds. Then it's time to add the flour.

PREPARATION TIME: 25 minutes
COOKING TIME: 25–30 minutes

4 extra-large eggs
½ cup plus 2 tablespoons (125 g)
    superfine sugar
heaping ½ cup (75 g) chickpea or gram
    flour
¼ cup (50 g) cornstarch
4 tablespoons (50 g) butter, melted
To serve:
jam, whipping cream (optional), and
    confectioners' or superfine sugar

Preheat the oven to 375°F/190°C. Butter a 9-inch (23-cm) springform cake pan and line the bottom with parchment paper. Using a handheld electric mixer, beat the eggs and sugar in an ovenproof glass bowl over a saucepan of simmering water until thick and mousselike. This should take about 10 minutes.

Sift together the chickpea flour and cornstarch and fold into the egg mixture, one-third at a time, until completely incorporated. Then fold in the melted butter.

Transfer to the prepared pan and bake until risen and golden, about 25 minutes. Let cool slightly, then remove from the pan and leave to cool on a rack. When cold, split in half and spread jam and, if desired, whipping cream between the layers. Dust the top with confectioners' or superfine sugar.

Walnut macaroons

These cookies are good with coffee. If desired, put walnut halves on only half of them, then put together in pairs with coffee, chocolate, or orange buttercream, or whipped cream. Store in an airtight container and fill just before serving.

PREPARATION TIME: 15 minutes
COOKING TIME: about 45 minutes
MAKES: 24 macaroons

rice paper
2 large egg whites
1 cup (100 g) confectioners' sugar
1 cup (100 g) finely chopped walnuts
finely grated zest and juice of ½ small, unwaxed lemon (if waxed, wash the lemon well in hot water)
24 walnut halves

Preheat the oven to 300°F/150°C. Line a large baking sheet with rice paper. In an ovenproof bowl, beat the egg whites until stiff peaks form, then fold in the confectioners' sugar, chopped walnuts, grated lemon zest, and lemon juice. Place the bowl over a saucepan of simmering water and stir until the mixture is slightly stiffened, about 10 minutes.

Drop spoonfuls of the mixture onto the rice paper, spacing them apart. Top each with a walnut half. Bake until risen but still slightly chewy, about 45 minutes. Leave to cool on the baking sheet, then trim away the excess rice paper.

Lemon surprise pudding

The surprise is in the two layers. You end up with a creamy lemon sauce topped with a delicate sponge cake.

PREPARATION TIME: 20 minutes
COOKING TIME: about 45 minutes
MAKES: 4–6 servings

4 tablespoons (50 g) butter
½ cup plus 2 tablespoons (125 g) granulated sugar
2 extra-large eggs, separated
¼ cup (25 g) cornstarch
¼ cup (25 g) fine cornmeal
finely grated zest and juice of 2 unwaxed lemons (if waxed, wash lemons well in hot water)
1 cup (250 ml) milk
To serve:
confectioners' sugar

Preheat the oven to 350°F/180°C. Put the butter and sugar in a bowl and add 1 tablespoon hot water. Cream until pale and fluffy. Beat in the egg yolks, then the cornstarch and cornmeal. Slowly stir in the grated lemon zest, lemon juice, and milk. The mixture may appear to have curdled, but this is normal.

In a separate bowl, beat the egg whites until soft peaks form, then fold into the lemon mixture. Transfer to a 1-quart (1-liter) dish and place in a roasting pan. Pour boiling water around the dish and bake until risen and just firm to the touch, about 45 minutes. Dust the top with confectioners' sugar and serve immediately.

Eve's apricot and apple pudding

PREPARATION TIME: 30 minutes
COOKING TIME: about 45 minutes
MAKES: 4–6 servings

14-oz (400-g) can apricot halves in fruit juice
2 medium-size apples, peeled and thickly sliced
¼ cup (50 g) granulated sugar
Topping:
½ cup/1 stick (125 g) butter, softened
½ cup plus 2 tablespoons (125 g) granulated sugar
2 extra-large eggs
1½ cups (125 g) ground almonds
1 teaspoon wheat-free baking powder
½ cup plus 2 tablespoons (50 g) sliced almonds
To serve:
light cream or whipped cream

Pour the juice from the apricots into a pan, add the apple and sugar, and cook gently about 5 minutes, until the apple is soft. Remove from the heat and stir in the apricots. Transfer to a 1-quart (1-liter) baking dish.

Preheat the oven to 350°F/180°C. Cream the butter and sugar together until pale and fluffy, then beat in the eggs one at a time. In a separate small bowl, stir together the ground almonds and baking powder, then fold into the butter, sugar, and egg mixture. Spread over the fruit. Sprinkle the top with sliced almonds and bake until risen, golden, and just firm to the touch, about 45 minutes. Serve with light cream or whipped cream.

Avoiding milk and lactose

Fruit lassi

There are two quite distinct reasons for avoiding milk: either to avoid **milk proteins** or to avoid **lactose**, the sugar found in milk. It is important not to confuse these two because the details of the avoidance diet required are different. Only a few people need to avoid both milk proteins *and* lactose.

Diarrhea and gas in response to drinking milk, but few other symptoms, usually indicates a reaction to lactose—but a response to milk proteins could be an alternative explanation. If it is a reaction to lactose, this may be due to either primary lactase deficiency or secondary lactase deficiency—your doctor can order tests to make an exact diagnosis (see p. 79). Note that a bout of diarrhea, however caused, often produces a *temporary* lactose intolerance (secondary lactase deficiency).

Any symptoms other than (or in addition to) diarrhea and gas strongly suggest a reaction to milk proteins. This might be a true allergy, another type of immune reaction to milk (see pp. 72–73), or an idiopathic intolerance reaction (see pp. 76–77). In theory, skin tests should identify true allergic reactions to milk proteins. Unfortunately, skin tests are not infallible, and it is possible to have a genuine allergy but give negative skin tests. This is especially common with babies (see p. 65 and p. 69). There are no accurate tests that can confirm intolerance reactions to milk proteins.

It is possible to have sensitivity to both milk proteins *and* lactose.

If tests do not give you a definitive answer, you may have to try both types of diet and see which one works. Remember that lactose intolerance may be only temporary.

Avoiding milk proteins

If you have a sensitivity reaction to cow's milk proteins, then you need to avoid
- milk and all milk-based drinks including Lactaid and Lacteeze milk; drops and tablets to reduce lactose (see Using lactase replacers, p. 183) are safe and could be used with a tolerated milk (for example, goat's milk)
- cream and yogurt
- all kinds of cheese, including cottage cheese and cream cheese (some people may be able to tolerate Norwegian brown cheese called Gjetøst, which is made with milk whey)
- white sauce, béchamel sauce, and other creamy sauces
- custard, rice pudding, and other milk-based puddings
- almost all homemade cakes, cookies, pancakes, and pastry
- some bread, rolls, waffles
- almost all chocolate
- casein, caseinate, and lactalbumin in packaged foods (see p. 173); you may be able to tolerate whey but experiment cautiously

Unless your sensitivity is fairly mild, you will also need to avoid
- butter
- most kinds of margarine (they generally contain milk derivatives, but some, for example canola and corn oil margarines, are milk-free—health-food stores and most supermarkets carry these.)

As long as you do not have a severe allergy to milk, you should be able to tolerate clarified butter. Make this by melting butter over a low heat, pouring it into a glass jar, and leaving it to cool in the refrigerator. The milk proteins will settle to the bottom, and be visible as whitish granules—eat only the clear butter above this level.

Alternatively, put olive oil into a wide-necked container and place in the freezer. It will solidify and can be used as a spread in place of butter.

A few people with cow's-milk allergy can tolerate sheep's milk and possibly (but less commonly) goat's milk. However, most people must avoid these as well. (There are also rare individuals who are allergic to goat's and sheep's milk but not to cow's milk.)

There are many substitutes for cow's milk now available, such as soy milk, almond milk, rice milk, and hazelnut milk. Your local supermarket may carry these, if not, try a health-food store. All can be used in place of ordinary milk when cooking.

Milk-free margarine can be used in recipes that call for butter. Soy yogurt and cream make reasonable substitutes for ordinary yogurt and cream.

Avoiding lactose

If you have lactose intolerance, you must either avoid (if very sensitive) or limit
- milk, unless lactose-reduced (Lactaid, Lacteeze, for example); milk-based drinks
- cream
- most kinds of yogurt, especially mild yogurt. A very strong, acidic yogurt may contain little lactose. (The bacteria that make the yogurt turn lactose into lactic acid, so the more acidic it is, the less lactose it contains.)
- cottage cheese and Norwegian brown cheese, or Gjetøst. Other kinds of cheese are usually so low in lactose that they are tolerated. Only those people with extreme lactose intolerance need to avoid all cheeses.
- white sauce, béchamel sauce, custard, rice pudding, and other milk-based puddings
- lactose in medicines. Lactose powder is used in many tablets and capsules, to add bulk. The amount used can be sufficient to provoke symptoms in some people with lactase deficiency. Certain dry powder asthma inhalers also contain lactose (see p. 162), and a small amount may be swallowed: this will affect you only if you have *severe* lactase deficiency.

Soy-based products, rice milk, and nut milks are lactose-free. Sheep's milk, goat's milk, and other milks (including human breast milk) all contain lactose.

Using lactase replacers

Many people with lactose intolerance are able to eat a more varied diet by using **lactase replacers**. These provide a temporary supply of the missing enzyme, lactase (see p. 79), which helps out by digesting the lactose in milky foods. Lactase replacers must be taken at the same time as the milky food, and are effective only for that one meal. The more lactose there is in the meal or snack, the more of the lactase replacer you need—trial and error is the only way of working out how much you need for a particular food. The replacer can also be added to milk and left overnight. There are a number of different brands of lactase replacers now available, and it is worth trying out several. Some people find that they are sensitive to an added ingredient in some brands. Sources of lactase replacers include pharmacies, health-food stores, and specialist suppliers—these can be located through the Internet (see p. 255).

White sauce

A white sauce is the base of many dishes. In this recipe the flavor of the wine and stock goes well with chicken, vegetables, or fish.

PREPARATION TIME: 5 minutes
COOKING TIME: 7–8 minutes
MAKES: about 2½ cups (600 ml)

4 tablespoons (50 g) milk-free margarine
⅓ cup (50 g) all-purpose flour
¾ cup plus 2 tablespoons (200 ml) hard cider or dry white wine
1¾ cups (400 ml) vegetable or chicken stock
1 bay leaf, salt and pepper

Melt the margarine in a small saucepan and stir in the flour. Cook, stirring, over low heat for 1 minute, then stir in the hard cider or wine followed by the stock. Add the bay leaf and simmer 5 minutes, stirring occasionally, until thickened and smooth. Season to taste.

Variations: Add about 6 tablespoons finely chopped herbs, for example parsley, chives, tarragon, or chervil; or add English or French mustard and lemon juice.

Sweet white sauce

PREPARATION TIME: 5 minutes
MAKES: about 1¼ cups (300 ml)

2 tablespoons (25 g) cornstarch
2 tablespoons (25 g) granulated sugar
1¼ cups (300 ml) apple cider or white grape juice
4 tablespoons soy milk
2 tablespoons (25 g) milk-free margarine

In a saucepan, stir together the cornstarch and sugar with a little of the juice to give a smooth paste, then stir in the rest of the juice and bring to a simmer over low heat. Simmer 1–2 minutes, stirring all the time, then stir in the soy milk and margarine.

Variations: Add milk-free chocolate to taste, or rum or brandy; or add 4–6 pieces finely chopped preserved ginger and 1–2 tablespoons of the syrup.

Crêpes

Soy milk has a slightly thicker consistency than cow's milk and therefore more is used in this crêpe recipe than would be needed in a traditional one.

PREPARATION TIME: 25 minutes

MAKES: about 16 small crêpes

1 cup (150 g) all-purpose flour, sifted
2 extra-large eggs
pinch salt
scant 2 cups (450 ml) soy milk
vegetable oil or milk-free margarine, for
    frying
To serve:
top with lemon juice and granulated sugar,
    or maple syrup

Put the flour, eggs, salt, and soy milk in a food processor and process until smooth. Alternatively, place the flour, eggs, and salt in a bowl, and slowly beat in the soy milk to form a thin batter.

Heat 1 teaspoon oil or margarine in a 7-inch (18-cm) nonstick skillet and swirl until hot. Pour in just enough batter to cover the bottom of the pan and cook until golden. Turn and cook on the other side until golden. Repeat this process until all the batter is used up.

Serve topped with lemon juice and sugar, or with maple syrup.

Apple and frangipane tart

The combination of apple and almond is delicious. Serve freshly baked. It can also be eaten cold, but if possible, warm it a little before serving.

PREPARATION TIME: 30 minutes

COOKING TIME: about 1 hour

MAKES: 8 servings

Pastry dough:
1¼ cups (175 g) all-purpose flour, sifted
7 tablespoons (100 g) milk-free margarine,
    softened
2 tablespoons (25 g) granulated sugar

Filling:
4 tablespoons (50 g) milk-free margarine
1 heaping cup (100 g) ground almonds
½ cup plus 1 tablespoon (100 g) granu-
    lated sugar
2 large egg yolks
2 tablespoons dark rum, brandy, or
    orange juice
2 large apples
4 tablespoons apricot jam

In a bowl, combine the flour, margarine, and sugar together with 1 tablespoon cold water to make a soft dough. Roll out and use to line a deep 8-inch (20-cm) fluted tart pan. Chill while you prepare the filling.

Preheat the oven to 375°F/190°C. Beat together the margarine, ground almonds, ½ cup (100 g) sugar, egg yolks, and rum. Peel, core, and roughly chop one apple and stir into the mixture. Spread this in the tart shell. Core and thinly slice the remaining apple and arrange the slices on top. Sprinkle the top with the remaining sugar and bake about 1 hour until risen and golden. Let cool slightly, then warm the apricot jam gently in a saucepan and brush over the top.

Coconut rice pudding with mango

Based on a Thai recipe, this is an excellent flavor mix. The rice pudding will become thicker the longer it cooks and also as it cools. Make sure the mango is ripe.

PREPARATION TIME: 45 minutes

COOKING TIME: 30–40 minutes

MAKES: 6 servings

1⅔ cups (175 g) short-grain rice, rinsed
4–6 tablespoons (50–75 g) sugar
1 quart (1 liter) rice milk
1¾ cups (400 ml) coconut milk
Serve with:
1 extra-large ripe mango, peeled and diced
toasted coconut shreds

Put the rice in a large saucepan with 4 tablespoons (50 g) of the sugar and the rice milk and coconut milk. Stirring, bring to a simmer. Simmer gently 30–40 minutes, stirring occasionally, until the rice is cooked and the milk absorbed. Add the extra sugar if desired. Serve warm or cold, topped with mango and toasted coconut.

Variation: Replace the mango with the seeds from 1–2 pomegranates and the toasted coconut with skinned pistachio nuts.

Baked strawberry custard with strawberry sauce

This recipe is originally from Spain. Use very ripe strawberries for an intense flavor.

PREPARATION TIME: 30 minutes

COOKING TIME: 20–25 minutes

MAKES: 6 servings

½ cup (100 g) granulated sugar
4 tablespoons Muscat or other sweet wine
1 teaspoon lemon juice
12 oz (350 g) strawberries, hulled and
    sliced (about 2 cups)
4 extra-large eggs, beaten
whole strawberries, to decorate
Sauce:
8 oz (225 g) strawberries, hulled and
    chopped (about 1½ cups)
2 tablespoons confectioners' sugar
2 tablespoons Muscat or other sweet
    wine

Preheat the oven to 325°F/170°C. Place six 5-fluid-ounce (150-ml) ramekins in a small roasting pan. If you plan to unmold the custards, oil the ramekins lightly.

Put the sugar, wine, lemon juice, and sliced strawberries in a saucepan, and heat gently to dissolve the sugar. Bring to a boil and cook, uncovered, for 5 minutes. Let cool slightly, then purée in a food processor. Beat into the eggs. Press through a strainer, then pour into the ramekins. Pour boiling water around the ramekins and bake in the center of the oven 20–25 minutes until lightly set. Remove the ramekins from the pan and leave to cool. Chill if desired.

Combine all the sauce ingredients and process until smooth. Pass through a fine strainer. Serve in the ramekins with a little sauce poured on top and decorated with a whole strawberry; or carefully unmold, pour a little sauce on top, then decorate with a whole strawberry.

Variation: Oil the ramekins. Dissolve ½ cup (100 g) granulated sugar in 4 tablespoons water over gentle heat, then cook to a rich caramel without stirring. Pour a little caramel into each ramekin, then continue as above. Pour the wine for the sauce into the pan used to make the caramel and warm gently to dissolve any leftover caramel, then continue with the sauce as for the main recipe.

Frozen vanilla dessert
A cross between sorbet and ice cream.

PREPARATION TIME: 30 minutes, plus
    freezing time
MAKES: 4–6 servings

1 vanilla bean, split
¾ cup (150 g) granulated sugar
2 cups (500 g) plain soy yogurt

Place the vanilla bean and sugar in a saucepan with 1¼ cups (300 ml) water. Dissolve over gentle heat, then bring to a simmer and simmer 20 minutes. Leave to cool. Remove the bean, scrape the seeds from it, and return them to the syrup. Beat in the soy yogurt and freeze.

You will get the best texture by using an ice-cream machine. Alternatively, freeze in a plastic container, then remove from the freezer and beat the mixture until smooth (you can do this in a food processor). Return to the freezer. Repeat this process once or twice.

Baked strawberry custard

Variations: Add 3½ oz (100 g) melted semisweet chocolate, or 2 tablespoons instant espresso coffee dissolved in 2 tablespoons hot water. Alternatively, melt ½ cup (100 g) granulated sugar over a gentle heat until it turns to a rich caramel. Then add ⅔ cup (100 g) unblanched almonds and stir with a metal spoon until they start to pop. Transfer to an oiled pan and leave to set. Crush roughly and add to the basic mixture.

Fruit lassi
Make this refreshing Indian drink with frozen fruit if you wish, in which case don't use ice water—cold water will do.

PREPARATION TIME: 10 minutes
MAKES: about 6 cups (1.5 liters)

2 cups (500 g) plain soy yogurt
4–6 tablespoons (50–75 g) sugar
8 oz (225 g) berries (raspberries, straw-
    berries, blackberries, or blueberries), or
    equivalent weight chopped mango,
    peach, or papaya
2½ cups (600 ml) ice water

Put all the ingredients in a food processor and process until smooth.

Frozen vanilla dessert

Banana and strawberry shake
A special treat for a child who cannot have milk.

PREPARATION TIME: 5 minutes
MAKES: about 2½ cups (600 ml)

2 large, very ripe bananas
6 oz (150 g) fresh strawberries
1½ tablespoons olive oil
pinch of nutmeg or other spice
about ¾ cup (200 ml) water

Peel the bananas and roughly chop. Place all the ingredients in a blender and process until very smooth. Add more water if mixture is too thick. Serve immediately, or cover tightly and store in the refrigerator.

Variations: Use a nectarine or a peeled peach instead of strawberries; or use coconut milk (available in cans) instead of olive oil, and the flesh of a small mango, or half a large mango, instead of the strawberries.

Egg-free diets

Tempura-style vegetables

There is nothing quite like an egg, especially when it comes to baking. Egg protein is the magical ingredient that holds together a pancake and creates the light and delicate structure of layer cakes, soufflés, mousses, and meringues.

Unfortunately, egg protein is also a potent allergen for some people and a cause of intolerance reactions for others.

Egg replacers, designed mainly for cake making, are one answer. They can be purchased in grocery stores or your local health-food store. These are protein-rich mixes that aim to simulate the structural properties of eggs, not the flavor. Recipes are usually supplied with the replacer, and it is best to follow these recipes at first for guaranteed results. Once you have the feel of using the egg replacer, you can experiment with substituting it for eggs in other cake recipes.

Note that these egg replacers make no attempt to simulate the richness and characteristic taste of eggs. You may need to add extra butter or other fats to your cake mix if using egg replacers. Vanilla extract can also improve the flavor of an egg-free cake.

Can cooking make eggs safe?

When a hot oven turns liquid egg white into a hard meringue, or a sloppy cake mix into a firm sponge cake, the visible effect is due to the egg protein being fundamentally changed.

Heating changes the basic molecular structure of the egg protein in a process called **denaturing**. Whereas natural egg protein is liquid, denatured egg protein is solid.

When the structure of the molecule changes, *some* of the epitopes (the key features recognized by allergy antibodies—see box on p. 15) are obliterated. For a few allergy sufferers—those who react only to the epitopes affected by denaturing—thorough heating can therefore turn the egg allergen into a harmless substance.

If eggs are hard-boiled, the denaturing process occurs to the fullest possible extent. Consequently, some people with egg allergy can eat hard-boiled eggs without ill effects. However, the same people still react badly to lightly cooked eggs, such as those in a soufflé or omelette, because with partial cooking the denaturing process is incomplete.

Cakes made with eggs pose an interesting question—given that the cooking process for cakes is prolonged and at a high temperature, could they, too, be safe? This is something that medical researchers have not so far investigated systematically. In practice, however, it has been observed that many children with egg allergy can tolerate traces of egg in baked goods. Your allergist can advise you about this.

If you want to test your response to hard-boiled eggs, you must do so under full medical supervision with resuscitation equipment available. Those who find that they can tolerate hard-boiled eggs might then want to test their reaction to cakes made with eggs. Again, there must be medical supervision for the test in case of severe life-threatening reactions. You will, of course, have to convince your allergist that such a test is worthwhile.

Egg protein is not unique in being susceptible to denaturing—most proteins can be denatured: some by heat, some by other means. But only in a few cases (tuna fish, and fresh fruits and vegetables—see p. 110) does denaturing tend to destroy the allergenic epitopes.

Very rarely, changing the structure of a protein by cooking may actually *create* an allergenic epitope where none exists in the raw protein. There have been cases of individuals with an allergy to cooked fish but not raw fish, and to pecans in cookies but not uncooked pecans. Roasting peanuts makes them much more allergenic.

Tempura-style vegetables

Beer is a good alternative to eggs for making a batter that is light and crisp in texture. Have all the vegetables prepared and ready, so you can cook and eat the tempura as quickly as possible.

PREPARATION TIME: about 45 minutes
MAKES: 4–6 servings

about 1 pound (400–500 g) prepared vegetables, cut into bite-size pieces—choose from red bell pepper, asparagus, broccoli, scallion or red onion, carrot, zucchini, baby corn, small white mushrooms, eggplant
vegetable oil, for deep-frying
1 cup (150 g) sifted self-rising flour, plus extra for coating vegetables
1 teaspoon salt
2 tablespoons sesame seeds
1 cup (250 ml) Japanese beer
Serve with:
soy sauce and dry sherry mixed together, or sweet chili sauce

Toss the prepared vegetables in flour until lightly coated, then shake off the excess. Heat the oil in a large, deep saucepan over medium heat until a cube of bread dropped in turns brown in 30 seconds.

In a bowl, stir together the measured flour, salt, and sesame seeds. Then quickly stir in the beer—don't worry if the mixture is slightly lumpy. Dip the vegetables in the batter, a few pieces at a time, and then immediately into the hot oil. Cook until crisp and golden.

Drain on paper towels, and keep warm in a hot oven until all the vegetables are cooked.

Serve with a dipping sauce made of equal quantities soy sauce and dry sherry, or sweet chili sauce.

Caramelized onion quiche

Feta in a crisp cornmeal jacket

Caramelized onion quiche

This makes a good substitute for egg-based quiches. The long, slow cooking of the onions is important to bring out their natural sweetness.

PREPARATION TIME: 45 minutes
COOKING TIME: 30 minutes
MAKES: 6–8 servings

2¼ pounds (1 kg) onions, thinly sliced
4 tablespoons olive oil
1 cup (125 g) finely chopped bacon
1 teaspoon caraway seeds
salt and freshly ground black pepper
12 oz (350 g) prepared bread dough or puff pastry dough

Put the onions in a very large saucepan with the oil, bacon, and caraway seeds and cook over medium heat, stirring occasionally, for about 30 minutes until the onions are soft and lightly caramelized. Season generously with salt and pepper.

Preheat the oven to 450°F/230°C. Roll out the dough thinly and use to line a deep 9½-inch (24-cm) fluted quiche pan. Prick the base with a fork, then fill with the onion mixture. Bake on a baking sheet for 30 minutes or until the dough or pastry is crisp and golden.

Variations: For a vegetarian version, replace the bacon with 4½–6 oz (125–175 g) crumbled goat cheese, or 4½–6 oz (125–175 g) diced smoked tofu, or a handful of pitted black olives.

Feta in a crisp cornmeal jacket

The oil must be very hot to ensure a crisp crust for these delicious croquettes.

PREPARATION TIME: 15 minutes
MAKES: 4 servings

vegetable oil, for deep-frying
7 oz (200 g) feta cheese, cut in 8 fingers
⅓ cup (40 g) cornmeal
To serve:
salad of your choice, for example, tomato, cucumber, red onion, and flat-leaf parsley, or roasted and peeled red bell peppers and arugula

Pour the oil into a deep, heavy saucepan and set over high heat. Meanwhile, soak the cheese fingers in ice water for about 1 minute, then roll in the cornmeal until evenly coated. Deep-fry 1–2 minutes until crisp and golden. Drain on paper towels, and serve at once on top of the salad.

Egg-free crêpes

Lemon cake

Tofu filling for a quiche

This very simple mixture makes an egg-free, milk-free substitute for a quiche filling. It can be flavored with a variety of tasty ingredients. This recipe makes enough filling for an 8-inch (20-cm) pastry shell.

PREPARATION TIME: 5 minutes
COOKING TIME: about 25 minutes

9 oz (250 g) tofu, natural or smoked
1 tablespoon wine vinegar or lemon juice
1 tablespoon dried mixed herbs
¾ cup plus 2 tablespoons (200 ml) soy milk

Blend all the ingredients together in a blender and pour into a prebaked pastry shell. Bake in a preheated oven at 375°F/190°C for about 25 minutes until set.

Variations: Add flavoring ingredients of your choice, such as sautéed chopped onion; chopped cooked ham with scallion; roasted vegetables, such as carrot, bell peppers, and tomatoes; or cooked spinach, beet, or broccoli.

Tofu mayonnaise

This mayonnaise can be flavored with chopped herbs, roasted garlic purée, or tomato paste. It will keep, covered, in the refrigerator for 3–4 days.

PREPARATION TIME: 5 minutes
MAKES: about 1 cup (250 ml)

3½ oz (100 g) silken tofu
½ cup (100 g) thick plain yogurt
1 teaspoon English mustard powder
1 tablespoon Dijon or grainy mustard
salt and pepper
ice water

Put all the ingredients, except the salt and pepper, in a food processor and process until smooth. Season to taste with salt and pepper, and thin as required with ice water.

Avocado dressing

Avocado's rich texture makes it an excellent dressing. This one is delicious with tomato salads, shrimp, and grilled steak. Always keep it tightly covered, otherwise it will discolor quickly.

PREPARATION TIME: 5 minutes
MAKES: about 1 cup (250 ml)

1 medium-size ripe avocado
4 tablespoons vegetable oil
2 tablespoons white wine vinegar, lemon juice, or lime juice
salt and pepper
ice water

Halve, seed, peel, and chop the avocado. Put all the ingredients, except the salt and pepper, in a food processor and process until smooth. Season to taste with salt and pepper, and thin as required with ice water.

Variation: Replace the avocado with a mango or 2 red bell peppers.

Egg-free crêpes

Crêpes can be served with both savory and sweet fillings.

PREPARATION TIME: 25 minutes
MAKES: about 10 small crêpes

¾ cup (100 g) all-purpose flour
2 tablespoons arrowroot
1¼ cups (300 ml) milk
vegetable oil or melted butter for frying
Serve with:
maple syrup, jam, or lemon juice and granulated sugar

In a bowl, stir together the flour and arrowroot. Then stir in the milk to make a smooth batter. Leave to rest, ideally for 20 minutes.

Heat 1 teaspoon oil or butter in a 7-inch (18-cm) nonstick skillet and swirl until hot or melted. Pour in 2–3 tablespoons batter or enough just to cover the bottom of the pan, swirling it as it falls into the pan to make a thin layer. Cook until golden on one side, then carefully turn and cook the other side until golden. Repeat this process until all the batter is used up. Make sure the oil is hot to ensure a crisp result every time.

For a sweet crêpe, serve topped with maple syrup, jam, or lemon juice and granulated sugar.

For savory crêpes, fill with a white sauce flavored with smoked fish and shrimp, or ham and parsley; or a ratatouille mixture with goat cheese.

Raspberry and sherry syllabub trifle

Syllabub makes an unusual topping for this trifle with its egg-free shortbread base, but if you prefer, top with vanilla pudding and whipped cream. Vary the fruit with the seasons—poached pears, fresh oranges, cooked cranberries will all be suitable.

PREPARATION TIME: 15 minutes
MAKES: 6–8 servings

6 oz (175 g) shortbread cookies
6 tablespoons medium or sweet sherry
8 oz/about 2 cups (225 g) fresh rasp-
    berries, or frozen raspberries, thawed
1¼ cups (280 ml) whipping cream
¼ cup (50 g) granulated sugar
Serve with:
¼ cup (25 g) toasted sliced almonds

Roughly break up the shortbread and put in the bottom of a clear glass bowl or any decorative serving bowl. Sprinkle with 2 tablespoons of the sherry, then top with the raspberries. Whip the cream and sugar with the remaining sherry until it holds its shape, then pile on top of the raspberries. Chill until required, then, just before serving, sprinkle with sliced almonds.

Lemon cake

This cake has a tangy lemon flavor and a slightly dense texture. Serve it plain or with fresh berries and whipped cream or crème fraîche. Try replacing the lemon with orange. Any leftovers can always be used for trifle.

PREPARATION TIME: 15 minutes
COOKING TIME: about 1 hour

7 tablespoons (100 g) butter, melted
1 cup (200 g) granulated sugar
1⅔ cups (250 g) self-rising flour, sifted
1 tablespoon baking powder
1 cup (250 g) plain yogurt
finely grated zest and juice of 1 small
    lemon

1–2 tablespoons milk (optional)
Serve with:
confectioners' sugar

Preheat the oven to 350°F/180°C. Butter an 8-inch (20-cm) springform cake pan and line the bottom with parchment paper. Put all the ingredients in a large bowl and beat to a firm dropping consistency. You may need to add 1–2 tablespoons milk, depending on the type of yogurt you have used. Transfer to the prepared pan and smooth out the batter. Bake 50–60 minutes until risen and just firm to the touch.

Let cool in the pan about 30 minutes, then transfer to a rack to cool completely. Dust the top with confectioners' sugar.

Fig, orange, and pear shortcake

PREPARATION TIME: 20 minutes
COOKING TIME: 45 minutes
MAKES: 8–10 servings

1¼ cups (250 g) chopped dried figs
finely grated zest and juice of 1 medium-
    size orange
1 ripe pear, chopped
1⅔ cups (250 g) all-purpose flour, sifted
¾ cup/1½ sticks (175 g) butter
½ cup (100 g) firmly packed light brown
    sugar
1 teaspoon ground cinnamon
Serve with:
confectioners' sugar (optional)

Put the figs, grated orange zest, orange juice, and chopped pear in a pan and cook over medium heat until the figs and pear are soft and all the juice has been absorbed. Preheat the oven to 350°F/180°C. Put the flour, butter, sugar, and cinnamon in a food processor and blend (or rub together with your fingertips) until the mixture resembles fine crumbs. Add 1 tablespoon cold water and blend

until the mixture forms rough lumps. Press half the shortcake mixture onto the oiled bottom of a 7½-inch (19-cm) springform cake pan. Spread the fruit mixture on top, then finish with the remaining shortcake mixture, pressing down lightly.

Bake 45 minutes. Let cool in the pan, then remove. Dust with confectioners' sugar, if desired, and serve in wedges.

Variations: Replace the figs and pear with dried apricots and an apple; or replace the figs with prunes, dried pineapple, or dried mango.

Date and walnut loaf

PREPARATION TIME: 15 minutes
COOKING TIME: about 45 minutes
MAKES: 1 large loaf

1¼ cups (250 g) chopped dried dates
½ cup (100 g) firmly packed light brown
    sugar
2 tablespoons (25 g) butter
2 teaspoons apple-pie spice
1 teaspoon baking soda
1 cup (250 ml) boiling water
about 2 cups (275 g) self-rising flour,
    sifted
¾ cup (100 g) walnut pieces
Serve with:
butter (optional)

Preheat the oven to 350°F/180°C. Grease a large bread pan and line the bottom with parchment paper. Put the dates in a large bowl with the sugar, butter, spice, and baking soda and mix together. Then stir in 1 cup (250 ml) boiling water. Let cool slightly, then beat in the flour and stir in the walnuts. Transfer the mixture to the prepared pan and smooth out. Bake until risen and just firm to the touch, about 45 minutes.

Let cool in the pan about 30 minutes, then transfer to a rack to cool completely. Serve in slices, with or without butter.

Yeast-free diets

Raisin, hazelnut, and rosemary bread

In terms of its traditional use, yeast is not really a food at all—it is a hardworking microscopic fungus that has helped us with the complex business of food preparation for many thousands of years. The ability of yeast to turn sugar into alcohol and carbon dioxide has long made it a valuable ally in the manufacture of both bread and alcoholic drinks.

In addition to this traditional use, yeast has, in the past 50 years, found a role as a true foodstuff in the form of yeast extract. This derivative of yeast, with its strong flavor, has also become an ingredient of stock cubes and "meat extracts."

These are the most concentrated sources of yeast—foods to which yeast has been deliberately added (such as bread and wine), plus the modern extracts of yeast.

People with an intolerance reaction to yeast usually need to avoid only these concentrated sources of yeast.

In addition to foods containing domesticated yeasts, there are many foods that become naturally colonized by wild yeasts, invisible scavengers whose spores are in the air all around us, like microscopic wasps, just waiting for a jar of jam to be opened.

Wild yeasts quickly multiply on fruit, fruit juice, jam, or any other sweet food, but unless the food is obviously fermenting (that is, it smells "yeasty"), the levels of yeast it contains are relatively low. However, there are also some foods that contain wild yeasts in quite significant numbers even before you buy them. They include dried fruits, such as raisins, and manufactured foods that are fermented or that take a while to mature, such as soy sauce, yogurt, and cheese. In all cases, the slow production process inadvertently encourages the growth of wild yeasts. Again, the amount of yeast in the food is far less than that in bread, wine, or yeast extract.

Do these wild yeasts matter? For people with yeast intolerance, probably not. In the case of true allergies to yeast, however, wild yeasts might be sufficiently numerous in some foods to evoke a reaction from the most highly sensitive individuals.

Wild yeasts may also be significant for anyone with the controversial condition known as yeast overgrowth (see p. 82). Some people suffering symptoms that suggest this condition, and who are following a no-yeast-no-sugar diet (see p. 205), may need to avoid all sources of yeast for a while, including foods containing wild yeast.

Concentrated sources of yeast include
- beer, wine, hard cider, and vinegar
- all brands of yeast extract
- yeast-based vitamin tablets; also most B-complex vitamin tablets unless specified as "yeast-free"
- stock cubes, gravy powder, and "meat extracts"
- bread (except unleavened breads such as soda bread, pita bread, matzos, and chapatis)
- all other forms of leavened dough, including breadsticks, pizza, rolls, croissants, English muffins, doughnuts, Danish pastries, and coffee cake
- some packaged food labeled with synonyms for yeast (see p. 174)

Low-level sources of yeast include
- distilled drinks such as whisky, gin, brandy, and vodka
- spirit (distilled) vinegar
- yogurt, sour cream, buttermilk, cheeses
- dried fruits and vegetables
- sauerkraut and possibly other pickled vegetables
- soy sauce, miso, tofu
- black tea (but not jasmine tea or other green teas)
- any fruit if unpeeled; very ripe fruit even though peeled
- jam, fruit juice, or wine that has been open for a while; many commercial fruit juices contain a significant amount of yeast—dead but still allergenic—at time of purchase
- leftovers that have been in the refrigerator for more than two days

Note that some of the ingredients in the recipes that follow, such as raisins, yogurt, and sun-dried tomatoes, may contain wild yeasts and therefore are not suitable for people on a strict yeast-avoidance diet. You should adjust the recipes to suit the kind of diet you are following.

Homemade stock

A good stock is essential for many recipes. As well as being yeast-free, this homemade stock tastes a great deal better than canned bouillon.

PREPARATION TIME: 10 minutes
COOKING TIME: about 2 hours (or 45 minutes in a pressure cooker)
MAKES: about 4 cups (850 ml)

1 carrot
1 onion
1 celery stalk
fresh thyme or other herbs, or a bouquet garni of dried herbs
remains of a carved roast chicken
6 cups (1.5 liters) water
salt and pepper
dry sherry (optional)

Peel and slice the vegetables. Tie the fresh herbs together with fine string. Put the chicken in a large saucepan, cover with the water, and add the vegetables and herbs. Bring to a boil, then cover and simmer for 2 hours. (Or cook in a pressure cooker at high pressure for 45 minutes using only 4 cups [1 liter] water.)

Allow to cool a little, then pass through a coarse sieve and discard everything except the liquid. When cold, skim off the fat from the surface. Heat until liquid again, then add salt and pepper to taste, and a dash of sherry.

This stock will keep in the refrigerator for 2–3 days or in the freezer for 3 months. When freezing, allow room in the container for expansion. If space is limited in the freezer, simmer the stock further until very concentrated, then freeze in an ice-cube tray to make frozen stock cubes. Once frozen, transfer to a plastic freezer bag.

Easy brown bread

This yeast-free brown bread is based on a traditional Irish soda bread recipe.

PREPARATION TIME: 10 minutes
COOKING TIME: about 45 minutes
MAKES: 2 small loaves

4 cups (450 g) whole-wheat bread flour
1½ cups (225 g) white bread flour
2 teaspoons baking soda
1 teaspoon salt
2–2½ cups (500 ml) buttermilk, or plain yogurt thinned with a little milk to make the same volume

Preheat the oven to 400°F/200°C. Put the whole-wheat flour in a large bowl. Sift the white flour, baking soda, and salt into the bowl and mix well. Stir in the buttermilk and enough cold water to make a fairly soft dough. Divide the dough in half and put into two small buttered bread pans. Bake until risen and firm to the touch, about 45 minutes.

Remove the loaves from the pans and tap the bottoms—they should sound hollow. If not, put back in the pans and return to the oven for 5–10 minutes more. Turn out onto a rack and let cool.

Corn bread with chilies

Seeded muffins

Layered potato pizza

Corn bread with chilies

If you need to avoid wheat as well as a yeast, try replacing the wheat flour with rice flour or soy flour—or use all cornmeal.

PREPARATION TIME: 20 minutes

COOKING TIME: about 45 minutes

MAKES: 1 large round loaf

1 cup (150 g) all-purpose flour, sifted
1¼ cups (150 g) fine cornmeal, sifted
3 tablespoons (40 g) granulated sugar
½ teaspoon salt
4 teaspoons baking powder
2 large mild fresh chili peppers (red or
    green), seeded and finely chopped
4 tablespoons olive oil
1 extra-large egg, beaten
⅔ cup (150 ml) plain yogurt
⅔ cup (150 ml) milk
¼ cup (25 g) grated Cheddar cheese
    (optional)

Preheat the oven to 400°F/200°C. Stir all the dry ingredients together in a large bowl. Then stir in the chilies and remaining ingredients, and mix to a soft dough. Transfer the dough to a buttered 8-inch (20-cm) round cake pan, sprinkle with cheese if desired, and bake until risen, golden, and firm to the touch, about 45 minutes.

Let cool in the pan 15–20 minutes.

Turn out onto a rack and let cool completely.

Variations: Add ⅔ cup (100 g) sautéed chopped bacon, ⅔ cup (100 g) corn kernels, or 4 finely chopped scallions.

Raisin, hazelnut, and rosemary bread

This bread is delicious with cheese. It is best eaten within a day or two of making. Store in a cool place.

PREPARATION TIME: 1 hour soaking time plus
    15 minutes

COOKING TIME: about 45 minutes

MAKES: 1 large loaf

⅔ cup (100 g) golden raisins
⅔ cup (150 ml) hot tea
about ¾ cup (175 ml) plain yogurt
⅓ cup (50 g) skinned hazelnuts
1⅔ cups (250 g) all-purpose flour, sifted
2 cups (250 g) whole-wheat flour
3 tablespoons (40 g) granulated sugar
2 teaspoons baking powder
1 teaspoon baking soda
1 teaspoon salt
1 extra-large egg, beaten
4 teaspoons freshly chopped rosemary

Soak the raisins in the hot tea for about 1 hour, then drain, reserving the tea. Add

enough yogurt to make 1¼ cups. Preheat the oven to 400°F/200°C.

Roughly chop the hazelnuts and toast in a dry skillet. Mix the dry ingredients together in a large bowl, then stir in the egg, yogurt mixture, raisins, and rosemary. Work to a firm dough. Knead lightly and shape into a long loaf. Transfer to a greased baking sheet and cut slashes in the top of the loaf. Bake until risen and firm to the touch, about 45 minutes. Turn out onto a rack and let cool.

Mediterranean scones

Serve fresh with butter or cream cheese.

PREPARATION TIME: 15 minutes

COOKING TIME: 15 minutes

MAKES: 9 scones

1 extra-large egg
5 tablespoons milk
1⅔ cups (250 g) self-rising flour
1 teaspoon baking powder
¼ teaspoon ground black pepper
4 tablespoons (50 g) butter
⅓ cup (50 g) chopped sun-dried
    tomatoes
⅓ cup (50 g) chopped pitted green olives
1 tablespoon freshly chopped basil,
    or 1 teaspoon dried basil, or other
    herbs to taste
milk, for brushing (optional)

3 tablespoons grated Parmesan cheese
(optional)

Preheat the oven to 425°F/220°C. Beat the egg and milk together in a bowl and set aside. In a separate bowl, sift the flour and baking powder together, then add the pepper. Using your fingertips, rub the butter and dry ingredients together until the mixture resembles fine crumbs. Stir in the tomatoes, olives, basil, and egg-and-milk mixture, and mix to a fairly soft dough.

Roll out the dough to about 1 inch (2–3 cm) thick on a lightly floured surface. Stamp out 2½-inch (6-cm) rounds and place on a baking sheet. If desired, brush the top of each scone with milk and sprinkle with 1 teaspoon grated Parmesan before baking. Bake until risen, golden, and firm to the touch, about 15 minutes. Let cool on a rack.

Seeded muffins

These seeded muffins make an excellent breakfast.

PREPARATION TIME: 15 minutes
COOKING TIME: 20 minutes
MAKES: 12 muffins

2 cups (300 g) self-rising flour, sifted
2 teaspoons baking powder
pinch salt
½ cup (100 g) firmly packed light brown
  sugar
⅓ cup (50 g) pumpkin seeds
⅓ cup (50 g) sunflower seeds
2½ tablespoons sesame seeds
2½ tablespoons flax seeds
4 tablespoons vegetable oil, or 4 table-
  spoons (50 g) butter, melted
2 extra-large eggs, beaten
¾ cup plus 2 tablespoons (200 ml) milk
Serve with:
marmalade or jam

Preheat the oven to 400°F/200°C. Put all the ingredients in a large bowl and beat

until evenly mixed. Line muffin cups with paper cases and spoon in the batter until two-thirds full. Bake until risen and just firm to the touch, about 20 minutes. Serve warm (not hot) with marmalade or jam.

Spinach and cheese polenta

Polenta can be served warm with a "sloppy" consistency to go with broiled or stewed meat or vegetables, or left to set firm—as in this recipe—then sliced and fried. Delicious served with baked ham, bacon, or tomatoes.

PREPARATION TIME: 30 minutes
MAKES: 10–12 slices

9 oz (250 g) fresh spinach (about
  2½ cups)
2 tablespoons (25 g) butter
1 small onion, finely chopped
3¾ cups (850 ml) boiling water
1½ cups (175 g) cornmeal
1 teaspoon salt
½ teaspoon ground nutmeg
2 egg yolks
¾ cup (40 g) mixed freshly grated
  Parmesan and aged Cheddar cheeses

Wash the spinach, remove the stems, squeeze out the excess water, and finely chop. Heat the butter in a skillet, then add the onion and sauté over medium heat for 5 minutes until soft. Increase the heat and add the spinach. Cook until the spinach has wilted and the liquid has disappeared. Add 3¾ cups (850 ml) boiling water, then slowly stir in the cornmeal, salt, and nutmeg. Cook over low heat 10 minutes, stirring frequently, until thickened. Remove from the heat and stir in the egg yolks and cheeses. Let cool slightly, then transfer to a small plastic-wrap-lined bread pan. There should be sufficient plastic wrap to allow it to be folded over the top of the pan. Shape the mixture and cover it with the plastic wrap. Leave until cold, then slice, and fry or broil.

Layered potato pizza

Layered sliced potatoes form the base for this "pizza."

PREPARATION TIME: 40 minutes
COOKING TIME: 25 minutes
MAKES: 3–4 servings

2¼ pounds (1 kg) waxy boiling potatoes
2 cloves garlic, minced (optional)
1 teaspoon finely chopped fresh rosemary
  or thyme
salt and freshly ground black pepper
3 tablespoons olive oil
14-oz (400-g) can crushed tomatoes
4½ oz (125 g) mozzarella cheese,
  thinly sliced
To serve:
fresh basil or arugula leaves

Peel and thinly slice the potatoes. Preheat the oven to 450°F/230°C. Then toss the potatoes with the garlic and herbs in a bowl, and season very generously with salt and pepper. Pour 2 tablespoons of the olive oil into a 12-inch (30-cm) nonstick skillet, and arrange the potatoes in overlapping slices. Cook over medium heat 10 minutes until lightly browned. Do not move the potatoes around, but allow them to stick together in a big, circular "pizza" base. Brush the remaining oil onto a baking sheet. Place the pizza base on this and bake 15 minutes until tender.

Meanwhile, cook the tomatoes over medium heat until all the liquid has evaporated, and season generously with salt and pepper. Spread the tomatoes over the potato base and top with the mozzarella. Return to the oven and bake about 10 minutes more. Sprinkle the top with fresh basil or arugula leaves, and serve.

Variations: After adding the mozzarella, top with classic pizza combinations, for example, anchovies and olives, pepperoni, or mushrooms and ham.

Elimination diet

An elimination diet is a method of diagnosing idiopathic food intolerance (see p. 74) and certain other forms of food sensitivity where indirect tests, such as skin tests, are unhelpful. The principle of the elimination diet is very simple. It begins by removing from the body every food that could possibly cause a reaction and seeing if this produces a symptom-free state. If it does, the elimination diet then presents the body with different foods, each in its pure form, to see which ones cause symptoms.

While the principle is simple, the practicalities of the elimination diet can be much more complex, and it is vital to understand all the details before you start. There is absolutely no room for "cheating" when following an elimination diet—one mouthful of cake is enough to ruin the whole thing. You need forward planning and a lot of self-discipline, backed by a good stock of the permitted foods for moments when hunger overcomes you. Some cooked foods, stored in the freezer in individual portions for quick defrosting, are a great help.

Doing an elimination diet incorrectly is not just a waste of time. Some people acquire new sensitivities during the diet, which may make it much more difficult to do a second elimination diet. So plan ahead, and get it right the first time.

The planning stage

First of all, start an accurate symptom diary. This will give you a precise picture of how bad things are now, before you try any dietary measures. A detailed daily record, covering a period of about two weeks, can be very useful, whether or not you actually do an elimination diet. It can serve as a baseline against which to judge the effects of any future treatment.

Before you begin an elimination diet, ask your doctor if the diet is safe for you. The more you know about elimination diets before talking to your doctor, the better. Read the next few pages before your appointment.

An elimination diet should never be tried during pregnancy or acute viral illness, and prescription medications should be continued unless your doctor advises otherwise.

There are some conditions in which, although an elimination diet can be very helpful, it should not be attempted without full medical supervision. Two main causes for concern exist:

- For people who are undernourished to start with, the elimination diet may be too demanding—it is difficult to eat enough calories during the first few weeks of the diet, unless an elemental diet is used as a supplement (see box on p. 196). If you are underweight, or have rheumatoid arthritis or Crohn's disease, the possible use of elemental diets is something you should discuss with your doctor.
- With certain diseases (see list that follows), *the testing stage may induce severe symptoms*. Sometimes these can be life-threatening and need immediate medical attention.

Medical supervision during food testing is recommended for anyone with these conditions:

- Crohn's disease—testing can bring on a prolonged relapse. Very small amounts of food should be tested initially, and the quantity slowly increased.
- brittle asthma—a culprit food can bring on a severe life-threatening asthma attack if it is eaten again after a period of avoidance.
- atopic eczema—after food avoidance, some children with eczema suffer quite severe immediate reactions on testing a food (see p. 198.)
- chronic urticaria (hives)—occasionally there is an immediate reaction to an offending food. It is advisable to test foods in very small portions (just a mouthful) at first. If there is no reaction whatever after four hours, a normal portion can be tested.

Note that an elimination diet is not suitable for anyone with true food allergy (see p. 62). If you have ever had an immediate reaction to any food, or any symptoms in the lips or mouth, testing foods can be dangerous. Caution is also necessary if you have ever reacted to a food with violent vomiting and/or diarrhea some hours after eating. This could be due to an infection, of course, but such symptoms can also, very rarely, result from true food allergy (see p. 64). Finally, if you have ever suffered anaphylaxis from any cause—not just food—the testing phase of an elimination diet might be risky. Ask your doctor's advice.

Once you have your doctor's permission to try the diet, work out how the stages of the diet will fit in with your life over the weeks or months ahead. Until it is over, eating food made by other people is virtually out of the question.

When eating away from home, you must either take prepared food with you or just eat very simple foods—such as permitted fruits or nuts. Think about the practicalities of carrying food for meals away from home.

Finally, devise the diet you will follow during the exclusion phase (see right), locate stores that sell the more unusual foods, and stock up on everything required. You will continue to eat a lot of these foods for the first few weeks of the testing stage, so

you may want to buy extra stocks and refrigerate them for longer storage, especially if the sources of supply are some distance from your home.

Note that food ingredients in medication could interfere with the results of the elimination diet. For example, if you are very sensitive to corn, the cornstarch that is added to many antihistamines and other drugs could generate some confusing reactions. Food-free medicines are available—talk to your pharmacist about this initially, then to your doctor if you need a different prescription.

The exclusion phase

During the first part of an elimination diet, you exclude all the foods that you normally eat, plus any closely related foods. For example, if you normally eat oranges, you should avoid all other citrus fruits, including lemons, limes, and grapefruit, even though you do not normally eat these. If you normally eat plenty of broccoli, you should omit all its relatives, such as cabbage, kale, and collard greens.

The best way to conduct the exclusion phase is not to follow a set menu, but to draw up your own list of permitted foods. This can include foods you have never eaten before and those you eat only infrequently.

The list should run to at least 10 items. One problem with an exclusion phase that consists of only two foods (as in the "lamb-and-pears" diet) is that you are bound to eat a huge amount of these foods. This is asking for trouble if you have a tendency to food intolerance, because you can quite quickly become sensitive to new foods if eating them in large amounts.

Your list of permitted foods should include:

Some starchy items. These are essential for keeping hunger at bay. Try some of the more exotic root crops, such as sweet potatoes, yams, taro, and cassava. They are available in some large supermarkets and in small stores catering to Indian, African, Chinese, and Caribbean communities. (Cook them as you would potatoes. In the case of cassava, it must be boiled, not baked.) You can also eat parsnips, turnips, chestnuts, and pumpkin. Tapioca, sago, buckwheat, millet, quinoa, and sorghum are other possibilities; a health-food store is a good source of some of these. Use rice, if it is not normally part of your diet. Do not include corn or cornmeal, even if you do not normally eat these—corn products are very widely used in packaged food, and sensitivity to corn is not uncommon.

Several fruits and vegetables that you don't normally eat. Exotic produce such as mangoes and okra can help a lot in keeping the diet tasty. Avocados, which are very rich and nutritious, can be included if you don't eat them often.

Some protein items. For meat eaters, this is the easy part—any meat that you don't normally eat is suitable. Consider turkey, duck, rabbit, or game, for example. (Soak rabbit meat in salt water overnight to get rid of the strong taste, if you dislike this.) Strict vegetarians have more problems here, since goat's milk, sheep's milk, and all birds' eggs are disallowed—their proteins are much too similar to those of normal milk and eggs. Soy products such as tofu should definitely be avoided, as should other legumes (beans and lentils) initially. Fortunately the exclusion phase is fairly brief, so a low intake of protein will not be disastrous. Including some nuts on your list of permitted foods will help, as these contain protein. If nuts are part of your normal diet, you may have to resort to rarely eaten kinds such as macadamias, cashews, or pistachios.

Elemental diets

An elemental diet is a powder that contains all the nutrients the human body needs but is free from the substances in food that provoke allergic and intolerance reactions. It is mixed with water to create a complete substitute for food. Originally designed for space travel, this totally synthetic form of sustenance is also known as "the astronaut's diet."

Used alone during the exclusion phase, elemental diets are the basis for the ultimate—and theoretically foolproof—elimination diet. They sustain you through the exclusion phase and continue to provide your basic diet during the testing phase.

For anyone with multiple food sensitivity, using an elemental diet circumvents the problem of finding 10 or more safe foods with which the elimination diet can begin.

Those who are underweight can also benefit from using an elemental diet, simply as a calorie-boosting supplement during the exclusion phase and testing phase.

Unfortunately, elemental diets taste fairly unpleasant and are quite expensive. You may need a prescription, so talk to your doctor. Ideally you should get an elemental diet that does not contain sucrose (sugar).

Some items that make good snacks. Nuts, pumpkin seeds, sunflower seeds, fresh fruit, and dried fruit are all useful for times when you are away from home or feel hungry between meals. At the outset of the diet, use only sulfite-free dried fruit—available from health-food stores. At a later stage, you can test ordinary dried fruit (all of which is treated with sulfite preservatives—see box on p. 207).

A cooking oil, preferably one that you have not used much in the past. Use this fairly liberally, to keep the calorie content of your diet at a reasonable level.

Note that this is a very plain diet—you eat the permitted foods and absolutely nothing else. You cannot use spices, herbs, or other flavorings. Salt is allowed, but sugar is out, as are tea, coffee, alcohol, and all soft drinks. You must drink only mineral water and pure juices from permitted fruits.

Don't use canned or precooked packaged versions of the permitted foods. Buy raw food and cook it yourself. The idea is to avoid food additives and other contaminants, such as those from the linings of cans.

Throughout this phase, and the next, you must be very careful not to eat too much of any one food. Never eat any food every day, and stay away from any food that you begin to develop a real passion for—this is often a bad sign in people with food intolerance. It is better to go a little hungry (as long as you are not underweight to start with) rather than binge on any of the permitted foods. Acquiring new sensitivities is all too easy.

Assuming you do have food intolerance, and you have excluded all the foods that affect you, there should be a complete clearance of symptoms within 7–10 days. The response is usually unmistakable. A partial or slight response is probably just a coincidence and should be discounted, except for people with rheumatoid arthritis (see below).

Be warned that you may feel a great deal worse before you get better. For those who do have food intolerance, the first 5–6 days of the diet can be very unpleasant—usually they suffer the same symptoms as before the diet, but far more severe.

Some conditions, such as Crohn's disease and rheumatoid arthritis, may require a longer exclusion phase, but there is no point in continuing beyond three weeks. Bear in mind that, if you have had rheumatoid arthritis for some years, structural damage to the joints may prevent a complete recovery. A partial but sustained improvement in the joints, accompanied by a distinct improvement in general health, suggests that food could well be playing a part in causing the disease and that it is worth going on to the testing phase.

Symptoms that are only intermittent, such as chronic urticaria or migraine, pose a special problem. You need to decide, before starting the diet, how long the exclusion phase should continue in order to give you a clear sign that your state of health is improved. A symptom diary is vital here. If, for example, your symptom diary shows that you sometimes have a week that is symptom-free but you never get through two weeks without an attack, then your exclusion phase should continue for two weeks.

You should go onto the testing phase only if you improve during the exclusion phase. If you do not improve, you have excluded the possibility of food intolerance, and can give up the diet.

The testing phase

This part of the diet, which is sometimes called the reintroduction phase, takes about 8 weeks. It requires careful observation of your symptoms, and constant self-discipline about everything you eat. You should not stop or delay the testing unless you are ill—it is vitally important to complete it as quickly as possible.

Foods have to be reintroduced one at a time, with a space between in which symptoms can be observed. It sounds simple, but this is where errors can easily occur.

During this phase, besides noting your symptoms daily, you should also record absolutely everything you eat.

For the first 2–3 weeks you should test foods that are unlikely to cause symptoms. Start by testing fruits, vegetables, and meats that you do not eat very often normally, but which you do like. If they pass the test, you can use them to vary your diet. This will make life much easier and reduce the risk of developing new sensitivities.

Next, test foods that you do eat reasonably often but not every day. Leave the most likely culprits—the foods you eat very regularly, such as wheat and milk products—until you have established a safe diet that contains at least 25 different foods. This safe and relatively varied diet should be the backdrop against which you test staple foods.

The testing procedure changes over time, because your sensitivity may decline as the diet progresses. During the first 8 weeks, you should test one food each day, eating a normal-sized portion for lunch or supper. A reaction to the food might occur quite soon after the meal, or some hours later. Any symptoms that occur within the following 24 hours should be provisionally attributed to that food.

Unfortunately, bowel symptoms can sometimes take longer to develop—up to 48 hours. This can confuse things when a new food is being tested every day.

There may also be uncertainty about intermittent conditions such as chronic urticaria. You may not be absolutely sure that the problem really responded to the exclusion phase. If so, when the symptoms recur during the testing phase, this may be due to a food, or it may just be a coincidence.

Should there be any doubt about which food caused a particular set of symptoms, cut out all the suspect foods for now, and retest them after a couple of weeks, using a three-day testing procedure (see below).

When a reaction does occur to a food, stop all testing and go back to the safe diet until you feel completely better. But don't wait too long before resuming testing. You need to get through most of the testing within eight weeks because, for some people, intolerance to the foods begins to fade after that. This does not mean that the intolerance has been "cured," unfortunately. A period of eating the food regularly will soon bring the problem back.

If you are still testing foods after eight weeks, you should change to **three-day testing**—eat a normal portion of the food every day for three days, stopping only if you get symptoms. Should you have no reaction to the food by the end of the fourth day, you can consider it safe. (But leave it out of your diet for at least another four days.)

There are some special procedures for testing certain foods:

• When you test wheat, even if it is quite early on, use the three-day test procedure (see above). Reactions to wheat can be very slow. (If you have rheumatoid arthritis, you should spend a full five days testing wheat, and eat it at least twice a day.) Don't use bread to test wheat because it contains yeast and other ingredients. A pure wheat cereal such as Shredded Wheat is good for testing—moisten it with fruit juice if you cannot have milk. Note that some people who react to whole-wheat bread or cereal are sensitive to the wheat germ, and can tolerate refined wheat, as in white bread and flour. For others, only white flour is a problem—they are usually reacting to additives in the white flour. Careful testing will sort out these issues.

• Test milk before cheese and butter. You may react to one but not the others. If you react to fresh milk, wait a few weeks, then test evaporated milk. Later, you can test goat's milk and then sheep's milk. Some people can tolerate these but must be very careful not to consume too much of them.

• You can test yeast using yeast extract or yeast-based B-vitamin tablets. Do this before you test mushrooms.

• At some point, test a canned food. This is to check for reactions to the lining material used on cans. Choose something that contains no other ingredients or additives, such as carrots. Test it first in a frozen or fresh form, so that you are sure you don't have a reaction to the food itself.

• Throughout the testing period, continue cooking all your own food from scratch. At a fairly late stage in the testing, when you have tested most foods, spend three days eating packaged food. The idea is to eat a wide range of different food additives all at once. Read the labels carefully (see p. 172) to check that all the food ingredients are ones that you have already tested and found safe. You are unlikely to react to these packaged foods, but if you do, you should then conduct tests with all the individual food additives. You may need some help from a dietitian for this (see p. 201).

Testing becomes more and more uncertain after 12 weeks. If you have not completed it by then, reintroduce all the untested foods. Should your symptoms come back, cut all those foods out again, then test them individually.

What next?

For anyone who recovers during an elimination diet and successfully identifies their problem foods, a period of complete abstinence from those foods follows. After about a year, it is worth testing the foods again, as the sensitivity may have subsided.

If, after a year or two, you find that a food no longer makes you ill, don't go back to your old ways—remember that you must eat the food only occasionally. Once every three or four days is a good rule of thumb for a food to which you were previously intolerant. You might get away with having it slightly more often than this, but never go back to eating it daily. If it starts to become your "favorite food" again—the thing you crave more often than anything else—watch out.

Good nutrition is an important issue for anyone avoiding certain key foods. If you have cut out all milk products, for example, you should probably be taking a calcium supplement, unless you eat a lot of other calcium-rich foods. Ask your doctor to refer you to a dietitian if you are on a restricted diet and feel you need help.

An elimination diet for children with eczema

Before putting your child on any kind of restricted diet, it is vital that you talk to your doctor. The risks of malnutrition are far higher for children, and there can be serious long-term consequences, such as stunted growth or impaired intelligence. You must therefore have medical consent and supervision for an elimination diet.

For young children with atopic eczema, there is rarely any need for a stringent elimination diet, such as that described on pp. 194–7. Children are usually sensitized to only one or two commonly eaten foods.

In the case of recently weaned infants, it is enough simply to cut out individual foods, one at a time. Avoid each food for two weeks, while observing symptoms carefully.

For older children a simple elimination diet, with an exclusion phase that avoids just the most likely culprits, works well.

The foods that you should exclude at the outset are
• any food that has given a positive prick test (see p. 69)
• any food that you think may have caused digestive symptoms, such as diarrhea, either now or in the past
• milk and all milk products
• eggs
• beef
• chicken
• citrus fruits (oranges, lemons, limes, grapefruit, and all similar fruit)
• food additives

If the child's skin is no better after a week of this diet, cut out the following foods also:
• peanuts and other nuts
• soy
• fish
• wheat
• tomatoes
• lamb
• corn

If there is no response after another week, food is unlikely to be contributing to the eczema.

For the testing phase, use three-day testing as described on p. 197 if you have fewer than 10 foods to test. Use one-day testing if you have more than 10 foods to test.

You should begin by testing a very small amount of the food, waiting 10 minutes for any symptoms (not just skin symptoms—the mouth or stomach may also be affected), then giving a little more if nothing has happened. Build up to testing a normal portion of the food.

A more cautious approach is required for children who give positive prick tests to foods or have a history of symptoms in the mouth or digestive tract. They are more likely to suffer severe symptoms in the lips, mouth, and throat—the type of reaction associated with food allergy. Emergency medical treatment may

Rare reactions

Very occasionally, atopic eczema sufferers on milk-avoidance diets develop a sensitivity reaction to calcium supplements. There is no scientific explanation for this, but it has been very well documented in two children. Should you encounter this problem, the answer may be some alternative natural source of calcium: sardines or other small fish, eaten whole, are one possibility, assuming your child will eat fish. A dietitian can advise on how much is needed per day.

There has also been one well-documented report of a child reacting to mineral water. When the water she usually drank was changed to another brand, her eczema cleared up. This is very unlikely to be a common problem.

be needed. You can see if there is any likelihood of a severe immediate reaction to foods by starting with a test on the face, and then the outer lip (see box on p. 23). If nothing happens, it is probably safe to go on to the next stage—giving the child a very small amount of the food to eat. However, you should have medical supervision for this procedure in the case of foods that gave positive skin tests. If your child has both *severe* eczema and additional symptoms (such as hives, or symptoms in the mouth or digestive tract) it may be advisable to have medical supervision when testing *all* foods.

Bear in mind that atopic eczema naturally fluctuates a great deal. To observe the effects of trying out a food, the child's skin should be in a steady state. That means being absolutely consistent about applying steroids and moisturizers, avoiding (for the period of testing) any stressful situations that could provoke a flare-up, not exposing the skin to sudden doses of irritants or airborne allergens, and keeping scratching under control. Be aware of other factors that could muddy the waters by provoking a flare of eczema—such as teething or a cold (see p. 44).

If certain foods are identified as provoking eczema symptoms and you cut them from your child's diet, a nutritional supplement may well be needed. Ask your doctor to refer you to a dietitian.

Other diagnostic diets

These diets are not used by (or even known to) the majority of doctors. While some, such as the low-nickel diet, have been subjected to rigorous scientific testing and shown their worth, others have not been tested scientifically. The evidence in their favor is purely anecdotal—in other words, a few doctors have used these treatments repeatedly and observed good results with some patients. That is not hard science, but it is how innovations in medicine often begin.

There are few risks with any of these diets—you are most unlikely to become malnourished. Your doctor should not object to your trying any of these diets, however skeptical he or she may be about its possible benefits.

Low-nickel diet

This diet is sometimes of benefit to adults with eczema who are sensitized to nickel. There are various pointers that indicate that the diet may help, as described on p. 55.

Make sure that you have absolutely no contact with any nickel (for example, in jewelry, jeans studs, watches, or hair clips) throughout this diet and for at least two weeks before starting it.

Ideally you should also stop treatment with steroids or antihistamines a week or so before starting the diet. This allows any improvement to be easily observed. Obviously you should get your doctor's permission to do this.

The diet could require anything from 6 weeks to 6 months to take full effect. Some people have a complete clearance of their eczema, while for others there is a partial improvement.

The foods with a high nickel content, (which should be avoided as much as possible) are:

- shellfish
- green beans and peas
- dry beans and lentils (legumes) of all kinds
- soy protein and products containing it (for example, vegetarian sausages and burgers)
- bean sprouts and alfalfa sprouts
- spinach and kale, lettuce, leeks
- wheat bran (avoid bran cereals and other products; replace whole-wheat bread with white bread, or eat it in moderation only—you can get plenty of fiber from fruits and vegetables; do not eat multigrain breads at all)
- oatmeal, millet, and buckwheat
- raspberries, prunes, pineapple, figs
- chocolate and cocoa
- tea from drink dispensers (restrict intake of other tea and coffee, and don't make them too strong)
- peanuts, hazelnuts, almonds, and marzipan
- licorice
- sunflower seeds, flaxseed

- baking powder, in large amounts
- vitamin and mineral preparations that contain nickel (check the label carefully).

Nickel is also found in drinking water, and absorbed from certain cooking utensils, so
- do not use items plated with nickel (for example, tea balls, some tea strainers, eggbeaters). Nickel's extremely shiny appearance makes it easy to recognize.
- do not cook acid fruits in stainless-steel pans, since the acid leaches some nickel out of the stainless steel. An enameled cooking pot is safe.
- minimize the amount of canned food that you eat.
- in the morning, let the faucet run for a few minutes; water that has been in the faucet overnight may contain nickel.

Several other foods and drinks seem to irritate the skin of nickel-sensitive people, even though the foods are not rich in nickel. These foods should also be avoided:
- beer, wine
- herring, mackerel, tuna
- tomatoes, carrots, onions
- apples and citrus fruits, including their juices.

Low-chromium and low-cobalt diets
Skin sensitivity to chromium or cobalt can, very occasionally, result in a tendency to react to these same metals when consumed in food or drink (see p. 55).

Unfortunately, both chromium and cobalt are essential for good nutrition, so avoiding them is fraught with problems. You would need the help of a really good dietitian, or a doctor with a particular interest in nutritional problems, to guide you through a diet of this kind.

The only measure you can safely take at home is to cut down on excessive consumption of these metals, *for three weeks only*, to see if this produces any improvement in your symptoms. If it does, that should encourage you to seek expert help for a more thorough avoidance diet.

In the case of cobalt sensitivity, avoid all canned and bottled beer. With chromium sensitivity, avoid
- beer, wine, and hard cider
- yeast extract and yeast tablets
- black pepper
- calf's liver
- wheat germ and whole-wheat bread
- cheese

If you also have nickel sensitivity, avoid nickel-rich foods (see p. 199) at the same time.

Low-histamine diet
Histamine in food is produced mostly by bacterial action. The majority of people can break down any histamine they eat, as long as the amount is not excessive (see box on p. 67).

Temporary susceptibility to histamine may accompany viral hepatitis or other liver conditions.

A permanently impaired ability to detoxify histamine is relatively unusual. When it does occur, it can result in symptoms such as chronic urticaria (hives), migraine, or recurrent headaches. A low-histamine diet may help in these cases. All of the following should be avoided:

Very high histamine content:
- red wine, champagne
- tuna, sardines
- Emmenthal and Camembert cheeses

High histamine content:
- beer, white wine
- anchovies
- Gouda, Roquefort, Stilton, and all other well-aged cheeses
- salami and other well-aged sausages, Westphalian ham
- sauerkraut
- spinach
- tomato ketchup (catsup)

If you improve only partially on this diet, this may indicate that you are on the right track (histamine is indeed the problem) but that the bacteria in your gut are undermining your efforts with the additional histamine that they generate. You can investigate this possibility by trying a low-carbohydrate diet, as described on p. 53.

Low-amine diet
Naturally occurring substances called amines, found in many different foods, can have a druglike effect on the blood vessels, making them open up a little and so increasing the blood flow. The effect is usually small, but some people are more susceptible than others. A low-amine diet is worth trying if you have chronic urticaria or migraines and have not improved with other treatments.

A low-amine diet can also be useful in atopic eczema: amines in food are not a basic cause of eczema, but they can aggravate the rash by increasing blood flow to the skin.

To begin with, cut out all foods listed below:

Very high amine content:
- all cheeses except cottage cheese
- dark chocolate
- yeast extract, miso, tomato paste, tandoori spice mix, stock cubes, ready-made sauces
- cola drinks, orange juice, tomato juice
- any dried, pickled, or smoked fish
- sausages, smoked meats, beef liver, chicken skin
- broad beans (fava beans), sauerkraut, spinach, almonds

High or moderate amine content:
- milk chocolate, soy sauce, beer, wine, and hard cider
- pork, including bacon and ham, salami, liver (especially chicken liver), and non-muscle meats
- all fresh or canned fish, except white fish
- all nuts, except chestnuts and cashews
- sesame seeds, sunflower seeds
- avocados, eggplants, mushrooms, tomatoes, broccoli, cauliflower, olives, and olive oil
- oranges, lemons, and other citrus fruits
- pineapples, bananas, raspberries, strawberries, plums, grapes, dates, figs, kiwi fruit, passion fruit

Continue for at least three weeks, longer if your symptoms are normally intermittent. If you improve, you can then experiment with reintroducing small portions of foods from the second list, three or four times a week. Gradually build up to a higher intake, but cut back if your symptoms return.

Organic diet

The objective here is to avoid pesticides; that is, chemical sprays applied to kill fungi and insect pests. This may be helpful for people with chemical intolerance (see p. 84.)

"Chemical-free" or "unsprayed" food (crops grown without pesticides) will do just as well as 100-percent organic food (which is grown without either pesticides or artificial fertilizers).

The highest intake of pesticides is from fresh fruits and vegetables, so if your budget is tight, concentrate on buying organic or chemical-free versions of these. If you have a garden, growing some of your own food will reduce the cost.

You can also reduce the pesticide content of ordinary fruits and vegetables by
- storing them for as long as possible before using them, because the pesticides break down quite quickly
- always peeling them. With difficult-to-peel items such as peaches and tomatoes, pour boiling water over them and leave them to stand for a few minutes first, as this loosens the skin.
- washing them very well with soap or detergent (if peeling is not possible), then rinsing them thoroughly.
- cooking them, as this drives off some of the pesticides; avoid inhaling the steam and ventilate the kitchen thoroughly while doing this.

You should drink mineral water from a reputable source, or use a very high quality water filter (not a jug filter).

Additive-free diet

Food additives are occasionally the culprit in chronic urticaria (see p. 53). As well as avoiding additives, people with this condition should cut out alcohol, spices, and all aspirin and aspirin-like drugs (see box on p. 151).

An additive-free diet may also be of value for some people with chemical intolerance (see p. 84). In the case of children with attention deficit disorder (ADD), the role of additive-free diets is a contentious issue (see p. 81).

An additive-free diet is very healthy but quite hard work. It means making all your own food from 100-percent fresh, unmodified produce (you cannot have bacon or ham, and even things like cooked chicken and ready-to-eat salad can contain some additives; so does most restaurant food). Note that wines, beers, and other alcoholic drinks may contain additives not declared on the label. (German bottled beer is an exception.) Baked goods sold unwrapped can also contain additives that are not declared.

Stop using toothpaste unless it is an additive-free brand. You can buy such toothpaste from a health-food store—or use baking soda instead. Drink mineral water or filtered water (you need a good-quality filter for this, not a jug filter).

Medicinal drugs can contain colorings and other additives, so you should try to get additive-free versions. Talk to your pharmacist about this initially.

Assuming that the symptoms clear up, testing can begin, but you will probably need medical help to work out exactly which additives are at fault. It is difficult to organize these tests at home, because most foods contain a mixture of additives.

With chronic urticaria, testing can produce quite severe reactions, so medical supervision is advisable. You can undertake cautious testing with *small* amounts of tap water, spices, and alcohol at home, but make sure you are in a position to get emergency medical help if you need it. ***Aspirin or aspirin-like drugs should not be tested at home.*** Life-threatening reactions are common in sensitive individuals, and temporary avoidance can heighten your reaction.

Investigating food intolerance

IN COLICKY BABIES

If you have followed the measures described on pp. 78–9 but have had little or no success in reducing colic symptoms so far, it makes sense to look into the possibility of a food sensitivity reaction (either intolerance or a mild allergy) to food *proteins*. This is a very different problem from lactose intolerance (an inability to digest the milk *sugar*, called lactose, due to a shortage of lactase—see p. 79), although the two can get entangled, creating a complex and confusing set of responses.

The complications arise because, when there is diarrhea as a result of allergy or food intolerance (or from any other cause, including infections), it temporarily strips the gut of its lactose-digesting capacity. This problem is called **secondary lactase deficiency**, and it will correct itself quite quickly once the real cause of the diarrhea is eliminated.

Unfortunately, the routine medical tests for lactase deficiency do not distinguish between this temporary problem and the less common **primary lactase deficiency**, which is inherited and therefore lifelong.

So if your child has had these routine tests, and you have been told that they show primary lactase deficiency, it remains possible that the real problem is a reaction to milk proteins (or proteins from other foods), and that the lactose intolerance is an *effect* of this, which adds to the diarrhea, but is not the root cause of it. If so, eliminating the offending food from the baby's diet (or the mother's) will produce impressive results, whereas reducing or eliminating lactose only helps a little.

The purpose of the dietary investigations described here is to discover which foods are causing problems for your baby. In the case of bottle-fed babies, the answer is usually cow's milk—and this is often the culprit for breast-fed babies too—but not necessarily.

For a breast-fed baby it can be any food that the mother is eating. A tiny proportion of what the mother consumes passes into the breast milk, and these few molecules of food are enough to provoke a reaction in the child.

Bottle-fed babies

For bottle-fed babies, proceed as follows:
- Change to an alternative milk-free formula (see box on p. 66). Wait two weeks before concluding that there is no improvement—recovery can take time—and try another type of formula before you decide this is not the answer.
- If there is no success with alternative infant formula, consider the possibility of relactation: stimulating the flow of your own breast milk once again. Breast-feeding support groups (see p. 255) can give you advice. Avoid all dairy products while breast-feeding, and take a calcium supplement.

For babies who are old enough, and who have severe symptoms, early weaning is one option, but this must be done very carefully:
- Keep all dairy products out of the diet—read labels carefully on prepared foods, and know all the different names used for milk (see p. 173). Test beef cautiously, as it shares some proteins with milk.
- To avoid the onset of new food sensitivities, keep eggs, wheat, chocolate, and oranges off the menu until the child's first birthday; then introduce them gradually. Avoid peanuts, other nuts, fish and shellfish for three years, if possible.

• Keep corn out of the diet for the first six months because it is a common ingredient in formulas and the child may have become sensitive to it. Note that some medicines contain corn syrup, but this will affect only those who are very sensitive. A pharmacist can check the full list of ingredients and suggest alternatives.

• No food should be given to the baby every day or in large amounts. You can use unusual starchy foods, such as sweet potatoes, yams, quinoa and millet (see p. 195), to vary the menu. These all make excellent baby foods.

• Never force a child to eat any food that is disliked. Try serving it again, once or twice, but give up if there are still fierce objections to the smell or taste—these are often a sign of intolerance or allergy.

• Ask your doctor to refer you to a pediatric dietitian so that the diet can be checked. A calcium supplement will probably be needed, and other vitamins or minerals may also be lacking.

Breast-fed babies

For breast-fed babies, the approach is quite different—the main focus here is on what you, the mother, eat and drink.

Start keeping a food diary and a record of the baby's symptoms. Are there any detectable patterns? Does the colic get worse if you have had a glass of red wine on the previous day, for example? Note that sometimes the time gap is more than a day, but it should be reasonably consistent for any one food.

At the same time, eliminate all items other than breast milk from the baby's diet, including

• any solids (for example, baby foods)
• fruit juice
• medicines or vitamin drops that contain other ingredients (for example, coloring or corn syrup)
• nipple creams containing peanut oil (the label may say "arachis oil")

Ask your doctor or pharmacist for alternative versions of medicines or vitamins, without added ingredients. Give boiled water to make up for fruit juice. Wait a week or so to see if things improve.

For the next stage, cut out coffee, tea, and all alcoholic drinks. Allow a week for this, and continue with the food/symptom diary meanwhile. If there is no improvement, go on to the next stage, while still avoiding coffee, tea, and alcohol.

For the next stage, compile a list of suspect foods, based on your food diary. Add to this list

• cow's milk and all milk products
• any foods that you craved when pregnant
• any foods that you normally eat in large amounts

• anything you dislike but have been eating because it's "good for you" or "good for the baby"

• any of the following foods if you eat them regularly: eggs, wheat, oranges and other citrus fruits (such as lemons, limes, satsuma mandarins, clementines and grapefruit), tree nuts, peanuts, fish, chocolate, chicken, and beef

Once you have your list prepared, talk to your doctor. Say that you would like to try eliminating cow's milk for two weeks to start with, and then—if the colic has not cleared up—all the other foods on your list as well (again, for two weeks). You will need a calcium supplement. If your doctor fears that your diet will be inadequate, ask for a referral to a dietitian. This needs to be arranged promptly. The fear of undernutrition, which is dangerous for both yourself and the baby, is a very reasonable one; but with sensible precautions, any mother can safely carry out this investigation.

Eat at home during this time, as you cannot possibly know all the ingredients in restaurant meals. Read the labels on packaged meals, and watch out for ingredient synonyms (see pp. 172–4).

If your baby recovers, and you want to pinpoint the problem food so that your diet becomes less restricted, you can test foods individually. Wait until there has been no sign of colic for a week. Choose one food and eat a portion every day for a week. If the colic does not reappear, cut this food out again and choose a second food to test—again, eat this daily for a week. Stop eating the food sooner if the colic returns. (Foods that proved safe can be reintroduced again later, but you need a break after the testing week.) Test cow's milk last.

Some babies get better during the exclusion phase but do not respond to any of the foods when tested. The temporary break from the problem food seems to be all they need to lose their sensitivity. In such cases, the mother can go back to an unrestricted diet, but not to exactly the kind of diet she ate before—no food should be eaten every day, or in large quantities, or the colic may return.

Many babies get over their sensitivity after one or two months without the problem food, so it is worth testing again after a while, especially if you are eating a very restricted diet.

Where cow's milk turns out to be the offender, pasteurized goat's milk or sheep's milk might be tolerated, but wait until the baby is completely free of symptoms, and experiment cautiously. Alternatively, drink one of the new milk substitutes now available (see p. 183).

If the baby clearly responds to a food in the mother's diet (for example, cow's milk or peanuts), this food should be given cautiously when first introduced to the child after weaning, in case he or she has a true allergy to it. An allergy test may be helpful in deciding whether to introduce the food at all.

Rebalancing the gut flora

The **gut flora** are a large collection of bacteria and yeasts living, usually without harmful effects, in our intestines. Some of these microbes are acquired by a baby during birth—several of the most useful kinds live in the vagina too, and the baby swallows them *en route* to the outside world. Recent research shows that babies delivered by cesarean section take much longer to acquire the normal gut flora. However, they catch up eventually because, like other babies, they pick up bacteria in the months immediately after birth, mainly from the mother.

There are hundreds of different species of microbe in the gut flora, with the exact mix varying from one person to another. These microbes eat the remains of our meals and provide certain benefits in return:

- They make some useful vitamins that we can then absorb.
- They keep disease-causing bacteria at bay simply by taking up all the potential "parking places" on the lining of the gut, so that alien bacteria can't find a foothold.
- They may also aid digestion in some way, although this is less certain.

On the downside, the gut flora also produce toxins, but we have had eons of evolution to get used to these, and the liver normally breaks them down quite easily. Only if the liver is badly diseased (as in cirrhosis) do these toxins become a problem.

The immune system is familiar with these longtime companions and tolerates them, while ensuring that they do not invade the body any further. However a loss of immune competence, as in AIDS, can allow them to become invasive and cause disease.

Studies of the gut flora are a relatively new field of medicine and most have been published in rather obscure medical journals. According to these studies, abnormalities of the gut flora—the increase of some species at the expense of others—are found in patients with rheumatoid arthritis, atopic eczema, irritable bowel syndrome, and Crohn's disease. The relationship between these abnormalities and the disease process is unclear at present, and is not necessarily a cause-and-effect relationship. The implications, as far as treatment is concerned, are also far from clear.

The controversial condition known as "candidiasis" seems to be a particular form of gut-flora imbalance, in which yeasts are overly successful. It is called **yeast overgrowth** in this book (see p. 82).

Among the factors that can cause an imbalance in the gut flora are

- prolonged or repeated treatment with antibiotics; also a single high-dose treatment, as may be given before a hysterectomy operation (see p. 76). Such treatment kills off the beneficial bacteria in the gut flora, allowing others to flourish.
- severe diarrhea, which can deplete the normal community of bacteria. Usually the effect on the gut flora is temporary, but it can sometimes be long-lasting and may lead to food intolerance (see p. 76).

Additional factors that might contribute to a disturbed gut flora are

- a diet that is high in sugar and refined carbohydrates. This is thought to give yeasts an unfair advantage over other members of the gut flora by providing yeasts with their preferred food
- the contraceptive pill. This is very controversial, but some doctors believe there is a link between the widespread use of the contraceptive pill and the number of cases of suspected yeast overgrowth in young women

Probiotics

Probiotics, also known as bacterial replacers, supply live bacteria to replenish the gut flora with favorable species.

Experimental trials suggest that taking probiotics may be a useful treatment for irritable bowel syndrome and atopic eczema. This approach may also be of value in yeast overgrowth, when combined with dietary treatment (see below). There have been no trials of probiotics in other diseases.

All probiotics have to be taken every day: the bacteria do not seem to establish themselves permanently in the gut flora. And any benefits from taking them vanish within a few days of stopping the treatment. This is, therefore, quite an expensive option.

Unless the bacteria in the product are alive—and alive in considerable numbers—the probiotic is of no value. Refrigeration is the key to keeping the bacteria alive, since after three days at room temperature, their numbers start to decline steeply. Probiotics purchased from a health-food store may have been kept at room temperature for some time and so contain very few live bacteria. Buying by mail, directly from the supplier, is a good plan; ask how long the delivery usually takes.

Many different brands of probiotic are now available. To locate companies selling by mail order, see p. 255.

The no-yeast-no-sugar diet

Although this diet has not been tested scientifically, it is widely used by doctors interested in gut flora disturbances and often produces strikingly good results with people who had previously intractable health problems. This is not hard scientific data, but the impressive results with certain patients (see p. 82) suggest that the diet is sometimes worth trying. Those with symptoms ascribed to yeast overgrowth or "candidiasis," especially bowel problems and an itchy anus (see p. 82), most frequently benefit.

The best way to carry out this diet is to start with a relatively low-key approach (Stage 1). Progress to more stringent dietary measures only if you don't improve adequately. If there is no improvement at all, even at Stage 4, then you can be reasonably sure that yeast overgrowth is not the cause of your problems.

Stage 1

If you are taking the contraceptive pill, talk to your doctor about changing to another form of contraception. Although the link between yeast overgrowth and the pill is not in any way established, stopping the pill often seems to be beneficial.

Cut out sugar and all sweet foods, including honey, syrup, jam, chutney, pickles, cakes and cookies, and soft drinks. Note that "no-added-sugar" jam should also be excluded—it is very rich in fruit sugars. Also avoid dried fruits, and talk to your doctor about changing any medicines taken as syrups to tablet form. Do not eat peanut butter, canned corn or baked beans, except sugar-free brands. Avoid sweet potatoes, and any vegetables that become very sweet when cooked, such as baked parsnips and caramelized onions. Your sweet tooth should be your guide here—if it tastes sweet, it's off the menu. Only artificial sweeteners are allowed.

Not eating sugar is thought to deprive the yeast of much of its food supply. Persist with this diet for 4–6 weeks. If you are no better, or only partially better, go on to Stage 2.

Stage 2

In addition to the restrictions of Stage 1, cut all fruit out of your diet, except for pure, unsweetened lemon juice and lime juice. These juices, plus salads and lightly cooked vegetables, should give you enough vitamin C—or you could take a supplement.

Cut out white bread and anything made with white flour (pancakes, pastry, noodles, and other pasta, for example). Small servings of whole-wheat bread, potatoes, and brown rice are allowed. Your staple diet should be vegetables and high-protein foods such as meat, fish, and eggs.

Do eat herbs, spinach, and fresh garlic, as these may help to curb the growth of yeast. Don't eat cheese or anything fermented.

Stick with this diet for at least 4 weeks, longer if you begin to feel partially better. If you feel a lot better, continue for several weeks, then gradually reintroduce fruits and other excluded foods—but not sugar, honey, jam, syrup, or similar foods.

Stage 3

In addition to all the restrictions of Stages 1 and 2, cut out any foods containing yeast (see p. 190). Why this should work is not entirely understood (see p. 83).

A response to this diet, even a partial response, is a good sign. Consider going on to Stage 4.

Stage 4

Your doctor must agree to your trying this diet, as it is not safe for everyone.

Avoid all starchy foods including bread, flour, potatoes, rice, pasta, cornmeal, parsnips, beans, lentils, and so forth. Nuts can be eaten in small quantities, but not cashews. This is an extreme diet that gives the yeast almost nothing to live on. No one should stay on this diet for more than a few weeks: it is used only to confirm the diagnosis or to get the problem under control before tackling it with other treatments.

If there is any improvement with the Stage 4 diet, talk to your doctor about antifungal drugs (see p. 83).

A DIET TO PROTECT
against asthma

There is growing evidence that several aspects of the modern Western diet make asthma more likely to develop. Parts of this evidence are very convincing, while other findings are less conclusive. Some people might argue that, until all the facts about diet and asthma are firmly established, no dietary changes should be recommended. However, all the dietary changes that might protect against asthma are also valuable for general health and help protect against heart disease and some cancers.

This diet is potentially useful for:
- atopic families who wish to reduce the chance of their children developing asthma. Other preventive measures, such as allergen avoidance and exercise (see Chapter 8), are obviously important as well.
- people who already suffer from asthma. With this diet, their symptoms may diminish.

The main elements of the antiasthma diet are
- A high intake of **fresh fruit**. Researchers in several different countries have shown that people who eat more fruit have better lung function and are less likely to develop asthma or bronchitis. Apples have a particularly good effect on the airways according to one recent study. Many other studies show a link between **vitamin C**—the major vitamin in fruit—and asthma prevention. This makes sense because vitamin C is an **antioxidant** which inactivates the pro-inflammatory substances (called oxidants) that are found in cigarette smoke and other polluted air. In addition to vitamin C, many fruits contain beta-carotene (see below)—mangoes and apricots are the richest sources.
- Regular helpings of **carrots**, which contain the orange pigment **beta-carotene**. This is another antioxidant that can help prevent inflammation in the airways. It should be obtained from food, not supplements (see p. 207).

- A high intake of **fresh green vegetables**, especially broccoli, collard greens, dark green cabbage, peas, parsley, and zucchini. One Australian study has shown that children who eat fewer vegetables are more likely to wheeze. The benefits of vegetables may be partly due to the fact that they contain beta-carotene and (if eaten raw or only lightly cooked) vitamin C. However, dark green vegetables are also a good source of **magnesium**, and researchers find that people with a higher magnesium intake have healthier airways. Magnesium is believed to protect against asthma by helping the muscles of the airways to relax.
- Plenty of **tomatoes and tomato products**, such as tomato juice, tomato sauce, ketchup, and tomato paste. The special protective effect of tomatoes is not entirely explained by their vitamin C or beta-carotene content—another antioxidant, called lycopene, may be the crucial component here. Good news for fast-food fans: the benefits of tomato paste are seen among dedicated pizza eaters, who are significantly less vulnerable to asthma.
- Daily intake of **sunflower seeds**, or sunflower oil and margarine. These are by far the best natural sources of **vitamin E**, another antioxidant (see left) that helps to reduce the risk of becoming asthmatic. Vitamin E taken in supplements seems to have a much less beneficial effect than natural vitamin E from food.

• A good intake of the essential minerals **zinc**, **manganese**, and **selenium**, as well as **magnesium** (see p. 206). Shortage of any of these minerals may be linked with asthma. It is important not to eat too much wheat bran or whole-wheat bread made without yeast (unleavened bread, soda bread, for example), especially with main meals, as these block the absorption of several minerals.

Good sources of zinc include meat, shrimp, clams, and oysters, with smaller amounts in cheese and egg yolks. Nuts, lentils, and beans are fairly good sources of zinc, while soy protein blocks its absorption.

Besides being found in dark green vegetables, magnesium is plentiful in sardines, peanuts, hazelnuts, walnuts, and lentils. Other fish, lean meat, milk, cheese, and bananas contain smaller amounts of magnesium.

Manganese is found in eggs and milk, and though the amounts are small, these are good sources because the mineral in them can easily be absorbed. Green leafy vegetables, whole grains, and tea apparently contain more manganese — and are frequently recommended as a source of this mineral — but in fact, very little can be absorbed from those foods. Lentils are a moderately good source of manganese.

Selenium is most plentiful in fish and meat. It may be scarce in home-grown plant foods in areas of the world (notably Finland and parts of New Zealand) where selenium is lacking in the soil.

• A limited intake of **meat**, especially red meat, plus complete avoidance of kidney, liver, and other non-muscle meats. An entirely vegetarian diet poses a risk of mineral deficiencies, however (see above). On balance, it is probably best to eat meat once a week or less.

• A low intake of **salt**. Researchers in Kenya found that children eating a high salt diet (which equals the *average* salt intake in most parts of the developed world) were at greater risk of becoming asthmatic. For existing asthmatics, increasing the amount of salt eaten can make asthma worse, while reducing salt can lessen symptoms. Male asthmatics seem to be more vulnerable than females. Salt probably affects the muscles of the airways, making them more likely to contract.

The role of supplements

Try to get all the nutrients you need from food. However, there are situations when a supplement can be useful.

Any asthmatic who has to cope with the effects of high air pollution, especially ozone and sulfur dioxide (see pp. 130–31), may find a vitamin C supplement beneficial. Avoid very high doses of vitamin C (for example, 1 g/day) as they can cause disturbed sleep.

If possible, use natural sources for vitamin E (see p. 206), but a supplement is better than nothing.

Vegans (vegetarians who abstain from eggs and milk as well as meat) should think about taking a multi-mineral supplement, given the difficulties of ensuring an adequate intake of zinc, manganese, and selenium from vegetable food. Vegetarians may also benefit from a mineral supplement.

Some supplements can do more harm than good. **Omega-3 oils** (also called w-3 oils, concentrated fish oils, or EPA and DHA) may make asthma worse for some people (see box on p. 221). **Beta-carotene** (sold alone and as part of mixed antioxidant supplements) may, according to some studies, promote cancer at the high doses used in some supplements. It should be obtained only from food.

Foods and drinks that bring on asthma attacks

By tackling the inflammation of the airways and the underlying tendency of the airway muscles to go into spasm, the antiasthma diet is concerned with the *long-term* treatment or prevention of asthma. In addition, you should obviously avoid any foods that aggravate asthma *in the short term*. Various foods and drinks can bring on an asthma attack:

• foods and drinks containing sulfur-based preservatives tend to give off the irritant gas sulfur dioxide while being chewed or swallowed. Some asthmatics are more sensitive to sulfur dioxide than others. The foods that most commonly cause problems are dried apricots and other dried fruit (except those labeled "unsulfited"), shellfish, french fries, ready-made salads, and fruit salads. Sulfur-based preservatives are used widely in the catering industry. On packaged food, look for the words "sulfite" and "metabisulfite." Wine, beer, and cider almost always contain sulfur-based preservatives.

• Foods that cause heartburn (GER—see p. 38) can aggravate asthma for some people.

• Alcoholic drinks may make the airways contract for some asthmatics (see box on p. 160).

• Some asthmatics need to avoid foods containing histamine (see box on p. 67).

• A few asthmatics respond badly to the smell of food cooking. The most severely affected can suffer an asthma attack from *any* food aroma. Cromoglycate-type drugs (see p. 148) or anticholinergics (see p. 156) may block this reaction.

Needless to say, if you have a sensitivity reaction to any food listed for the antiasthma diet you should not eat this food.

Chapter 7
complementary therapies

"I always wanted to be a doctor, and I enjoyed medical school immensely, but once I went into family practice, I no longer felt quite so sure about what I was doing. It seemed clear to me that there were a lot of people coming to my office who I couldn't do much for. And there were others who, although I could treat their obvious medical problems with some success, remained distressed and were not coping well with life. Once I became a senior partner in this practice, I experimented with having a counselor come in for one session a week, and then a chiropractor for the bad backs. It was popular with the patients, and I saw some people improve enormously. Now we have stress-management classes too, and one of my colleagues has trained in acupuncture, which he uses for selected patients. We also use elimination diets for patients with a lot of long-term problems, like migraine. Overall, I think of it in terms of having more tools at our disposal—being able to tackle things from a different angle when standard medicine isn't hitting the spot."

Geoffrey, a family doctor with a busy practice, exemplifies the synergy that is now beginning to occur between conventional medicine and alternative medicine.

But he also has plenty of criticisms to make of the alternative scene. "The idea that alternative medicine is 'holistic' while conventional medicine isn't, really raises my hackles. Most family physicians could be magnificently holistic if they had an hour with each patient as alternative therapists usually do. We have just 15 minutes, on average, and we have to pack a lot into that—including our basic duty to eliminate the possibility of serious organic disease such as cancer. Time pressure is everything now, and it has squeezed the humanity out of medicine, to a very large extent.

But the potential for a holistic approach is there—most doctors have a tremendous store of wisdom and life experience at their disposal, which could form the basis of a holistic approach to treatment if only there were more time to spend with each patient."

It is in search of a more unhurried and all-embracing approach to treatment that many people turn to alternative medicine. Frequently, what they get out of the therapy has less to do with the actual methods used, and still less with the theories behind those methods, but everything to do with spending a quiet hour with someone supportive and caring who listens to all the complex concerns that surround any illness, gives reassurance or advice, or just offers a "safe space" in which to talk about life's difficulties.

Other people turn to alternative therapies due to a more serious disillusionment with orthodox medicine. When patients with inscrutable medical problems—such as persistent unexplained diarrhea, joint pain, or chronic urticaria (hives)—are given a succession of different diagnoses by different doctors, they may reject orthodox treatment in favor of alternatives. This is a great—and potentially dangerous—mistake. Modern medicine isn't perfect, but that is only to be expected, because it is not a fixed body of knowledge but a *process*—a continuing journey of questioning, investigation, discovery, and improvement. Scientific medicine has come a tremendously long way from the state of ignorance that prevailed two centuries ago, and it will undoubtedly go further.

Conventional medicine has a great deal going for it—ask anyone over 50, with severe lifelong asthma, what they think of treatment now compared to treatment in the 1950s or early 60s. You will hear a hymn of praise to the improvements in both drugs and drug delivery systems. Asthma is just one example—

conventional medicine has a lot to offer for all the classical allergic diseases. Alternative medicine should always be regarded as an adjunct to conventional treatment, not a replacement. That is why many doctors prefer the term **complementary medicine**.

A third reason for using alternative medicine is a more philosophical one, a need to understand illness in some larger sense, often part of a general search for meaning in life. Some types of alternative treatment attempt to offer metaphysical reasons for allergy— rather than the scientific explanations of antibodies and immune cells that are given in this book—and this can be attractive to some people. There is no harm in this approach, which can prompt you to make a critical review of your life, look at unresolved emotional issues, or reassess choices that are making you unhappy.

But not all illness, or worsening symptoms, can be explained by emotional causes, and the rigid belief that every illness must have a meaning can be damaging. It easily degenerates into the wholesale psychologization of illness, the kind of blame-the-victim mentality that can attribute hay fever to "Emotional congestion; fear of the calendar; a belief in persecution; guilt" and asthma in babies to "Fear of life; not wanting to be here." Both these diagnoses are taken from the best-selling *You Can Heal Your Life*, by Louise Hay, which is very influential among some alternative therapists. This compulsive psychologization of illness can be profoundly damaging, and if your complementary therapist is preoccupied by ideas of this kind, you could find yourself on a very long guilt trip indeed.

Apart from the psychological aspects of alternative medicine, there is the question of whether it actually works in a practical sense—whether it provides more than just emotional support and placebo effect (the benefit that comes from any treatment that you believe

in). This is always the central question for scientific medicine in relation to its own treatments, and conventional doctors naturally apply the same criteria to alternative medicine. Most of this chapter is concerned with trying to answer that question.

Unfortunately, there are so many different kinds of alternative therapy available today that it is impossible to cover all of them in this book. To complicate matters further, many complementary therapists now practice two or more different techniques, mixing them to produce their own unique cocktail of diagnosis and treatment. This eclectic approach can span a remarkable range—you may find a therapist doing distinctly whacky stuff such as iridology (looking at the eye to diagnose all illness—it has been tested and definitely doesn't work), combined with something perfectly rational such as an elimination diet.

With new forms of therapy springing up all over the place, a healthy skepticism is a distinct asset for the consumer. Be skeptical about any diagnostic test or treatment that is being practiced by only one person in the country, or in the world—when doctors hit on something that works, they want other doctors to try it out. World exclusives in medicine are usually suspect.

Avoid any practitioner who tells you to stop using your drugs without your doctor's consent. Likewise, avoid those with an evident disregard for logic or reasonable discussion, or an amazing cure that fixes everything from acne to AIDS. Very few of those who sell bogus cures and phony diagnostic tests are complete rogues. Most are nice people who are quite genuinely convinced that they have indeed found the answer to people's problems. The powers of placebo effect (see p. 233) can sustain such a conviction for a very long time.

ALTERNATIVE FORMS OF
desensitization

When Leonard Noon reported his first tentative experiments with immunotherapy for hay fever, in 1911 (see p. 164), he believed that pollen contained a toxin. Most people were "immune" to this toxin, he said, in the same way that people might be immune to measles or diptheria, but hay-fever sufferers lacked this immunity. Noon thought that his steadily increasing doses of pollen, injected just under the skin, were inducing immunity to the pollen toxin, in the same way that a smallpox vaccine could induce immunity to smallpox.

Noon's theory was all wrong, as we now know, but the important thing was that the treatment seemed to work. In fact it transformed the lives of some patients, especially those who were very severely affected by hay fever. One spoke of a "marvelous cure," another of "going for walks to kick my old enemy the hay."

So doctors kept using Noon's treatment, and in time—when it became clear that Noon's theory was flawed—medical researchers began trying to figure out how the injections *really* worked.

Surprisingly, they have still not succeeded, even though a great deal is now known about the changes that can occur in people undergoing immunotherapy. Despite a wealth of detailed knowledge (see pp. 165–6), it remains impossible to say exactly how conventional immunotherapy reduces allergic reactions. Surprising discoveries about the effects of conventional immunotherapy are being made all the time.

New methods of immunotherapy are still being devised today, and there are three different approaches being taken.

First, there are doctors experimenting with modifications of the technique devised by Noon. For example, instead of injecting the allergen extract, some doctors are giving it to their patients in capsule form, to be swallowed. Others are giving it as a liquid, to be placed under the tongue and held there for a few minutes, then spat out. Sound scientific trials show that both these methods work well, at least with certain allergens. Surprisingly, some trials show that certain allergens, when held under the tongue, are not absorbed into the bloodstream, but simply stay stuck to the surface of the mouth—somehow exerting an effect on the immune system in this way. There are also experiments with speeded-up immunotherapy, called **ultrarush** techniques; at the outset, injections are given at hourly intervals, or even more frequently (in a hospital, of course, where severe reactions can be dealt with immediately). Doctors have found that they can induce a remarkably rapid tolerance of the allergen in this way.

The second approach is to apply modern medical knowledge about allergic reactions and so develop entirely new methods of immunotherapy. Such research involves working out, from first principles, novel ways of modifying the immune response in general, or the reaction to one allergen in particular.

This theory-led approach is certainly successful for classical allergies such as hay fever and perennial allergic rhinitis, where there is a good understanding of the basic mechanism (that is, the malfunctions of the immune system that produce the disease). But for those diseases where the underlying mechanism is only partially understood, such as atopic eczema, this approach is not necessarily the best one. And for diseases such as food intolerance, where the cause of the illness remains largely unknown, it is entirely useless.

The third type of approach is to devise a technique by trial and error, and then puzzle out the "how" question later. This is the same kind of path as Noon originally took, and some people believe that this kind of pragmatic experimental approach—practicing a method that seems to be effective, even though it's a mystery how it works—is as valid now as it was in 1911. Others disagree.

The two most widely used methods that have been developed in this way are provocation-neutralization and enzyme potentiated desensitization. Although these techniques are practiced by doctors with a conventional medical training, they remain "outside the pale" as far as orthodox medicine is concerned. The controversies that surround them are discussed below.

Enzyme potentiated desensitization (EPD)

This technique has been developed by a British doctor, Dr. Len McEwen, who began work on it in the 1960s. It is now practiced in many parts of the world, including the United States, Germany, and Italy.

EPD is used for a far wider range of problems than conventional immunotherapy, being given to people with food intolerance and chemical intolerance, as well as to those with true allergies. This—along with the fact that it is unclear how it works—contributes to the controversies that surround it, because these conditions do not have the same basic causes.

Dr. McEwen began with the observation that when immune cells are aroused during inflammation—whether caused by allergy or some other stimulus—they release large amounts of an enzyme called beta-glucuronidase. This enzyme increases the immune response to the allergen or antigen that provoked the inflammation.

Dr. McEwen experimented with injecting beta-glucuronidase into the skin, along with very small amounts of allergen, believing that in such circumstances the enzyme might have the opposite effect and reduce the immune reaction to the allergen. Eventually he discovered a combination of enzyme and allergen that seemed to have the desired effect.

EPD has been tested, in a rigorous scientific manner, and the results suggest that it can work for hay fever and asthma, as well as for childhood migraine and hyperactivity in children when these are triggered by foods.

In one trial with hay-fever patients, researchers measured the levels of anti-pollen IgE following EPD treatment, and it did not rise during the pollen season as it normally does in those with hay fever. This kind of finding is impressive because it is unlikely to be due to placebo effect.

In addition, doctors using EPD claim that it is very effective for patients with allergies who have not done well on the standard course of immunotherapy injections (see p. 164) and for those suffering from atopic eczema—a condition that rarely responds well to conventional immunotherapy. This fits in with other studies suggesting that the immune changes brought about by EPD are fundamentally different from those induced by the traditional form of immunotherapy.

Patients with true food allergy have been given EPD, and while it does not enable them to eat their culprit food, it does seem to reduce the reaction to accidental exposures.

Doctors in the Netherlands are using EPD as a treatment for people with chronic fatigue syndrome (CFS) also known as myalgic encephalomyelitis (ME), and report that it helps about 50 percent of patients.

Unfortunately, the number of good scientific trials that have been carried out for EPD is relatively small (thorough and convincing scientific trials cost a lot of money, and this is not easy to obtain in the case of nondrug treatments, especially speculative ones). It would require a great deal more evidence to convince the majority of doctors that EPD works, and despite the current evidence in its favor, there is tendency against it among orthodox allergists.

One point in favor of EPD is that it uses very small amounts of allergen and is therefore safe—anaphylaxis has never occurred with this technique.

Provocation-neutralization

"After following conventional methods [of immunotherapy] for thirteen years, I heard Carleton H. Lee deliver a paper on provocative testing in 1965, at a meeting of the American College of Allergists in Chicago. I was naturally skeptical, but tried his suggestions when I returned to my office. The results can only be described as astounding. Many patients with unresolved allergic problems responded markedly and rapidly. Many with resistant asthma or perennial allergic rhinitis improved greatly or cleared completely when food injection therapy was added to their inhalant injection therapy." So wrote Dr. Joseph B. Miller—a distinguished allergist and pediatrician and a Professor of Medicine at the University of Alabama, in 1972.

The technique that he learned from Carleton H. Lee was controversial then, and although Miller developed it with great care and precision during the years that followed, it remains controversial now.

There are two elements in provocation-neutralization: testing and treatment. Both are used for a wide range of problems—not just classical allergic diseases but also food intolerance and chemical intolerance. As with EPD (see left), this is one of the controversial aspects of the technique.

Although provocation-neutralization involves an injection technique that looks superficially like conventional immunotherapy (see p.165), there are several important differences.

First, the allergen extract used (in the case of true allergies) is a very dilute extract, so that far less of the allergen is injected than in conventional immunotherapy. Likewise, in the case of food intolerance and chemical intolerance, the extracts of the offending substance are used in highly dilute form.

Second, the idea of the **neutralizing dose**—which is the central plank of provocation-neutralization—is quite different from anything in conventional immunotherapy. Broadly speaking, the conventional technique (see pp.165–6) works by slowly reeducating the immune system, with a gradually increasing dose of the allergen. Only after a succession of injections does the immune system start to behave differently on encountering the allergen. By contrast, in provocation-neutralization treatment, the neutralizing dose is claimed to have an instantaneous and direct effect on the body, "turning off" symptoms that have already begun. This is the **neutralization** aspect of the technique. The doctors who practice this technique do not claim to know how the neutralizing dose might work.

According to the theory of provocation-neutralization, the strength of the extract that acts as a neutralizing dose is specific for a particular allergen and a particular person. It can be worked out only by a rather slow procedure involving a series of injections. These are **intradermal injections**—they place the allergen extract in the skin, at a slightly deeper level than a prick-puncture test. (For treatment, rather than testing, **subcutaneous injections** are used—these go deeper than intradermal injections, placing the allergen extract just underneath the skin. Neither hurts very much.)

Ideally, the neutralizing dose should be decided on by measuring the size of the **wheal** (a raised area of skin around the injection site), and whether it grows, stays the same size, or disappears. The doctor or nurse carrying out the procedure can, in theory, work out the neutralizing dose just by careful examination of the skin wheals. However, it is part of the tradition of provocation-neutralization techniques that verbal feedback from the patient is also taken into account—so if the patient says that an injection has turned off the symptoms, that reinforces the belief that the neutralizing dose has been found.

The problem with this aspect of provocation-neutralization is that expectations, and the power of suggestion, can become involved. So if the doctor or nurse says, "you may find that this next injection makes the symptoms go away," that is often exactly what happens—because the forces of placebo effect (see p. 233) come into play. Unfortunately, verbal interactions such as this are a key aspect of the provocation-neutralization procedure in many clinics.

Just the same hazard besets provocation-neutralization if it is used to *test* for the existence of allergy or intolerance, because it is quite common for practitioners to tell patients which allergen (or other offending substance) is being injected and ask if any symptoms are provoked by the injection. This is not a good practice— if someone expects to react to a particular substance, they are quite likely to produce symptoms through purely psychological mechanisms (see pp. 232–3).

Quite apart from this, the question of allergy testing with provocation-neutralization techniques is contentious, because the pioneers of the technique, such as Professor Miller, never advocated using provocation-neutralization in this way. Using it as a routine test for sensitivity reactions was a later development, and there are many doctors today who, while they practice provocation-neutralization as a treatment, say that it does not work well as a test for sensitivity reactions. While they agree that injecting a dose that is either stronger or weaker than the neutralizing dose may provoke actual symptoms (this is the **provocation** aspect of the technique), they don't think the reaction is reliable enough to form the basis of a test for allergies. Nor do they think that using skin-wheal measurements alone (silent testing) turns the technique into an accurate test for allergies.

The evidence from research

Recent research from the Nova Scotia Environmental Health Centre confirms that testing by provocation injections is not reliable. The subjects in this study were all suffering from multiple chemical intolerance, a condition that—for one reason or another—makes patients likely to develop symptoms at any time. No less than 70 percent of these patients experienced symptoms in response to a dummy injection which contained none of the offending substance. Indeed, 15 percent also produced a skin wheal in response to some of the dummy injections, confirming that even this reaction may be subject to the power of suggestion (see pp. 232–3).

Looking just at the patients who did *not* react to the placebo injection (in other words, those least susceptible to suggestion), the test still did not yield any reliable result—a person might react to one injection with a particular substance but fail to react to a subsequent injection with the same substance. The authors concluded that their patients were "in a state of heightened sensitivity as the result of the chronic irritation by various environmental components and other external and internal stressors." In this state of sensitivity, symptoms can be triggered by the smallest thing. So the apparent reactions to the test injections were actually caused by other factors—some psychological factors (including a psychological response to the prick of the needle) and some external ones, such as exposure to smells or tiny amounts of airborne chemicals.

Another recent research study, carried out by scientists at the University of California, confirmed the finding of the Nova Scotia team as regards testing. Although this study did not set out to look at the use of the neutralizing dose for treatment, some of the patients were given neutralizing doses during the testing process, and the researchers observe that "in most cases a single neutralizing injection relieved the symptoms." This casual observation clearly needs to be confirmed by more rigorous testing.

Oddly enough, despite this positive observation about the neutralizing doses, the overall conclusion of the researchers was to completely dismiss *all* aspects of provocation-neutralization as "the result of suggestion and chance." This conclusion has been very widely publicized in North America as part of a general campaign against provocation-neutralization and those doctors who practice it.

Other researchers have looked at treatment with neutralizing doses, using stringent scientific methods (a double-blind placebo-controlled trial—see p. 90), and found that they *do* work. In one such trial, patients with asthma and allergies to dogs or cats were treated with injections of the neutralizing dose and showed a reduction in the sensitivity of their airways, as measured by objective tests. In another experiment, patients with perennial allergic rhinitis and an allergy to dust mites were studied, and the neutralizing dose was given as drops of allergen extract placed under the tongue (**sublingual drops**)—an alternative to injections. The blockage of the nose, as measured by scientific tests, was reduced by the neutralizing dose.

A great many more trials of this kind would be required to convince most doctors that provocation-neutralization works.

Furthermore, the recent study in California—which observed a number of practitioners of provocation-neutralization at work with their patients—showed that these practitioners need to be a lot more rigorous and objective in their approach. However, the fact that provocation-neutralization is often practiced badly does not necessarily mean that the basic technique is without any value. There are many levelheaded doctors and patients who, while initially very skeptical about provocation-neutralization, have found it surprisingly effective—just as Professor Miller did back in 1965.

Deciding for yourself

So is provocation-neutralization an option that is worth trying for your condition?

With respect to *testing*, the answer is probably "No." The most reliable tests are prick-puncture tests or RAST blood tests for true allergies (see pp. 91–2), an elimination diet for food intolerance (see p. 194), and avoidance followed by reexposure (a challenge test) for chemical intolerance.

With respect to *treatment* for true allergies, conventional immunotherapy has been far more thoroughly tested and the chances of it working effectively are probably better simply for that reason. It is definitely the best treatment for allergy to insect stings.

However, one major advantage of provocation-neutralization, in the case of true allergies, is that it is far safer. Because such small amounts of allergen are used, anaphylactic reactions (see p. 58) don't occur.

When it comes to treatment for food intolerance, complete avoidance of the problem food(s), for a period of a year or two, is usually a very effective treatment (see p. 77). Other forms of treatment are needed only for people who find that they have intolerance to many different foods (*on the basis of an elimination diet*, not hair tests, blood tests, and the like—see p. 93) and cannot devise an adequate diet from the foods they are able to eat. For such people, provocation-neutralization may be worth a try. Many patients feel that they have gained considerable help from this treatment. They report suffering fewer symptoms and being able to return to a more nutritionally balanced diet.

In the case of chemical intolerance, the first line of treatment should be to avoid the substances concerned as much as possible, eat a good balanced diet, and take a vitamin and mineral supplement if nutritional deficiencies are suspected. Treating any underlying hyperventilation (see pp. 226–9) can also help considerably. Only if there are persistent symptoms, and you are sure these are not due to psychological causes, might provocation-neutralization be worth a try. Some people with chemical intolerance do find it is helpful, but whether this is a real effect, or simply placebo, remains uncertain.

If you decide to give provocation-neutralization a try, find a doctor who has good medical qualifications, who seems objective and sensible in his or her approach, and who doesn't make implausible claims for the technique. Take note of what other treatments are practiced, and whether these seem rational or not—this is often a good guide to the care and objectivity with which provocation-neutralization is practiced.

Ask the doctor how he or she assesses the neutralizing dose, and avoid those who do not use the traditional method of a series of injections combined with wheal measurement. When the neutralizing dose is being assessed, say that you would like it to be done "single-blind"—that is, you don't want to be told anything about what is being injected. Reporting how you feel to the doctor or nurse during the assessment is fine, but only mention really significant symptoms, or a very definite clearance of the symptoms, if this occurs. These precautions will help you to be sure that you are getting something that is of genuine benefit, rather than just a very expensive form of placebo treatment.

Acupuncture

Acupuncture shot to fame in the West in 1972, when James Reston, a correspondent for the *New York Times*, fell ill with appendicitis while covering President Nixon's historic trip to China. Following the removal of his appendix, he received acupuncture treatment for pain, and was highly impressed with its effects.

His Chinese doctor invited Reston to witness the use of acupuncture in anesthesia, and he reported the remarkable fact that patients undergoing surgery could be free from pain with just a few tiny needles inserted into carefully chosen points on the body. They remained alert and talkative throughout the operation.

Traditional Chinese medicine has enjoyed a good reputation in the West ever since; but what few people realize is that acupuncture anesthesia is a very new invention. Surgery was not traditionally practiced in China, and it was only in the 1950s, after Chairman Mao had urged Chinese doctors to unify Western and Chinese medicine, that the anesthetic potential of acupuncture was discovered.

The remarkable effects of acupuncture anesthesia made a huge impression on doctors in the West—a high-profile success that has had both good and bad effects. On the positive side, conventional medicine has been prepared to take acupuncture seriously and to undertake some research into it. On the negative side, that research

has mostly concerned pain control—the effects of acupuncture on the nervous system and on **endorphins**. These are natural painkilling compounds made by the body (their effects are mimicked by opiate drugs such as morphine).

Western researchers have paid little attention to how acupuncture affects most other aspects of health, including the immune system and allergic diseases. One exception to this is asthma, in which certain nerves do play a large part in producing the symptoms (see box on p. 235).

Treating the person

Diagnosis and treatment are far more oriented toward the individual patient in traditional Chinese medicine, and diagnostic labels such as "allergy" or "hay fever" are less important than the particular character of a person's *qi* (vital energy—see box on p. 215), as detected by the acupuncturist. A traditional Chinese acupuncturist gives great attention to the quality of the different pulses, and takes them at the start of every appointment, and at intervals during treatment, to check how the *qi* flow has changed. Each treatment session is unique and tailored to the individual's condition at that particular moment.

This makes it very difficult to carry out conventional scientific research into traditional acupuncture.

In an effort to make acupuncture accessible to research, a more Westernized and formulaic approach has been developed, using orthodox medical diagnosis and needling a set of acupuncture points that are prescribed for that medical condition. Experts in traditional acupuncture feel that this approach—first name the disease, then apply a standard remedy—will often fail and is missing the whole point of acupuncture.

That is not the only problem with Westernized acupuncture, as Dr. David Eisenberg of Harvard University, a leading expert on acupuncture, points out. He describes a typical acupuncture session in China: "Each time the acupuncturist inserts a needle, he or she asks the patient, 'Do you have it or not?' referring to the patient's 'obtaining the *qi*' (*de qi*). The question asks whether the patient has felt a sensation of fullness, distension, pins and needles, or the like, from the insertion of the needle in the spot being used. . . . Most Chinese have experienced acupuncture, and they understand the phenomenon of *de qi*. . . . By contrast, most Western patients seeking acupuncture therapy know nothing of the phenomenon of *de qi*. Not knowing what sensations they should anticipate, they cannot tell the acupuncturist whether a needle is in the right place. When both therapist and patient know little about *de qi*, as frequently occurs in

Western acupuncture clinics, the result is bound to be disappointing." Fortunately it *is* possible to find acupuncturists who have been properly trained, and the sensation of "obtaining the *qi*" is perfectly detectable, even to a skeptical Westerner, so look for someone who pays attention to this.

There can be emotional and psychological reactions to acupuncture, so make sure that you also feel relaxed with your acupuncturist and that there is a certain empathy between you.

Does acupuncture work for allergies?

According to Chinese theories, acupuncture can have some benefits in any illness—if you are ill, your flow of *qi* must be disturbed, and acupuncture will help to put that right. Indeed, most people do feel a sense of well-being after an acupuncture session.

To look at this from a Western scientific perspective, acupuncture can stimulate your body to increase its production of endorphins (see p. 214). This gives you a mild high, similar to that you'd get from running for a couple of hours. Feeling relaxed and confident helps most people to cope better and gives them a new perspective on life's problems. Since the mind plays some part in almost all illness (if only to aggravate the effects of an underlying physical problem), inducing a more positive state of mind can be of benefit.

If you are looking for a more specific effect on your allergies, then it is hard to say what acupuncture can give you—there is little evidence simply because Western researchers have not investigated this, except in the case of asthma.

Several studies show that acupuncture can have a small but detectable short-term effect in opening up the airways of asthmatics. This is not surprising, because acupuncture affects the autonomic nervous system, the "autopilot" part of the nervous system (see box on p. 235). Besides controlling heart rate and breathing, the autonomic nervous system can tighten or relax the muscles around the airways.

A short-term effect is just that—it doesn't treat the real problem. What matters more in asthma is the long-term impact of any treatment on the underlying inflammation of the airways (see p. 36). Although some studies of acupuncture treatment have found a general improvement in the state of the airways and a reduction in inflammation, other studies have not. However, only one study to date used an individualized approach to acupuncture, as opposed to a same-for-everyone formula. It is interesting that this study *did* find good long-term effects on airway inflammation.

The larger picture

Acupuncture is just one element of Chinese medicine, which has several other techniques available. In China (and in some Chinese clinics in the West) these techniques are used together, as different ways of tackling the same problem. No traditional Chinese doctor would dream of trying to treat every patient with acupuncture alone, and in the case of a patient with allergies, herbal remedies would usually be a central part of the treatment. Eczema, in particular, may respond well to traditional Chinese herbal treatment, taken by mouth; but be very cautious about using Chinese herbal creams (see pp. 220–21).

The flow of energy

Acupuncture is rooted in ancient Chinese ideas of the human body, which are radically different from those of Western medicine:

- Invisible vital energy, called *qi* or *chi* (pronounced "chee"), is what distinguishes living bodies from dead ones. It should flow easily and harmoniously throughout the body, nourishing and protecting the organs. When the flow of *qi* is blocked, or becomes unbalanced, illness develops.
- Channels called meridians are the conduits for *qi* in the body. Most of these run vertically (from head to toe), and the points where acupuncture needles are inserted all lie on these meridians.
- The flow of *qi* can be measured by carefully taking pulses—not just one pulse, as in Western medicine, but several different kinds of pulse.
- By detecting disturbances in the flow of *qi* and correcting them, existing illness can be cured, and incipient illness prevented, before there are any obvious symptoms.

The nature of the meridians and the acupuncture points remains a mystery to Western doctors. Some parts of the meridians run roughly along the lines of certain nerves or blood vessels, but they do not follow them exactly. The acupuncture points have no anatomical reality—there is nothing to see either on the surface or under the skin. However, many are located near major nerve endings or over deep pressure receptors.

Homeopathy

"We believe that a serious effort to research homeopathy is clearly warranted despite its implausibility." That was the conclusion of a group of American and German scientific researchers who, in 1997, looked at every study of homeopathy they could find. This prestigious transatlantic team carefully assessed the scientific validity of each study, and then considered the data from studies that were of reasonably good quality.

This kind of study, in which all the available research data on a topic are combined, is called a **meta-analysis**. There were 119 research studies that were good enough to be included in this meta-analysis, and, taken together, these studies suggested that homeopathy does indeed have some real effects. In other words, it produces more benefits than simple placebo effect—the psychosomatic improvement that tends to occur with any treatment, even a dummy pill (see p. 233).

Some of the most convincing scientific studies included in the meta-analysis were those relating to homeopathic remedies for allergic conditions (see p. 217). But what exactly does this mean for allergy sufferers? Is homeopathy a treatment that is worth a try? Unfortunately, it is difficult to say.

First, the evidence from the homeopathy meta-analysis is far from overwhelming, as the researchers themselves point out. The observed improvements—the overall differences between the placebo and the homeopathic remedy—are not huge. Second, even if there are *some* homeopathic treatments that have real effects, it does not mean that *every* kind of homeopathic treatment works. Homeopathy is a very broad field, with a multitude of different approaches. The types of homeopathy that have been tested, and appear to help, may bear little or no relation to the homeopathic remedies that are generally available (see p. 217).

"Let like cure like"

The central idea in homeopathy— often known as the principle of **similars**—is that a substance that causes a particular set of symptoms can also, if handled in the right way, cure symptoms of a similar kind. In the words of Samuel Hahnemann, the German doctor who invented homeopathy at the beginning of the nineteenth century, "Let like cure like."

The natural substances that form the basis for homeopathic remedies are derived mostly from toxic plants or minerals. (Sometimes extracts from diseased tissue—called **nosodes**—are used instead, but this is a relatively recent development. So is the use of allergen extracts, such as pollen, described on p. 217.) Hahnemann himself began with the standard drugs of his own day, such as belladonna and arsenic compounds. His innovation was to use them in very much smaller doses than used by his fellow physicians and to apply them to entirely different diseases.

Hahnemann worked by first discovering what the effects of the drugs were when taken by a healthy person (he experimented on himself and his family for this). Then he tried to match the symptom pattern produced by the drug with the symptoms of a particular disease. For example, he observed that belladonna produces hallucinations and a hot, dry skin—symptoms that were seen also in children with scarlet fever. He claimed that by giving belladonna *in very small doses*, much less than was normally used, he could stimulate the body to heal itself of scarlet fever.

Hahnemann, unlike his medical contemporaries, also advocated a good diet, fresh air, and exercise. And he was heartily opposed to the conventional medicine of his day, a brutal business that involved a great deal of bloodletting and large doses of very toxic medicines. Considering how useless, and indeed dangerous, the orthodox medicine of the time frequently was, Hahnemann's successes were not really surprising.

"Less is more"

Homeopathy today is the ultimate version of the "less is more" philosophy. A homeopathic remedy is prepared by taking the basic ingredient, dissolving it in water, and then diluting that solution over and over again. Imagine pouring a bottle of wine into the Pacific Ocean, and you have a rough idea of how dilute homeopathic remedies are. Making extreme dilutions was an idea introduced by some of Hahnemann's followers after his death.

Dilution is only part of the story, however. With each dilution, homeopaths apply a special shaking-and-tapping technique known as **percussing**. This was originally done by hand, but now is often done mechanically. Homeopaths believe that percussing makes the active substance *more* powerful, despite the dilution. The term used by homeopaths is **potency**, and a homeopathic remedy of the highest potency is the one that has been most thoroughly diluted and percussed.

In fact, a simple calculation, using the basic laws of physics, shows that there is nothing there at all but water. Many homeopathic remedies are watered down so thoroughly that not one single molecule of the active substance is likely to remain. It is this that leads medical researchers to use words such as "implausibility" (see p. 216) when talking about homeopathy.

What homeopaths do

A homeopath starts by considering all your symptoms (not just allergies, but any other symptoms as well) and various other characteristics that conventional doctors do not usually consider, including physical appearance and psychological traits. The homeopath then chooses a substance that, if taken at full strength, would produce a comparable set of symptoms and characteristics. This approach is called **classical homeopathy.**

In addition, homeopaths often give advice on diet, sleep, exercise, and allergen avoidance. As in the early days of homeopathy, this may be the most important part of the treatment.

Like many other complementary therapists, homeopaths will listen if you need to talk about personal problems and emotional difficulties, and will offer reassurance or advice. This can be valuable, though not everyone would agree that a homeopath is the best source for such help. There are two distinct traditions within homeopathy—a scientifically inclined tradition (represented today by experiments with homeopathic immunotherapy—see right) and a highly metaphysical tradition. Among the many ideas floating around within the metaphysical tradition is the notion that all illness is a result of psychological or moral failings. Attitudes of this kind, which are quite common among complementary therapists, can be very damaging (see p. 209).

Sometimes homeopaths recommend avoiding certain foods, on the assumption that the patient suffers from food intolerance, though they rarely use an elimination diet (see p. 194), the only way to achieve accurate diagnosis.

In addition to all this, some homeopaths also give herbal remedies where they think it will help. This approach is called **complex homeopathy**.

A much more recent development within homeopathy is **homeopathic immunotherapy** or **HIT**, which uses an extreme dilution of an allergen (such as pollen or dust mite) to treat people who are allergic to that substance. While homeopathic immunotherapy was inspired by conventional immunotherapy, the relationship between the two is a very distant one indeed. The extensive dilution process means that the liquid used for homeopathic immunotherapy is unlikely to contain even one molecule of the allergen. This puts it in a completely separate realm from conventional immunotherapy, in which the presence of the allergen, and the steadily increasing dose with successive injections, is what produces the beneficial effect (see p. 165).

Does it work for allergy?

Two scientific trials suggest that HIT makes a difference, albeit a small one, for hay fever and pollen asthma. In the meta-analysis described on p. 216, one of these trials was given a good rating for scientific reliability, and the other was considered fairly good.

Another type of homeopathic treatment that appeared to be effective for patients with allergic asthma was one using a **nosode**—a diluted sample of the asthmatic airway itself. A small sample of the airway was taken from each asthmatic patient (as for a biopsy—see p. 90), diluted, and percussed, then given to the patient as a treatment. It seemed to work, and the scientific rating of this trial was very high.

The third homeopathic treatment that appeared to have an effect in valid scientific studies was Galphimia, used for symptoms in the eye caused by pollen allergy.

If you go to a local homeopath, it is very unlikely that you will be given either of the first two treatments—these are used only experimentally, in large research centers.

The Galphimia treatment (see above) might be available from a local homeopath, but it will not necessarily be in the same form as the treatment used in the scientific trial.

Herbal remedies
WESTERN AND EASTERN

Plants make a great many different chemical substances, mostly for the purposes of dissuading other living beings—fungi, insects, and grazing animals—from consuming their leaves, roots, and fruits. These chemical substances are extraordinarily potent and diverse. Many taste disgusting, some are virulent poisons, and many will induce vomiting or diarrhea. None of these effects are surprising, given that substances such as these are produced to defend the plant. However, some of the chemical substances produced by plants happen to have a beneficial druglike action for people suffering from certain diseases. This is the basis of **herbalism**, sometimes known as **botanical medicine**.

Over the millennia, herbalists have, through trial and error, tried to discover which plants have worthwhile effects. Indeed, this process probably began with our ape ancestors; chimpanzees have been observed, when they are ill with parasitic infections, for example, to carefully select and eat particular leaves that have therapeutic effects. If chimpanzees do this, it is a fair guess that the apelike ancestors of human beings also did so.

At some point in human history—or prehistory—this use of wild plants became a systematic and specialized activity, now known as herbalism. No doubt the patients who went to see herbalists (like patients visiting their doctors today) expected a cure for every ill, and no doubt herbalists felt bad about telling anyone that their problem was incurable. At this point, quite a bit of wishful thinking and placebo effect (see p. 233) probably found its way into herbalism. The outcome was a mixed bag of herbal remedies—some that worked, some that had no effect at all (apart from placebo effect), and a few that were positively toxic but whose bad effects escaped notice because of the seriousness of the diseases being treated.

In recent times, a few herbal remedies have been put through rigorous scientific tests. As one might expect, some work and some don't. More details of those that have been shown to work

for allergies are given on p. 221. First, however, it is important to consider some of the misconceptions that surround herbal medicine, especially those relating to side effects. These misconceptions are rooted in the basic philosophy of herbalism, so it is also important to look at this—and at other points of view about herbal treatment.

The "Mother Nature" viewpoint

Some modern herbalists maintain that for every human ill nature has created a complete cure somewhere in the plant world; the job of herbalists is simply to identify that cure. This belief is essentially religious and anthropocentric—that is, it assumes that the welfare of human beings is the central focus of the plant world. This goes against common sense, because it suggests that plants produce a complex array of chemical components, not for their own benefit but for ours. A brush with poison ivy should be enough to cure most people of such views.

A related idea, and more common belief, is that anything "natural" must automatically be either harmless or beneficial to human beings. This view is regularly promoted by advertisers of all kinds, whether they are selling face cream, shampoo, or breakfast cereal.

When the word "natural" is used as an endorsement of herbal remedies, it is generally understood to mean "therefore totally harmless." Nothing could be farther from the truth, as a quick survey of the plant world shows: hemlock is natural, belladonna is natural, and ricin—the most deadly poison known—is natural. All come from plants. Indeed, many wild plants are either poisonous to humans, or produce very unpleasant effects if eaten.

Belladonna, of course, while being deadly poisonous in sufficient quantities, is also a medicinal plant. Its most significant ingredient, atropine, is a useful druglike substance in small amounts, and a poison in larger amounts. There is no sharp dividing line between these positive and negative aspects—even a small beneficial dose will have some undesirable effects too.

In other words, herbs produce **side effects**, in just the same way that medicinal drugs do. This is almost inevitable—anything that alters body functions enought to act as a drug will usually have some other unwanted effects.

In the case of herbal medicines, there is an added complication. Plants contain dozens, even hundreds, of different chemical substances, many of which have no benefits for humans at all—they are just plain toxic. These plant toxins can produce various unpleasant effects of their own, to add to the side effects of the useful ingredients. So the possibility of side effects is actually *higher* with herbal medicines than with medicinal drugs.

The side effects that occur with herbal treatment are sometimes very serious. Deaths have occurred in some cases, and in others irreversible damage has been done.

The "pure is best" viewpoint

Many modern anti-allergy drugs were first obtained from plants—cromoglycate or cromolyn (see p. 148) for example, was originally extracted from the roots of an Egyptian plant called ammivisnaga. The ground-up roots of this plant contain many other things besides cromoglycate, whereas the pharmaceutical preparations of cromoglycate are pure and of known strength. This pure form of the drug has also been tested very thoroughly by pharmaceutical companies, in order to demonstrate its effectiveness to identify the correct dose, and to look for any serious side effects.

As modern science sees it, herbalism is just a very crude and primitive form of pharmacology (the study and use of medicinal drugs). Much of pharmacology originally developed out of herbalism and other folk cures, by analyzing the remedies used, identifying the active substances in them, then purifying these and—if possible—puzzling out how they work.

An advocate of scientific pharmacology would maintain that with modern drugs, the patient is just taking the substance that works, not a mysterious cocktail of unknown plant chemicals. In other words, you know what you are getting with a drug. You also know it has a good chance of working and a relatively small chance of causing serious side effects. With an herbal remedy, you are, to some extent, taking a leap in the dark.

Ephedra sinica, the herb known to the Chinese as Ma huang, illustrates this point well. It contains a mixture of substances, including the powerful drug called ephedrine—it was named after the plant. Ephedrine (see p. 156) can relieve the narrowing of the airways that occurs during an asthma attack. The presence of ephedrine gives Ma huang the ability to ease asthma, although it is more often recommended to help with weight loss. Unfortunately, overuse of Ma huang can cause a spasmodic contraction of the blood vessels in the brain, which can result in injury or death. Liver toxicity has also been recorded (see p. 220).

As for its antiasthma ingredient, ephedrine, although this drug was once important in conventional asthma treatment, it is rarely prescribed now. Ephedrine has long been superseded by asthma-relievers that have a more precise effect on the airway muscles and so produce fewer side effects.

The multiple-action viewpoint

Practitioners of Chinese herbal medicine, in preparing a treatment for atopic eczema, combine ten or more different herbs. There are some conditions, they say, that can be treated with a single plant, but atopic eczema is not one of those. It requires a mixture—and none of the ingredients of that mixture, taken alone, has any effect. What they are claiming is that the different druglike substances in the herb mixture have a **synergistic action**, working together to treat the disease.

This same idea is sometimes applied to the many different chemical substances found in a single plant. Some herbalists argue that an herbal remedy is better than a modern drug precisely because it contains a cocktail of different druglike substances, the effect of one substance augmenting or balancing that of another.

There is no actual evidence to support this claim, but the fact that Chinese herbal mixtures have significant success in treating very difficult cases of atopic eczema (see p. 221) demands that Western doctors at least take the possibility of synergistic action seriously.

It might seem that this multiple-action viewpoint goes against the whole grain of Western scientific pharmacology—the "pure is best" approach. However, Western medicine frequently treats certain allergic diseases, such as asthma and chronic sinusitis, with a mixture of drugs. The difference is that each of these modern drugs also works when taken alone, and each has a clearly defined and well-documented action.

The Chinese approach

One fundamental concept of Chinese medicine is that, instead of just matching the remedy to the disease, the treatment should also be based on the particular characteristics of the patient concerned. This idea is shared by some other Eastern systems, such as Ayurvedic medicine.

Whereas a Western doctor might see you as a person with atopic eczema, a traditional Chinese doctor sees you as a person with a certain constitution that has gotten out of balance and so produced symptoms in the skin. The constitution is usually the main focus of treatment, not the eczema. This approach means that different eczema patients get different herb mixtures, and the same is true for other allergic diseases.

A traditional Chinese doctor will assess your constitution by taking your pulses (there are several in Chinese medicine, not just one), asking various questions, and studying the appearance of your tongue—the same sort of diagnostic process that is used prior to acupuncture.

For the purposes of scientific investigations, where a uniform treatment is necessary, this traditional approach has been modified. A single standardized treatment is applied to a particular disease—and the disease itself is diagnosed by Western medical criteria. Whether this is really comparable with traditional Chinese herbal medicine is open to question. The same caveat applies to any ready-made Chinese herbal formula that is sold directly to the public, rather than being prescribed for an individual patient by a trained practitioner.

The traditional philosophy of Chinese medicine makes for a lot of variability in herbal preparations. That is why categorical statements about side effects cannot be made—while one mixture used for atopic eczema may contain a potentially toxic ingredient, another mixture may not.

Using herbal remedies safely

Always talk to your doctor before taking any herbal medicine, because of the risk of side effects, or interactions with any conventional drugs that you may be using.

If possible, get herbal treatment from someone who is also a doctor qualified in conventional medicine. Ideally, your herbalist should have access to laboratory facilities and should order blood tests to monitor your reaction to the herb(s). Monitoring every 1–3 months is necessary with some herbs, to check for serious side effects such as toxicity to the kidneys or liver (see right).

Before buying herbal remedies from a health-food store or via the Internet, contact the manufacturer and ask to see detailed reports of trials showing that the product is safe.

Think very carefully before taking an herb that has not undergone full safety trials. Find out all you can about the herb and discuss the matter with your doctor. Don't fall for the "it must be safe—people have been taking it for centuries" argument. If a herb is toxic only to a minority of people, and its bad effects are slow to emerge (so people don't get ill or die immediately after taking it for the first time), its deadliness can escape notice for a very long time, perhaps indefinitely. In the case of pharmaceutical drugs, highly sophisticated information-gathering systems are needed to ensure that such rare-and-slow effects are noticed (see p. 137), but nothing of the kind exists for herbal medicines.

Above all, do not neglect vital medical treatment (for example, inhaled steroids for asthma) while trying out herbal remedies, as this can be dangerous. Always follow your doctor's advice about your medication.

Risks to the liver

Among the side effects recorded for herbal treatment, liver damage is especially alarming. Deaths from liver failure have occurred with both Western and Chinese herbal treatment. Liver toxicity has been recorded with the following herbal remedies:

- blue-green algae, chaparral, germander, skullcap, mistletoe, senna, valerian
- Chinese herbal teas prescribed for atopic eczema; however, this is not true of all eczema preparations—several of the most widely used ones appear to be relatively safe.
- Jin bu huan, Ma huang or ephedra (*Ephedra sinica*)

If you feel ill while taking an herbal remedy, stop taking it immediately and see your doctor. The early symptoms of liver toxicity, which you should watch out for, include jaundice (yellow skin, and a yellowish tint to the whites of the eyes), pale feces and dark urine, nausea, and pain (usually in the region of the stomach).

Illicit steroids

Be very cautious indeed about jars of Chinese herbal cream sold for atopic eczema. Analysis of a selection of such creams obtained in London, England found that two-thirds illicitly contained powerful steroids—the very drugs that the people buying the creams were anxious to avoid. The dose of steroid in these herbal creams was alarmingly high, considering the purposes for which some of them had been supplied—such as for use on the face of a baby. A substantial risk of serious side effects existed with these adulterated creams. In Canada, look for creams that carry a Drug Identification Number (DIN). These have been authorized for sale and should not contain any steroid. Unfortunately, there is no way for U.S. consumers to be assured of the quality of Chinese herbal creams.

Sensitivity reactions to herbs

Like other natural products, herbs can provoke a true allergic reaction, and anyone with a tendency to allergies is at particular risk. Although any herb could, in theory, cause such a reaction, some seem especially likely to do so:

• The popular herb echinacea, which is said to promote healing and have antibiotic properties (an unproven claim) quite often causes allergic reactions. Like chamomile, goldenrod, and feverfew, it is a member of the daisy family (Compositae). Reactions to all of these are particularly likely in people with allergy to ragweed or sagebrush.

• Preparations containing pollen or royal jelly (obtained from honeybees) have sometimes caused near-fatal anaphylaxis in those allergic to pollen. Propolis, obtained from bees, should also be treated with caution.

Contact dermatitis often occurs with tea tree oil and some other plant-derived substances applied to the skin (see p. 55).

Herb-drug interactions

Using herbal remedies and taking medicinal drugs at the same time can be hazardous. The following herbs have been proven to interact with anti-allergy drugs:

• Aloe vera, buckthorn, cascara sagrada bark, ginseng, and senna pod or leaf can all interact with steroid tablets.

• Squill, lily of the valley, and pheasant's eye can increase the action and side effects of betamethasone (a steroid); rhubarb root also interacts with this drug.

• Kava and valerian, if taken with antihistamines can increase side effects such as drowsiness and poor coordination.

• Henbane may increase some of the side effects of astemizole (an antihistamine).

Note that many drugs prescribed for conditions other than allergies may interact with herbs. Some of these interactions can be serious, so check with your doctor before taking *any* herbal remedy.

Herbs that may work for allergies

Of the herbal treatments that have been tested, the following appear to have potential benefits for people with allergies:

• **Chinese herbal teas** for atopic eczema have shown substantial good effects in scientific trials with both adults and children. Patients with widespread and persistent eczema—the kind that is particularly difficult to treat—were chosen for these trials, which were all carried out in London, England. The puzzling thing is that when exactly the same herbal treatment was studied in Hong Kong, with Chinese youngsters suffering from eczema, there was no improvement. The reasons for this are as yet unclear.

If you are interested in trying Chinese herbal medicine for eczema, it is advisable to be monitored properly, as liver toxicity has sometimes occurred (see p. 220).

• *Euphorbia acaulis* has shown good effects with atopic eczema. Licorice root may also help, but can have serious side effects if taken in large amounts.

• **Evening primrose oil** taken in capsule form, is known to calm inflammation and might be helpful for atopic eczema. Don't chew the capsules, as irritation of the throat can occur. Epileptics should not take this oil.

• *Ginkgo biloba* seems to reduce the reaction to allergens. For people with asthma, it may also calm inflammation in the airways. Use only standardized extracts (GBE). Unprocessed ginkgo in any form, including teas, contains potent antigen sensitizers (see p. 54).

• **Ayurvedic medicine** utilizes two herbs, *Coleus forskohlii* and *Tylophora asmatica,* in the treatment of asthma. The former relaxes the airway muscles, in much the same way as beta-2 reliever drugs, making the airways open up. The latter has more general benefits in asthma but also some unpleasant side effects: it can cause nausea and soreness in the mouth.

Omega-3 oils

These oils are derived from certain types of fish. They are obviously not herbs, but they are often sold alongside herbal remedies in health-food stores, which is why they are included here. Generally speaking, omega-3 oils have a calming effect on inflammation, but asthmatics who are sensitive to aspirin may find that they gradually get worse if they take omega-3 oils. This is probably due to problems with the production of messenger chemicals called prostaglandins in people with aspirin sensitivity (see box on p. 151). The connection is that omega-3 oils can act as raw materials for the manufacture of prostaglandins and leukotrienes (see box on p. 151). The details of how omega-3 oils cause trouble for aspirin-sensitive people are not yet understood.

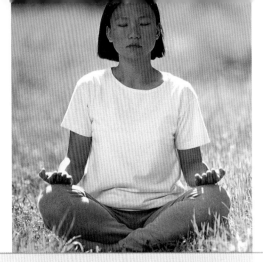

Therapies
THAT PROMOTE RELAXATION

Controversy abounds in medicine, especially when it comes to alternative forms of treatment, but there is one thing that almost everyone agrees on: feeling calmer and more relaxed is good for your health. There are many ways in which a person's mental and emotional state can affect their allergies or other sensitivity reactions (see pp. 232–7), and these help to explain the beneficial effects of relaxation.

There are several different types of approach that can help in the quest for a calmer state of mind and a more relaxed state of body:

• simple relaxation techniques that you learn and then practice for yourself, either on a daily basis or whenever you need them, or both. Examples include relaxation exercises of various kinds, biofeedback, autogenic training, and self-hypnosis.

• relaxation techniques that are rooted in spiritual practice, such as meditation, yoga, t'ai chi, or qi gong (pronounced "chee gong"). Some other martial arts, in addition to t'ai chi, also have a strong element of spiritual practice.

• treatment techniques, such as massage, aromatherapy, reflexology, and short courses of hypnotherapy, that are intended to help you feel more relaxed. Acupuncture (see p. 214) can also have this effect. Some therapists providing this type of treatment will also teach you simple relaxation exercises to use at home.

• investigative approaches that look into the fundamental causes of tension and attempt to deal with deep-seated emotional problems: psychotherapy (in its many different forms), psychoanalysis, long-term hypnotherapy when this has psychotherapeutic aims, and biodynamic massage.

In the long run, approaches that make you dependent on another person (an aromatherapist or reflexologist, for example) in order to feel relaxed, are usually less helpful than those that give you an active role. If you are learning and practicing a technique, as with relaxation exercises or yoga, this puts you in charge of your state of mind.

The techniques that are rooted in spiritual practice, especially meditation and yoga, are particularly helpful because they invite you to take a very broad view of the problems that face you and the situations that cause you stress. First, rather than focusing very narrowly on your own tense muscles and recurring difficulties, they look at the human situation as a whole—at the basic causes of tension and unhappiness in human beings. Second, rather than trying to graft a relaxed viewpoint onto a horribly unrelaxed daily existence (which is what most of us now endure) a regular meditation practice can result in a fundamental and long-lasting change in outlook, with a greater sense of wholeness, direction, and stability. This is something that happens naturally within the stillness of meditation practice, and it should be an individual process of change, not something imposed from outside. At a very practical level, a spiritual practice tends to improve relationships with other people, and since a great deal of our stress is caused by the people around us, any improvement in our social interactions can reduce stress enormously.

Some kind of psychotherapeutic approach may be the best choice for those who have tried and failed with other techniques, or achieved only a temporary reduction in stress levels. By tackling the problems at a deeper level, it is often possible to achieve a more profound and long-lasting solution.

Many people discover that whenever they try to relax or to meditate, they feel even more agitated and anxious. Others begin to cry or show other signs of distress. Not surprisingly, people who react in this way quickly give up their attempts to unwind, because their responses are so disturbing. Underlying these reactions to relaxation exercises there may be deep-seated problems, usually going back to childhood, which can be held at arm's length only with the help of a tense and always-busy approach to life.

Constant mental activity is part of this defensive strategy, which is why relaxing or meditating is such a frightening experience. Although it is tempting to run away from the problem, by plunging back into a life of frenetic activity, both mental and physical, this is ultimately no solution. Some form of psychotherapy is usually needed to deal with these long-standing problems.

Whatever you decide to try, make sure that the teacher or therapist seems like a calm and relaxed person. You should also look for someone who is sympathetic and supportive about your illness. Avoid those who attribute all allergies and other physical symptoms to mental or emotional problems (see p. 209). Such people can cause immense psychological damage.

Hypnotherapy

Hypnosis has a distinctly shady reputation, because of its use—or misuse—in stage and television performances. But hypnotherapy is also used by some entirely mainstream doctors, as a legitimate treatment for conditions such as atopic eczema, and the fact that it is used in this way, despite its dubious reputation, is a great testament to its effectiveness medically.

Hypnosis is certainly a mysterious phenomenon, and it is difficult to say exactly what happens when a person is hypnotized. Dr. Ruth Lever, a doctor who combines hypnotherapy with conventional medical practice, describes the hypnotic state as "not a form of unconsciousness but rather an altered form of consciousness, in which the patient is more open to suggestion than he would normally be, and in which a corridor is opened between the conscious and the subconscious mind."

It is certainly *not* true that the hypnotized person is under the control of the hypnotist or hypnotherapist. Autonomy is retained, and no one under hypnosis can be forced to do anything that is really against his or her will. While the person may experience a different state of mind, he or she remains aware of what is going on in the room and anything that is said.

The exact change in mental state during hypnosis varies greatly from one person to another. Some people respond far more readily than others and go into a deeper hypnotic state. (These same people are more susceptible to placebo effect, a psychological response to drugs or other treatment—see p. 233.)

At one time, it was thought that only adults could be hypnotized. Children seemed to be immune to hypnosis, but in fact they are just immune to the particular hypnotic techniques used for adults. With the right techniques, children can also be hypnotized.

Hypnotherapy treatment can be quite brief, taking only a few sessions. This approach relies on suggestions from the therapist to achieve relaxation, a change in perceptions (for example, that the skin feels cool and smooth, for someone with atopic eczema), and a beneficial change in habits (for example, stopping scratching).

Another approach is to use hypnosis as a means toward achieving personal insight into emotional problems by accessing suppressed memories. This is a more long-term treatment, which has much in common with psychotherapy. It should be practiced only by those who have full psychotherapy training.

Scientific studies show that hypnotherapy can be of benefit in both asthma and atopic eczema. Your best bet is to look for a hypnotherapist who also has conventional medical training, or psychotherapy training.

You may be given exercises in self-hypnosis to do at home, or tapes, possibly music tapes to be played at bedtime for children with eczema. These can be useful in reinforcing the messages about sleeping deeply and not scratching.

Relaxation exercises

Acquiring the knack of relaxing is a very personal thing—what works for one person will be useless for another. You may have to try several different techniques before you succeed in finding one that is right for you.

Guided imagery is often an effective method, and increasingly popular with the widespread availability of relaxation tapes. The tape will ask you to sit in an armchair, or lie down, and picture the scenes described ("waves are lapping gently on the golden sand..." for example). If you are able to visualize the scene, this should induce a more relaxed state of mind—somewhat like the relaxation you get from watching a good film.

There are also tapes of special music, or music combined with natural sounds (such as waves and seagulls), which are intended to produce a relaxed state of mind. Much of this music is incredibly banal, and it may irritate you more than relax you. However, there are also some excellent tapes available, so be prepared to shop around.

One time-honored method of relaxing is to sequentially contract, and then release, muscles in each part of the body, beginning with the hands or feet. This is known as Jacobsonian systematic relaxation training or progressive muscle relaxation. A study of children suffering from asthma found that this training increased the peak flow by an impressive 32 percent for some children, although others did not do quite so well.

Autogenic training

Based loosely on self-hypnosis, autogenic training is a very down-to-earth approach to relaxation which may be useful for anyone who is wary of things esoteric. You are taught to concentrate on different parts of your body in turn and imagine them growing warm and heavy. Beginning with "My right arm is heavy and warm . . ." (repeated three times, either out loud or in your head) you work your way through the rest of the body: "My left arm...," "Both my arms...," "My right leg...," and so forth.

You could, in theory, teach autogenic training to yourself, using a book; but it is helpful to go to a class. The teacher can encourage you to persist when you feel discouraged by your slow progress and can help with any problems that arise.

Teachers of autogenic training often add more specific lines at the end of the exercise, such as "My breathing is calm and regular" for asthmatics, or "My skin is soft and cool" for someone with eczema. A study of asthmatics found that they performed better in basic lung-function tests after eight months of regular autogenic training.

Autogenic training can sometimes evoke strong reactions, if there are longstanding problems or suppressed feelings and memories. In these situations, the training sessions may need to incorporate some elements of psychotherapy. Teachers vary in the extent to which they can offer this.

Yoga

Yoga, in its original form, provides a complex religious philosophy of life. If followed with dedication, it affects the whole person—physical, mental, emotional, and spiritual. Those who have practiced yoga seriously for many years achieve a great deal of mental focus and calmness, plus a surprising level of control over bodily functions such as blood pressure and heart rate. These profound changes are achieved through a combination of breathing exercises (*pranayama*), yoga postures (*asanas*), meditation, and careful attention to diet and way of life.

Yoga has now been practiced in the West for over a century, and during that time it has been watered down and very thoroughly Westernized. There are now forms of "yoga" that consist of little more than stretching and relaxation.

For the greatest benefits from yoga, look for classes with a more rigorous approach. If the particular kind of yoga is specified—Hatha Yoga or Kundalini Yoga, for example—the chances are that you'll be getting something more authentic.

Iyengar Yoga is a popular form taught in the West, but is rather narrow, concentrating almost entirely on postures. A form of yoga that includes breathing exercises (*pranayama*) is probably more useful, especially if you have asthma.

Before you sign up for a class, talk to the teacher and find out what it includes. If you are asthmatic, make sure the teacher is really experienced in working with asthmatics. It is all too easy to get the yoga breathing exercises wrong, making the breaths too deep. This can turn into a form of hyperventilation (see p. 226).

Approaching the breathing exercises with a "got to get this right" attitude is another pitfall for Westerners doing yoga. Most of us have the unfortunate habit—acquired in early childhood—of tensing up and "really trying" when we are taught anything. This is a major obstacle to doing yoga breathing correctly. Eastern attitudes are much more easygoing, and this helps asthmatics much more, because relaxing as you breathe is the key to it all.

Meditation

Basic meditation involves stilling the mind—either emptying it of all thoughts or focusing it on one very simple object. This is fantastically difficult for most people at first, but with time, and regular daily meditation, it gradually becomes easier.

Many different forms of meditation exist. Most are part of a spiritual tradition such as Hinduism, Sri Lankan Buddhism, Tibetan Buddhism, Zen Buddhism, or Taoism. Meditation also forms part of yoga, and it is a cornerstone of most martial arts, though this tends to be played down when these are taught in the West. In each case, meditation takes a slightly different form and has different psychological effects.

Biofeedback

This is the most thoroughly scientific, rational, and high-tech of alternative treatments. Biofeedback uses technology to measure the state of some part of your body—a part that is usually under automatic control, such as the electrical activity in your brain—and relays this information back to you (hence bio-feedback).

The feedback is shown by means of swinging needles on dials, flashing lights, or bleeping sounds. The idea is that you gradually learn to influence the signal, by noticing that it has changed very slightly in the desired direction, and then rerunning (in your head) the thoughts or feelings that apparently led to that change.

In quite a short space of time, you can, with this method, alter bodily states that are beyond voluntary control in most people. Scientific studies show that biofeedback can teach people to regulate their heartbeat, for example, or reduce the amount of acid produced by the stomach. Although yoga practitioners have long claimed to be able to influence such bodily functions, it was only with the invention of biofeedback that scientists accepted that this was possible.

Biofeedback can also teach asthmatics to relax tight airway muscles, something that has been demonstrated convincingly in scientific trials. Unfortunately, the specialized equipment needed for this particular form of training is not generally available.

If you sign up for biofeedback, you will probably be trained with equipment that measures the electrical resistance of the skin (this varies with how tense you are) or the electrical activity of the brain. This kind of equipment can help you learn to relax at will.

Massage and aromatherapy

There are many different varieties of massage, and most are relaxing to some extent. Regular massage treatments may improve your general sense of calmness and your ability to cope with life's stresses and problems. In the case of long-standing asthma, massage may also help with tension in the muscles of the chest, back and neck, which frequently develop during asthma attacks.

Aromatherapy is really a form of massage, with the use of scented oils derived from plants. For self-help, these oils are diluted according to instructions, and added to a steaming bowl of hot water, or a warm bath. You should bear in mind that the strong smell of some oils can provoke asthma attacks (see p. 39), while other oils can irritate the skin of people with atopic eczema or contact dermatitis. Never use undiluted aromatherapy oils on the skin. See a qualified practitioner if you are pregnant, have epilepsy, or high blood pressure.

Reflexology and zero balancing

Reflexology is based on the belief that specific zones on the soles of the feet correspond to particular parts of the body and that stimulating those zones on the feet (by gentle pressure) can induce a healing process at distant points in the body. It may or may not be true—certainly, having your feet massaged is immensely pleasurable and can induce a profound relaxation.

Zero balancing is a sequence of static touch, gentle holding, and light pressure, applied to specific parts of the body. It can induce a state of great well-being and calmness.

Psychotherapy

The basic tenet of psychotherapy is that it is much more painful and exhausting to keep on repressing bad memories than it is to bring them out into the open, in a safe therapeutic situation, which allows you to process them and move on. Dealing with deep-seated problems lets you relax and live life more fully. In some cases it may help with physical symptoms, such as allergies.

There is a bewildering choice here, with so many different varieties of therapy on offer. Fortunately, according to recent research, they *all* work to about the same extent, as long as you have a good rapport with the therapist.

But if you *don't* click, the therapy doesn't usually work, however expert the therapist might be. So make sure you have an introductory meeting before committing yourself to a course of therapy, and don't be afraid to say "No" and try someone else, if you don't feel quite right with the therapist.

Counseling can also be valuable, and again you will do much better with someone you feel at home with, but who is not afraid to challenge you when necessary.

Breathing exercises

Breathing is a delicate art, and it is possible to get it wrong, in a variety of ways and for a variety of reasons. A poor breathing pattern can gradually become habitual, without the person concerned being aware that their breathing is at all abnormal.

Allergy and sensitivity reactions sometimes play a part in causing abnormal breathing, and the symptoms produced by a poor breathing pattern may then augment the symptoms of sensitivity, creating a vicious circle. Correcting an abnormal breathing pattern, by means of breathing exercises and retraining, can produce remarkable improvements in health for some people.

Breathing too much

Taking in too much air, often called overbreathing or **hyperventilation**, is a common breathing disorder. It can produce a variety of rather strange symptoms (see p. 227) that are sometimes diagnosed correctly and treated appropriately, but often get overlooked or misdiagnosed.

The primary purpose of breathing is to obtain **oxygen** from the air and absorb it into the blood. The lungs are a crucial interface here, a trading post for gases that are exchanged between the bloodstream and the external air. The delicate, moist membranes that cover the inner surface of the lungs are accessed by millions of tiny threadlike blood vessels known as capillaries. Oxygen from the air seeps into the blood through the thin walls of these capillaries. At the same time, the lungs clean the blood of **carbon dioxide**, a waste gas produced by the body's metabolism. As oxygen seeps into the blood, carbon dioxide seeps out.

That is the school-textbook view of breathing, and it is correct up to a point. But it is oversimplified and misleading if it simply portrays oxygen as totally good and carbon dioxide as totally bad. In fact, there is a correct level in the blood for both gases, and too little or too much of either can cause problems.

Carbon dioxide plays an important role in the equilibrium of the blood because, when dissolved in any liquid, carbon dioxide makes a weak acid. So the amount of carbon dioxide present is crucial in deciding the acidity of the blood. Given that the blood reaches every part of the body, it is not surprising that any changes from its normal composition have far-reaching effects.

Normally, blood is very slightly acidic, and that is what the body is accustomed to. While some body parts can cope with small changes in the acidity of the blood, other parts respond very badly. The nerve cells are particularly vulnerable to changes in acidity.

Hyperventilation, or overbreathing, has relatively little effect on the level of oxygen in the blood, which is carefully controlled, but it can lower the level of carbon dioxide in the blood, thus making it less acid. More commonly, hyperventilation just makes the level of carbon dioxide vary a great deal.

When the carbon dioxide levels in the blood yo-yo around all the time, this has some unpleasant effects. In particular, it disrupts the smooth running of the nerve cells, which is why many of the symptoms of hyperventilation involve the senses, feelings, or behavior.

The symptoms of acute hyperventilation (that is, a short-lived attack of hyperventilation) can include
- numbness or pins and needles in the hands and feet, occasionally affecting the lips and tongue as well
- difficulty in swallowing
- aching muscles, cramps, tremors, and twitches
- sudden loss of strength in the muscles
- dizziness, confusion, unreal or spaced-out feelings
- blurred vision, ringing in the ears
- headache
- breathlessness
- aching in the chest
- abnormal heart rhythm
- sensitivity to bright lights and loud noises.

In the case of chronic (long-term) hyperventilation, there may also be some severe psychological symptoms:
- panic—a brief but intense state of anxiety
- prolonged anxiety, which can include an irrational fear of dying
- mood swings and phobias.

Each of these symptoms can, of course, be caused in several other ways, but when this whole cluster of symptoms—or a large number of them—occurs together in an individual, that person is very likely to be a "hyperventilator."

When there are short self-contained bursts of hyperventilation, the effects are often described as a **panic attack**. Doctors usually have no trouble recognizing this problem, but—not surprisingly— are often misled by the sustained psychological symptoms of chronic (long-term) hyperventilation. Many people with chronic hyperventilation are diagnosed as having some kind of mental illness, and they may go for years without getting the right diagnosis.

Hyperventilation and sensitivity reactions

The link between sensitivity reactions and hyperventilation seems to be a complex one. Unfortunately, very little research has been done in this area, so what follows is based on the case histories of patients and the collective experience of doctors, not on hard scientific data.

In some cases, a sensitivity reaction may directly provoke a change in breathing pattern. This is what appears to happen for some people with **caffeine sensitivity**. Cutting out all caffeine-containing drinks (coffee, tea, and colas) seems to put a stop to the hyperventilation symptoms, because the multiple symptoms promptly disappear.

In other cases, a severe sensitivity problem such as **multiple chemical intolerance** (see p. 236) results in an anxious state of mind, and the anxiety leads to hyperventilation. It is difficult to determine which comes first: psychological symptoms which then predispose to hyperventilation or hyperventilation causing secondary effects such as psychological symptoms.

Wheezy as a mountain breeze

Ionizers—devices that supposedly turn indoor urban air into a fresh mountain breeze—are often promoted as alternative devices that can clear allergens from the air. In the case of asthma, however, research shows that some ionizers can actually make symptoms *worse* by generating ozone, which irritates the airways. It is usually the cheaper ionizers that do this. More expensive models are less likely to produce ozone, but they are unlikely to help, either. Several scientific trials show that ionizers have no significant benefits when used by asthmatics.

Hyperventilation and asthma

While hyperventilation can develop in anyone, asthmatics are particularly vulnerable. During an asthma attack, especially a severe one, developing an abnormal breathing pattern is an entirely understandable reaction. In an attempt to get more air, you may start breathing more rapidly and taking air into the upper chest, using the accessory muscles of breathing (see p. 230). These muscles should not normally be used when one is at rest—they exist to give extra breathing capacity when running fast.

As long as the asthma attack lasts, this forced breathing does no harm, because its effects are cancelled out by the narrowing of the airways. But if this overbreathing persists after the attack has ended, then too much air is going in and out of the lungs, so carbon dioxide levels in the blood begin to fall.

Simply feeling anxious can also trigger off rapid upper-chest breathing. If you get very worried when an asthma attack starts, you may begin hyperventilating just out of anxiety.

For asthmatics, in addition to the usual symptoms of hyperventilation (see p. 227) there are some subtle effects of hyperventilation that can make asthma worse:

- The airway muscles (and all other muscles that are not under voluntary control) contract slightly when carbon dioxide levels in the blood fall.
- Mast cells are quicker to degranulate (see box on p.12) when there is less carbon dioxide, and this triggers allergic symptoms.

Just to complicate matters, one of the symptoms of hyperventilation is breathlessness. Sometimes this is the most prominent symptom in non-asthmatic hyperventilators, and the doctor may overlook the other symptoms and give a diagnosis of asthma. In such cases, people are told they have asthma when they are actually suffering from hyperventilation alone.

Testing for hyperventilation

You can do two simple tests for hyperventilation at home, if you think that it could be playing a part in your symptoms. (If you are asthmatic, do these tests only when you have no asthma symptoms and your peak flow reading is good. Make sure your reliever inhaler is nearby, in case of a bad reaction to the test.)

The first test should be done when you have some symptoms that might indicate hyperventilation (see p. 227).

Find a clean paper bag, and hold it over your nose and mouth while breathing normally. Any symptoms that are due to hyperventilation should clear up, because, by re-inhaling the air that you have just breathed out, you will increase the level of carbon dioxide in your blood.

The second test is done when you *don't* have any of the symptoms listed for hyperventilation.

Speed up your breathing, and inflate your upper chest with each breath. Do this for a few minutes. Do any of your usual symptoms appear? If they do, this suggests that they may be caused by hyperventilation.

If either of these tests indicates hyperventilation, make an appointment to see your doctor. It is important that you have a proper diagnosis, so that you get the right professional treatment.

Treating hyperventilation

If you hyperventilate, you could be taught a more healthy breathing pattern by a physiotherapist—ask your doctor for a referral. Certain complementary therapists, such as osteopaths and Feldenkrais practitioners can also teach good breathing patterns, and so can experienced yoga teachers (see p. 224). A teacher or therapist who takes their time, is not too dogmatic, and helps you to find your own way to healthy breathing is preferable to one who tries to impose a regimented breathing pattern on you.

On the assumption that most people who hyperventilate don't just overbreathe, but also breathe with their upper chest and underuse the diaphragm (see pp. 229–230), all these different practitioners will take a combined approach—tackling both sides of the problem at once. This represents an important difference from the Buteyko method (see below).

The Buteyko method

The stated aim of the Buteyko method (also called the Buteyko treatment) is to stop people from hyperventilating. However, Buteyko practitioners do not work with people who have the symptoms of hyperventilation, as recognized by conventional medicine (see p. 227). Instead they work with asthmatics—*any* asthmatics, not just those whose symptoms suggest that they might be hyperventilating.

The rationale for this is the claim, by the originator of the exercises, Professor Konstantin Buteyko, that asthma is actually *caused* by hyperventilation. (What is more, Professor Buteyko cites hyperventilation as the cause of no less than 150 different diseases, including allergies, eczema, migraines, insomnia, bronchitis, high blood pressure, and hemorrhoids. However, his treatment is marketed only for asthma.)

The claims made for the success of the Buteyko method in treating asthma are startling. According to one training center, it can get 97 percent of asthmatics off most of their drugs and able to control attacks within a week of starting.

Not surprisingly, this is a bit of an exaggeration. An Australian research study showed that during the course of Buteyko lessons, the overall use of reliever inhalers (for example, Ventolin) fell substantially and remained relatively low 3 months later.

However, the patients' average peak flow stayed the same, and 15 percent of those studied were admitted to a hospital with a severe asthma attack during the trial. In the 8 months that followed, 30 percent needed a course of steroid tablets—indicating a substantial worsening in their condition. In other words, the Buteyko method can give some help to many asthmatics, but the claim that it can get almost everyone off asthma drugs and free of asthma is just hype.

Professor Buteyko's claim to have discovered the *fundamental cause* of asthma is clearly untrue. What he seems to have discovered is that there is much more hyperventilation among asthmatics than was widely realized and that this can occur without bringing on the obvious symptoms of hyperventilation. His other important contribution is to suggest that mouth-breathing may create a lot more problems for asthmatics than previously recognized.

The Buteyko method has three aspects:
- unblocking the nose
- training to breathe through the nose, not the mouth
- training to take fewer breaths and pause between breaths.

Unlike other treatments for hyperventilation (both conventional and alternative), the Buteyko method pays no attention to teaching asthmatics to breathe with the diaphragm. However, a few Buteyko practitioners are now beginning to incorporate this aspect of treatment.

The Buteyko method is widely taught in Australia and Britain, but is not well known yet in North America. If you would like to try the Buteyko method, there are video cassettes and books that explain how to do the exercises (see p. 255).

Whichever option you choose, it is vital that you get your doctor's permission before starting. Make sure that your reliever inhaler is in your pocket while doing the exercises, because they could provoke an asthma attack. Keep taking your preventer drugs regularly throughout the treatment. If you start to feel much better and want to reduce your dose of preventer, you must talk to your doctor first.

Don't follow the Buteyko method blindly, because some of the advice given is dangerous. For example, some Buteyko publications advise you to refuse oxygen if you are taken to the hospital with a severe asthma attack. They claim that oxygen levels in the blood are not reduced during a severe asthma attack, but this is just not true. Measurements clearly show that the level of oxygen gets very low, **and this is frequently the cause of death**.

Another very peculiar Buteyko idea is that you should not try to shift mucus from your airways because mucus "protects you" against losing too much carbon dioxide. This too is dangerous advice. Accumulated mucus narrows the airways, adding to your asthma symptoms, and it can even block a small airway completely. The part of the lung served by that airway then collapses—a serious complication that no asthmatic would want.

Using the right muscles

Hyperventilation is often linked with an abnormal way of breathing, in which the wrong muscles are used. This is one common pattern that conventional doctors recognize for people who hyperventilate:
- The main muscle of breathing, the diaphragm (see below), is not used fully
- The muscles of the upper chest become involved in breathing, even at rest, when they should not be needed
- There are lots of rapid, shallow breaths
- The breathing is quite irregular, with deep, sighing breaths from time to time, or frequent yawning.

Even in those who do not hyperventilate, breathing with the upper chest and/or neglecting the diaphragm, can become a problem. This pattern of breathing is sometimes linked to anxiety and emotional problems (see p. 230).

To understand what goes wrong, you need first to know about the healthy way to breathe.

The **rib cage** and the **diaphragm** are the workhorses of breathing. You can feel your rib cage through your skin and feel its movements, but the diaphragm is far more inaccessible. It lies below the lungs, but above the stomach and intestines.

In its contracted state, the diaphragm becomes a thick slab of muscle, with a slight curve, like an inverted saucer. When it relaxes, it becomes far more curvaceous, changing to a shape like an inverted bell. In this shape, there is less space for the lungs above the diaphragm.

If you are breathing correctly, the diaphragm contracts when you breathe in and relaxes when you breathe out. The contraction lowers the dome of the diaphragm, pulling the base of the lungs downward and so making them expand.

Breathing out requires no muscular force whatever, as long as you are just sitting or walking around (and therefore not breathing hard). The lungs are naturally elastic, like balloons, so they automatically contract and force out the air, once the diaphragm relaxes into its bell-like shape and stops pulling them downward.

While you cannot feel the diaphragm itself, you can feel the effect of its in-breath contraction. As it contracts, the diaphragm pushes down on the stomach and intestines, so that your abdomen bulges out a little with each breath. Western women, conditioned to admire a flat-bellied body shape, often breathe badly because they are trying to "hold the tummy in." This steely tightening of the muscles across the front of the abdomen fights against the contraction of the diaphragm, and prevents a natural and relaxed in-breath.

The diaphragm should do virtually all the work of breathing in, when you are not exerting yourself much. The upper part of the rib cage should hardly expand at all, and the muscles that run between the ribs, called the **intercostal muscles**, should not be working as you breathe.

When you become more active, and therefore need more oxygen, the upper chest automatically starts to expand with each in-breath. At this point the intercostal muscles become involved, along with a whole team of other muscles in the chest region— these are known as the **accessory muscles of breathing**.

The effects of an asthma attack

In the grip of a severe asthma attack, you may well start using the accessory muscles of breathing to try to take in more air. If you have frequent attacks, or if this way of breathing gets to be a habit and goes on between attacks, then the chest may be distorted by the constant use of the accessory muscles, plus the overinflation of the lungs. Severe asthmatics often have high shoulders and a "barrel-chested" look as a result of this. Hyperventilation may also start in this way.

Observing how you breathe

To discover whether you are breathing with your diaphragm or your upper chest, lie on your back with your left hand on your belly, and your right hand on your upper chest. Just lie still for a few minutes, let your arms relax, then start to pay attention to your hands. When you breathe in, which hand rises? It should be the left hand, with little or no movement in the right.

Alternatively, bend over and hold the back of a chair with your hands. Your back, head, and arms should form a straight horizontal line, at right angles to your legs. Just stay quietly in this position for a while. It is very difficult to breathe with the upper chest in this pose, whereas breathing with the diaphragm is easy. If you feel fine in this position, then you are probably breathing well in normal life.

Correcting upper-chest breathing

Learning to breathe with the diaphragm is often an important part of correcting hyperventilation (see p. 228). It should also be taught to anyone who has the kind of chest deformities that develop in severe asthma (see above).

Diaphragmatic breathing, or **abdominal breathing**, as it is sometimes called, should help make you feel more relaxed because the in-breath can disperse tensions in your abdomen.

This is where many people "hold on" to their fears, with chronically tense abdominal muscles. When you start breathing into this area of tension, it is important to take things gently. Be aware of any resistance to the in-breath in the abdomen, and of any emotional reactions that occur when you challenge this resistance. It may be better to learn abdominal breathing from someone who has time to deal with such issues, and with whom you feel very comfortable and relaxed—for example, a yoga teacher or an alternative therapist whom you like and trust. Physiotherapists tend to take a brisk and practical approach to breathing, which may not be entirely appropriate or helpful when habitual ways of breathing are tied up with anxiety.

When learning to breathe with the diaphragm, be careful not to get carried away and become a "belly breather," whose every in-breath sends the abdomen bulging out like a mainsail. The abdominal muscles should be firm enough to counteract the downward movement of the diaphragm to some extent, without being too tense. In other words, the abdomen should expand a little with each in-breath, but not excessively.

Clearing the nose

Breathing through the nose, rather than the mouth, is beneficial for asthmatics, because it cleans and warms the air. It can also help those with chronic sinusitis, because it oxygenates the air in the sinuses, which discourages some of the more troublesome microbes responsible for sinus infections.

This technique for clearing a blocked nose, part of a set of breathing exercises for opera singers, is based on a time-honored yoga exercise called **alternate nostril breathing**:

- Sit with your mouth closed.
- Press your right nostril against your nose to close it, using the thumb of your right hand.
- Breathe out through your left nostril.
- Press your left nostril against your nose with the index finger of your right hand, to close it. (The hand makes only a very small movement from side to side.)
- Breathe in through your right nostril.
- Repeat the sequence

Once you have gotten the hang of this, do ten fairly rapid breaths in succession, with no pause between out-breath and in-breath. Pause and rest.

Repeat using your left hand, and reversing the flow of the breath: out through the right nostril and in through the left. Again, do ten breaths and then rest.

Alternatively, try the following exercise, which is recommend by Buteyko practitioners for unblocking the nose. This technique has not been tested scientifically, but the reports of asthmatics who have used it suggest that it often works wonders, even with children who could never breathe through their noses previously:

- Have your reliever inhaler at hand, just in case the exercise brings on an asthma attack.
- Breathe as you do normally, and at the end of a normal out-breath, close your mouth and hold your nose.
- Stay like this, without inhaling, for as long as you can without discomfort. Walk around the room while you are doing this, or, if you are young and fit, do something more strenuous—either walk upstairs or squat-then-stand several times.
- When you need to breathe in, keep your mouth closed but release your nose.
- Breathe in slowly through the nose.
- Repeat the exercise if your nose becomes blocked again.

Special exercises for asthma

In addition to tackling the problem of hyperventilation, if one exists, asthmatics can use other breathing exercises to tackle specific aspects of their asthma.

Clearing mucus from the lungs A physiotherapist can teach methods of clearing mucus from the airways which are suitable for asthmatics. Ask your doctor for a referral. You could also try the following exercises:

Huffing Take an in-breath, then tighten your abdominal muscles very sharply, to push the air out. Imagine there is a candle in front of you, and you are trying to extinguish it, but using your belly muscles only. Your out-breath should make a short soft "huff" sound—if it is more of a loud "wooosh," you are contracting the muscles in your chest as well as those in the belly. Try again, and focus your attention on your belly as you make the out-breath.

The in-breath should be effortless with this exercise—it just bounces back in. Do as many huffs as you can without feeling breathless. Rest and repeat. The aim is to build up stamina until you can do thirty or more huffs in succession.

Pursed-lips breathing Take a fairly deep in-breath, then purse your lips together. As with huffing, your belly muscles have to do all the work of the out-breath, but in this exercise they are working against the muscles of the lips. The aim is to divide the out-breath into as many fragments as possible—to push the air out through the lips in a succession of tiny, forceful blasts.

One objective of these exercises is to encourage mucus to start moving up to the top of the airways. From there, it can be cleared with a little throat-clearing cough. Note that the mucus will probably take a while to reach the throat—this may happen some time after you do the exercise. For maximum effect, repeat these exercises several times each day.

Coping with asthma attacks

The crucial thing during an asthma attack is to focus on your out-breath, not your in-breath. Of course this goes against the grain, because you feel so desperate for air, but remember that the central problem is stale air from your last in-breath, now trapped in your lungs by the narrow airways. If you can focus on exhaling this used air, you will have more space for fresh air to come in with the next in-breath.

At times when you are *not* suffering from an asthma attack, it is worth doing some exercises that improve the strength of your out-breath. The key problem during an asthma attack is that the natural elasticity of the lungs, which should power the out-breath, is not equal to the challenge of pushing out all that air through narrowed airways in a short space of time. In this situation, contracting your abdominal muscles so that they push upward and assist in emptying the lungs is helpful.

The two exercises described above for clearing mucus—huffing and pursed lips breathing—also strengthen those abdominal muscles that can assist you with your out-breath during asthma attacks.

Strengthening exercises

Several different exercises or pursuits that strengthen the breathing muscles seem to produce an improvement in asthma. The reasons for this are not understood.

Asthmatics who take up a wind instrument, such as the flute, often report that their asthma improves considerably. The same effect has regularly occurred with asthmatics who undertake classical training in singing. One set of exercises, taught to aspiring opera singers and designed specifically to strengthen the diaphragm has been scientifically tested and shown to improve asthma and reduce the need for drugs. These exercises can be learned at home (see p. 255). There are also some mechanical devices that can strengthen the breathing muscles (see p. 255).

The role of the mind
IN ALLERGY AND INTOLERANCE

"I get sick if I take a long bus trip—six or seven hours, say. I'm usually very nauseous at the end of the journey, and have a headache. The funny thing is, if I'm walking along the street and I happen to see a bus of the kind that I take long trips on, I feel a bit nauseous then too, just for a short while. It seems crazy, but I feel sick just from *seeing* the bus."

What Jake is observing is the powerful effect of the mind on the body, in the reaction known as **conditioning**. Some people are more susceptible to it than others, but no one is completely immune.

The Russian scientist Ivan Petrovich Pavlov first demonstrated conditioning in 1889, with his famous dog-and-dinner-bell experiment. Pavlov rang a bell every time he fed the dog, and eventually the dog would salivate each time it heard the bell, whether dinner was being served or not. Its stomach would also begin to secrete acid, in anticipation of the meal, simply on hearing the bell.

Modern-day experiments have shown that conditioning works with immune reactions, too. For example, rats can be conditioned by repeatedly giving them an immunosuppressive drug and always adding saccharin to their drinking water on the day the drug is given. Subsequently, just the taste of saccharin in the water is enough to suppress their immune responses.

This surprising discovery is partially explained by the finding that there are nerves running to the lymph nodes—key areas where the immune responses are coordinated. In other words, the immune system and the nervous system, once thought of as completely separate domains, are in conversation with each other. In fact this is a three-way discussion, because the hormones are also involved. The study of these complex interactions, which we are only just beginning to understand, is known as **psychoneuroimmunology**.

Even before Pavlov carried out his classic experiment, Dr. John MacKenzie, of Baltimore, Maryland, had discovered that an artificial rose, in the vase on his desk, would bring on an attack of rhinitis and asthma in one of his patients, who believed that she was allergic to roses. (In fact such an allergy is unlikely—see box on p. 127. It is usually the strong scent that triggers symptoms, the allergy being to something else, often grass pollen, which is in the air when roses flower.)

Much more recently, something similar happened—this time unintentionally—when a boy with severe hay fever and pollen asthma was undergoing hypnosis, aimed at helping him relax. Part of the hypnotist's standard technique was to describe an idyllic scene in an alpine meadow and ask the subject to imagine being there. For this boy, it worked all too well—the thought of the grass pollen in the meadow brought on a severe asthma attack. The hypnotist, with great presence of mind, asked him to imagine a helicopter suddenly appearing in the sky and rescuing him from the meadow—and the asthma attack subsided.

Scientific tests, carried out in a laboratory, back up these casual observations. For example, many people who are allergic to grass pollen will suffer an asthma attack if the experimenter says they are inhaling grass pollen through a mouthpiece—even though they are actually inhaling fresh air.

It can work the other way as well. Telling the same asthmatics that they are now inhaling a reliever drug alleviates the attack, even though they are still breathing the same air as before. This is the basis of **placebo effect**, the benefit that tends to occur with any treatment, even a dummy pill, as long as patients believe that the treatment will work.

Note that it is not necessarily the immune system producing all these reactions. There are also direct effects of the mind on the skin, in atopic eczema, on the airway muscles, in the case of asthma, and on the nose in rhinitis. Some of these are due to the autonomic nervous system (see box on p. 235), while others are less well understood.

The findings described above should be reassuring for anyone who has noticed that their allergy or asthma symptoms are sometimes affected by their thoughts and feelings. There is no need to feel bad about this, and it certainly doesn't mean that your allergies are "all in the mind." Conditioning and other psychological responses are an entirely natural reaction to a very real illness.

However, if psychological reactions are making a big contribution to your symptoms, and you would like to overcome this, you could try to address the problem directly. Hypnotherapy (see p. 223) can be particularly useful in this regard, because people who are most susceptible to conditioning are also very responsive to hypnotic suggestion—which can counteract the conditioning messages. Hypnotherapy can also help those asthmatics who become psychologically dependent on their inhalers—something that happens quite often, especially in people with severe asthma. In the words of one asthmatic "If I found that I'd left my Ventolin at home, that would sometimes start me off wheezing straight away. I was so afraid of being without it." Of course, it is important to carry your reliever inhaler with you at all times, but this kind of excessive psychological dependence is distinctly unhealthy. At worst, it can lead you to overuse your reliever inhaler, which can increase your risk of a life-threatening asthma attack (see pp. 153–4).

Sometimes the psychological effects involved in allergies and asthma are far more complex and deep-rooted than this, not just a matter of simple conditioning. It is not uncommon for asthma attacks, in particular, to be provoked by family tensions and anxieties. This can occur even though the asthma also has a clear-cut physical cause, such as an allergy to dust mites. Some people find that their asthma always gets worse when they are in a certain place, with a certain person, or in a particular situation. These problems are usually helped by psychotherapy (see p. 225).

While hypnotherapy and psychological treatments can sometimes be valuable, it is vital to remember that the mental factors in allergic reactions are always operating in combination with purely physical responses—such as the triggering of mast cells by allergen (see box on p. 12). Using psychological treatments alone is as much of a mistake as ignoring the mental and emotional dimension of ill-health completely. The two aspects of treatment—physical and psychological—should always go hand in hand. Be very wary of alternative therapists who overemphasize the psychological aspects (see p. 209).

Under the skin

To see a baby with severe eczema is heartbreaking for any parent—tormented by something it cannot understand, the child often experiences touch, not as a comforting and pleasurable contact, but as a further irritation. According to some psychologists who have studied eczema in depth, suffering from severely itchy skin in the early years of life may create long-lasting psychological problems. They believe that the discomfort associated with the skin, and especially with being touched, interferes with normal processes of relating to the world and developing loving relationships with others. That is why it is so important to get the skin symptoms under control, with the proper use of steroid creams, skin care, dietary changes if appropriate, and an anti-scratching program (see p. 46).

How allergies affect the mind

In studying the psychological aspects of allergy, researchers have discovered that some patients frequently have thoughts that catastrophize the situation. In the case of atopic eczema, these thoughts might go along the lines of "this terrible itching will never end" or "none of the treatments really make much difference."

Such thoughts may be just below the surface of the conscious mind most of the time, and it is only by developing the ability to notice what is going on internally that the allergy sufferer can become aware of them.

Researchers have also found that, when negative thoughts such as these arise, eczema sufferers are far more likely to scratch their skin and so make the eczema worse. Thus the thought becomes a reality—a self-fulfilling prophecy.

The tendency to catastrophize difficult situations is something that most people develop (or acquire from others) at a very young age, and it may take some effort to even become aware of this mental habit, let alone change it. Yet it is possible to start thinking about illness, and about life in general, in a different way—for example, as a difficult challenge but one that can usually be overcome.

Allergies are in no sense unique. Any long-term disease that causes intense discomfort, makes life unpredictable, or limits your activities is bound to have profound effects on your personality. However strong a person you are, it affects your life and influences you in a very deep way—shaping you as a thinking and feeling individual. This is especially true if illness begins at an early age, becoming part of your formative interactions with your parents (see box on p. 233) or marking you out as different from other children.

This shaping can have both positive and negative aspects, and it is important to recognize that there is a choice about which aspect you emphasize. It is never too late to try to change the emphasis. Counseling or psychotherapy (see p. 225) may help with this, especially if the counterproductive attitudes to the illness are deeply rooted in family experiences.

The role of the mind in asthma

The diagnosis of **intrinsic asthma**, commonplace in the 1950s and 1960s, has long since been abandoned. It technically meant "asthma with no external cause," but the widespread assumption was that the cause was psychological. As older asthmatics will tell you, this made their lives particularly miserable, because they were held responsible for their disease. Families were often ashamed of having an asthmatic child.

The injustice of this sweeping assumption is clear today. Modern research shows that an external stimulus which initiated the asthma, such as an allergen, can usually be found. Among asthmatic children, an allergic cause exists in 80–90 percent of cases. Even where no specific stimulus can be found, there is still a clear-cut state of inflammation in the airways. No one with any knowledge of asthma would now claim that it is an entirely psychosomatic disease, or even that it is predominantly psychosomatic.

Nevertheless, once asthma has begun, the mind may play an important role in bringing on attacks or making them worse, as many asthmatics know from their own experience. This is entirely understandable when you think how closely breathing is tied up with our emotional lives—fear, sadness, excitement, and anger all alter the usual breathing pattern in different ways, and any of these reactions may trigger an asthma attack.

The interactions between the mind and the airways are complex in the extreme, and vary from one person to another. Anxiety and tension can make asthma a great deal worse for some people, while others suffer an asthma attack only when the stress is over. A few people actually have *less* trouble with their asthma when under stress, and, oddly enough, this is the reaction that is easiest to explain. Stress activates the sympathetic nervous system (see box on p. 235), which produces epinephrine (adrenaline), and the epinephrine opens up the airways.

For stress to make asthma worse, as it frequently does, there must be some other reaction going on that overrides the effect of the epinephrine. Doctors don't know exactly what this is, but asthmatics who get worse when stressed could be hyperventilating (see p. 226) just a little—not enough for it to be obvious, but enough to make their airway muscles contract.

Breathing through the mouth, rather than the nose, can also occur under intense stress, and this is bad for the airways because the air they receive tends to be drier, dustier, and possibly colder, for not having passed through the nose. This raw air may irritate the sensitive airway linings of an asthmatic and so make the airway muscles tighten. Small local nerves, that run directly from the airway linings to the airway muscles, could cause this reaction.

Psychological symptoms from sensitivity reactions

"People thought that because the hospital could not find anything wrong with me, and because I wasn't terminally ill, there was nothing wrong with me at all. No one could understand how I was feeling, or even believed me. My friends and family lost patience with me. I overheard one member of my family saying they thought I was just attention-seeking. This hurt me so much. I hated being ill all the time. I wanted to go out and enjoy myself and do the things I'd always done, but I couldn't because I felt so bad."

Josie, who is now 27, was ill in this way for several years, and her symptoms were so incapacitating that she had to give up work and abandon any kind of social life. Now, as she puts it, "I have my life back again."

The cause of her symptoms—dizziness, confusion, panic attacks, prolonged anxiety, shortness of breath, and a conviction that she was dying—turned out to be a sensitivity to caffeine, which was overstimulating her nervous system and inducing hyperventilation (see p. 226). Giving up tea, coffee, and cola drinks restored her to normality very promptly, and she has not relapsed since, except on one occasion, when she unwittingly took a headache remedy that contained caffeine.

What is clear from Josie's story is how much the disbelief of those around her added to her problems. She felt trapped by her symptoms, which she could not overcome, while everyone around her assumed that the whole problem was in her head, and that she could "snap out of it" if she chose to.

Although Josie's case is extreme, her suffering (and the suffering of others who are less severely affected) could easily be avoided if more doctors knew how to recognize sensitivity syndromes that can induce hyperventilation.

Caffeine sensitivity leading to chronic hyperventilation is a condition that is well described in the medical literature but does not always get onto the curriculum in medical schools. As a result, many hyperventilating patients go through a lot of expensive investigations, and may not get a proper diagnosis even then. This is especially sad when hyperventilation is so easy to diagnose and treat (see p. 228).

The autonomic nervous system

The autonomic nervous system is a kind of "autopilot"—a set of controls that can keep you well adjusted to your external circumstances without your having to think consciously about the situation at all.

The autonomic nervous system controls all the involuntary muscles—those in the heart, around the digestive system, and around the airways. It also controls the state of the blood vessels, including those in the skin. The autonomic nervous system does its work by issuing two different sets of signals—one set that gears the body up for action and one set that calms the body down.

Two completely separate nerve networks, the sympathetic nervous system and the parasympathetic nervous system, issue these different signals. The target organs—the airways, heart, skin, and so forth—all receive input from both networks.

The "get active" signals are issued by the **sympathetic nervous system**, which comes into play at times of stress, excitement, fear, or anger. When you can hear your heart pounding or feel your pulse race, that is your sympathetic nervous system at work. It also makes your nasal passages and airways open up, because extra oxygen is needed for intense physical activity, and it tightens the muscles around the blood vessels, which raises your blood pressure.

"Chill out" messages are delivered by the **parasympathetic nervous system**. This network comes onstream when you know you can afford to relax. It slows down the heart, lowers the blood pressure, encourages the digestive system to do its work, and makes the airways grow narrower, because less air is needed when you are less active.

Epinephrine (adrenaline) is the messenger substance released by the sympathetic nervous system. Its action in tightening the muscles around the blood vessels allows epinephrine to be employed as a drug, which saves the lives of people affected by anaphylaxis (see p. 150). During anaphylaxis, there is a massive fall in blood pressure produced by histamine (see box on p. 12), but an injection of epinephrine can reverse this.

Both epinephrine and its derivatives, the beta-2 relievers such as Ventolin (see p. 152), also help in asthma attacks. They do this by making the muscles around the airways relax.

The messenger substance of the parasympathetic nervous system is **acetylcholine**. Drugs that *oppose* its action—the anticholinergics—can also help relieve an asthma attack (see p. 156) by blocking the airway-narrowing action of the parasympathetic.

One of the ways in which acupuncture appears to work is by adjusting the activity of the autonomic nervous system. When acupuncture is used to deal with the immediate symptoms of an asthma attack, this is probably how it makes the airways open up.

While the symptoms of hyperventilation are easy to spot, once you know what to look for, this is certainly not true of all sensitivity reactions. Food sensitivity can occasionally cause some unexpected psychological symptoms (see p. 80), that the majority of conventional doctors would never associate with food.

Inevitably, patients with sensitivity problems such as these will initially be diagnosed as having a psychological illness rather than a physical one. It may be a long time before the correct diagnosis is established.

Even if the patient works out the link between eating the food and experiencing the psychological response, the doctor may well remain unconvinced. What complicates matters for doctors is that quite a few people with genuine psychological problems would prefer to think that these have a nonpsychological cause, such as a sensitivity to food. (In the opinion of most doctors, patients of this kind are far more common than patients with psychological problems that are genuinely caused by food or chemical intolerance.) For such patients, accepting that their problems have a psychological cause means thinking about what that cause might be—and such causes are often something deeply distressing which the person would rather forget.

For people who get into this situation, unfortunately, the phony explanation doesn't actually help at all, though it can provide a temporary distraction. Ignoring unpleasant hidden memories is not the answer—the problem does not go away, it just festers. Facing up to the real underlying problem is the only way to get rid of the distress (see p. 225).

If you have psychological symptoms of any kind, bear in mind that psychological causes are by far the most likely cause. These causes can include difficult life circumstances, damaging experiences during childhood, loss of close relationships, or extremely traumatic incidents in the more recent past. Where there are long-standing problems, neurological factors (damage to the nerves or brain) or metabolic factors (something affecting the balance of chemicals in the brain) might also play a part, or sometimes be the sole cause.

For a busy doctor, without much time to spare, it is immensely difficult to distinguish patients who really do have psychological symptoms due to food or chemical intolerance, from patients with psychological problems that they have mistakenly attributed to an intolerance reaction.

What adds to the difficulty is that, with time, psychological causes can sometimes be grafted onto a straightforward intolerance problem. This occurs because illness of any kind can produce some psychological problems of its own, especially if the person affected cannot lead a normal life. The psychological effects of the illness invariably get worse if the person concerned has been treated with disbelief by other doctors, family or friends—as is frequently the case when a person has indefinite long-term symptoms that are due to food or chemical intolerance. Separating the secondary psychological reactions to the illness (or to the skepticism of others) from the primary psychological symptoms that are genuinely produced by the intolerance reactions is far from easy.

Hyperventilation and chemical intolerance

Hyperventilation (see pp. 226–9) and chemical intolerance (see p. 84) often go hand in hand. A person who is sensitive to airborne items that they cannot avoid inhaling, such as perfume or gasoline fumes, may well feel apprehensive when they catch a whiff of these and unconsciously alter their breathing in response. They may hyperventilate.

If they do, this can both aggravate the sensitivity symptoms and increase their anxious feelings—because one key symptom of hyperventilation is anxiety (see p. 227). In this way the problem begins to feed upon itself, and can spiral out of control.

Hyperventilation, pure and simple, may also *masquerade as* chemical intolerance. In these cases, a deep underlying anxiety probably exists in the person concerned, and one way in which this expresses itself as a fear of synthetic chemicals. The person's fear triggers hyperventilation, which is the initial cause of symptoms. That is not how the person interprets those symptoms, however—because the person was anticipating a reaction to synthetic chemicals, the symptoms seem to confirm that a reaction has occurred. Again, a vicious circle has been started which is hard to break.

Another possible scenario is that someone with a few sensitivity reactions—for example, a reaction to perfume and cigarette smoke—starts to feel concerned about other chemical substances and to suspect that these might also cause problems. If an anxious reaction to the presence of these suspects develops into hyperventilation, symptoms will ensue from the hyperventilation. These symptoms will appear to confirm the person's fears about yet more sensitivity reactions. In this way, people with relatively mild chemical intolerance can begin to believe that their chemical intolerance reactions are far more extensive and disabling than they actually are.

Where the symptoms of hyperventilation are all tangled up with symptoms due to genuine chemical intolerance, opinions tend to split. Some doctors will interpret all the symptoms as psychological, while some will attribute them all to the intolerance. Both are oversimplifying the problem and missing a crucial ingredient—hyperventilation. Recognizing and treating hyperventilation (see p. 228) can help a great deal to alleviate the illness.

The psychologization of illness

"From the moment Joanna was born, she was never hungry." Sandra recalls. "It took all day to force an ounce of milk down, and she seemed to have terrible stomach pains. At six months old, after countless trips to the doctor, she was admitted to the hospital. The doctors couldn't work out what was wrong, and in the end they said that she was just very independent and that she wouldn't eat until she could feed herself. I couldn't believe my ears—what a thing to say about a six-month-old baby!" But as far as the doctors were concerned, that was that.

As Joanna got older, the symptoms got worse. She developed severe constipation, moving her bowels only once every four weeks. Because her over-full bowel put so much pressure on her bladder, she wet herself several times a day. "She hated school, because the other children teased her, saying she smelled. And she had such awful stomach pains that she couldn't bend down to tie her shoelaces. When she was six she was admitted to hospital for a second time."

"Again they said there was nothing physically wrong with her and it was all in her head, and this time they decided that it must be because something traumatic had happened at home. They wanted her to see a psychiatrist. It was terrible. I knew nothing like that had happened to her at home, but it was impossible to convince them."

Two weeks before seeing the psychiatrist, something happened to change Joanna's life. Sandra saw an item on television about a book on food allergies. She bought the book, and, remembering how fiercely Joanna had rejected milk as a baby, she hazarded a guess that milk was the problem. She immediately took all dairy products out of Joanna's diet.

The effect was astonishing. "Within twelve hours her stomach pains had gone, and after six weeks she began moving her bowels almost daily. She stopped wetting herself, and was so much happier and healthier." In fact, all of Joanna's symptoms went away, and she has remained well on a milk-free diet.

Psychologization is most frequently encountered by patients with medical problems that are unrecognized by conventional medicine—Joanna is a typical example of such a patient. Occasionally, however, those with true allergies find themselves in the same situation. Take, for example, someone who has collapsed after being stung by a wasp but gives a negative skin-test result to wasp venom. In the case of insect-sting allergy, skin tests are supposed to give very few false negatives—so the doctor may be skeptical about the patient's observation of what happened. A RAST test (see p. 92) may be ordered, but sometimes this, too, gives a false negative.

Doctors are—not unreasonably—more inclined to believe that the patient is an unreliable witness (there was never any insect involved), or that the patient has a psychological problem which has led to this consultation, than that both these tests gave a false negative result. A patient in this position may need to be quite persistent to get proper treatment. The same goes for anyone else with unusual allergic reactions that are initially labeled "psychological" by their doctor. In such cases, good communication is everything.

Good communication with your doctor

Given the intense pressure under which they work, doctors often react badly to symptoms that don't fit into a neat diagnostic pigeonhole or don't respond to standard treatment. They simply don't have the time for unraveling complex problems, and there is a tendency to automatically "psychologize" such symptoms. This often does great damage to the patients concerned, boxing them into a corner from which it is difficult to escape—the more they try to convince the doctor their symptoms are genuine and request further tests or treatment, the more the doctor is likely to view them as difficult, demanding patients with psychological problems. Unfortunately, it is part of the dogma about psychosomatic illness that patients affected by it will object vehemently to such a diagnosis. So the more you insist that the symptoms are not psychological, the more this confirms the diagnosis as far as some doctors are concerned.

The psychologization of illness becomes a real nightmare where the patient is a child, and parents are suspected of actually causing the symptoms in some way (see Joanna's story, left). This has happened more than once to children with unusual sensitivity reactions.

Good communication with your doctor may stop you from sliding into this situation. First, avoid getting emotional, agitated, or angry, which may cause your doctor to suspect a psychological cause for your symptoms.

Second, be very open with the doctor, and don't conceal anything. Be clear about describing symptoms, and accurate about times, the intensity of the reaction, and any other details. Never exaggerate. If you are given to describing things quite colorfully in everyday life, tone it down.

Third, don't make your own diagnosis—there is a tendency for doctors to believe that patients who diagnose themselves may well be suffering from hypochondria. Present any medical knowledge you have acquired from books or the Internet as tactfully as possible. Finally, it will help to use the appropriate words to describe your illness when talking with your doctor (see pp. 6–7).

Chapter 8
protecting children against allergies

"Good health is one of the most important things we can give our kids," says Martha, now in her sixties with two grown-up children.

"When I see how bad my daughter's asthma is, and how hard her life is sometimes because of it, I do feel bad about the fact that I smoked when I was pregnant. But we just didn't know in those days. Even my doctor smoked. No one thought anything of it.

"I stopped when she was little, because it seemed to me that her wheezing got worse whenever I lit up. I'm sure that stopping then was better than nothing. It must have helped.

"In any case, there's no point feeling guilty about things now—that won't change anything. But if I'd known what damage it could do, I would have stopped sooner."

Martha's regrets stem from the discoveries made in the past decade about the effects of smoking on allergies. We now know that smoking during pregnancy increases the amount of IgE (the allergy antibody) in the blood of a newborn baby—an indication that he or she is at an increased risk of developing allergies. After the birth, exposing a child to cigarette smoke continues to encourage high levels of IgE in the blood, as well as irritating the airways and making asthma more likely to develop.

The research on smoking is just one part of a worldwide research effort during the past 20–30 years into the possible causes of the allergy epidemic. That research can help parents who are themselves atopic (allergy-prone) to reduce the risk of passing their allergy problems on to their children.

Who should be implementing these preventive measures? First, any prospective parents who have allergies themselves or had them as children. They are at higher risk (compared to a non-allergic parent) of producing a child who is susceptible to allergies. The risk is especially high if both parents have (or have had) allergies.

Second, these preventive measures could be worthwhile for parents who don't have allergies themselves but who come from atopic families (families with a tendency to allergy). If you or your partner have brothers, sisters, or parents with allergies, you are more likely than the average person to produce allergic children.

Finally, if you already have one allergic child—even though you and your partner don't have allergies yourselves, and no one else in the family does—there is a higher-than-average chance that subsequent children will have allergies. Your allergic child is a sign that the genes for allergy are there.

Given the important role that genes play in allergy (see p. 8), preventive strategies make a lot of sense for parents-to-be with allergies in the family.

Unfortunately, this is a topic which often generates confusion—some people assume that if a trait is genetic, it will inevitably come out in the child, and that nothing can be done to prevent this from happening. Although that is true for some inherited traits, such as metabolic abnormalities (see box on p. 75), it is not the case for allergy.

Developing allergic disease is not inevitable unless

a child has a very big dose of the genes that favor allergy. Only a few children—generally those whose mother and father are both badly affected by allergies—will fall into this category. Even with these high-risk children, following the measures described here will probably help to reduce the severity of their allergy.

For most children at risk of allergies, even though they have some pro-allergy genes, there has to be an unfavorable environment to actually produce allergic disease. "Environment" here means *everything* external that affects the child, including diet, air quality, allergens, diseases, and medical treatment. Factors occurring before birth, such as the mother's lifestyle during pregnancy, are also part of the child's environment. It is the interplay between genes and environment that will decide whether your child develops allergies or escapes them.

This interaction is not a simple one, however, and different aspects of the environment operate in different ways. First, there are some environmental factors that work at the most fundamental level—conspiring with the pro-allergy genes to make the overall tendency to allergy far stronger. These are factors such as cigarette smoking by the mother during pregnancy, or excessive hygiene during childhood, which influence the fundamental make-up of the child's immune system. Second, there are environmental factors, such as early exposure to dust mites or grass pollen, which can cause trouble by provoking specific allergic reactions. Note that factors like these will not become important unless the allergic tendency is already there.

Efforts to reduce the risk of allergy operate on both types of factor. On the one hand, there are measures such as quitting smoking or easing up on hygiene, which tackle the allergic predisposition itself. These measures are, in effect, trying to make a Western child's immune system more like the immune system of a child from a poor rural village in the developing world, whose chance of developing allergy is very low indeed. On the other hand, there are measures such as reducing dust-mite levels that try to stop the development of particular allergic reactions.

Obviously, if measures of the first kind could be truly successful, there would be little or no need for measures of the second kind. But this rate of success is very difficult to achieve in modern Western society. Although we can certainly improve matters a great deal, and lessen the tendency to allergy, the conditions that would completely reverse it are beyond our reach at present. So both kinds of preventive measure remain necessary.

In reading the pages that follow, it is important to keep things in perspective, and not feel excessively anxious about your child. Do what you can, but don't feel guilty if you can't manage everything that is suggested here. And if you already have a child with allergies, please *don't* feel guilty about things that might have contributed to this. Only hindsight is perfect, and you no doubt did the best you could, given the information you had at the time, and the many other constraints and difficulties that you faced. That is the best that any of us can do.

Pregnancy,
BREAST-FEEDING,
AND WEANING

Having a baby should, first and foremost, be a positive and enjoyable experience. Inevitably, there are also anxieties involved, and the huge amount of advice you receive while pregnant—from doctors, midwives, friends, relatives, and even well-meaning strangers—can add to these anxieties. You may feel that the last thing you need is any more advice. But if you are susceptible to allergies yourself, taking steps to avoid them developing in your baby could, in the long run, save you a great deal of time, worry, and expense—quite apart from the benefits for the child.

Most of the measures described here are based on strong scientific evidence, or on the long-term experience of doctors and midwives, so you can feel sure the effort is worthwhile. While taking these measures cannot absolutely *guarantee* that your child will grow up allergy-free, it will shift the odds in the right direction. And even if your child does not escape allergies entirely, you can feel confident that these protective measures will have made the child's problems less severe than they would otherwise have been.

Planning the pregnancy

As far as developing allergies is concerned, a baby is most vulnerable during the first year of life—especially the first few months. This is because the newborn's immune system is geared toward making the allergy antibody, IgE (see box on p. 12).

If a baby is exposed to a large dose of powerful airborne allergens during this first phase of life, he or she is at risk of making IgE to those allergens. (The same is true of food allergens—these are dealt with on pp. 241–3.) Although there will probably be no symptoms at the time, these can develop later, in the form of hay fever, perennial rhinitis (a year-round nasal allergy—see p. 28), or asthma.

As a parent, you should be focusing your efforts on reducing the allergen load for your baby during the first year, especially during the first 4–6 months.

Timing the birth

In the case of pollen, the best approach—if you can manage it—is to plan conception so that the birth occurs shortly after the season for the most troublesome allergenic pollen in your region. That way the baby will be over 6 months old by the time the next pollen season comes around.

Studies of birth month and allergy show that North American children are most likely to develop hay fever if they are born in mid- to late summer, just before the ragweed season. In Scandinavia, those born in early spring, shortly before the birch pollen season, are the most vulnerable.

Allergens in the home

In the case of household allergens such as dust mite and mold, the sooner you can begin work to reduce the level in your house (see pp. 244–5), the better. Recent research shows that a fetus may have its first encounter with the allergens of the dust mite as early as 16 or 17 weeks of age. By then, the fetus is already swallowing a little of the fluid that surrounds it in the womb—the amniotic fluid. This normal activity introduces any substances found in the amniotic fluid to the baby's immune system, via specialized areas of immune recognition in the gut. During the sixteenth or seventeenth week of pregnancy, the powerful allergens produced by dust mites begin to show up in the amniotic fluid.

How do these allergens get there? The dust-mite allergen was originally inhaled by the mother, then absorbed from her lungs into her bloodstream, and then passed from there into the amniotic fluid.

This is a controversial area, but some medical researchers believe that this early contact with allergen explains why a few infants are born with the ability to mount an allergic reaction to dust mites. Actual symptoms of allergy may not appear for several months or years, but the essential first step—making the allergy antibody, IgE (see box on p. 12)—has already occurred for some babies.

In situations where IgE does the job it is supposed to do—protecting against worms and other parasites (see p. 13)—this advance programming of the immune system before birth has definite advantages. A child whose mother is infected with parasites is born with the ability to make IgE against those parasites, even though he or she has had no direct contact with them before birth. The baby's immune system has been forewarned of the likely hazards of life in the outside world, and is armed to tackle them at birth.

While this is obviously valuable in conditions where parasitic infections are rife, emerging into the modern mite-infested world with IgE against dust mites already in the bloodstream is a serious disadvantage, because it can pave the way for perennial allergic rhinitis and asthma.

Given the trouble caused by dust-mite allergen, some doctors think that women should try to reduce their exposure to it during the second half of pregnancy, so that little or none reaches the unborn child. At present, it is not known for sure if this can make a difference to the risk of allergies developing in a child, but it seems plausible.

What is absolutely clear, from several previous studies, is that the level of dust mites in the home immediately after birth does have a distinct effect on the infant's chance of developing allergy. Minimizing a newborn baby's exposure to dust mites is definitely worthwhile, and the measures needed to achieve this are described on pp. 244–5.

Implementing these measures will raise the level of dust-mite allergen in the air temporarily, so it makes sense to do the work in the early stages of pregnancy (or—even better—before conception), rather than expose yourself and the fetus to a tremendous burst of allergen later on in pregnancy.

There may be other potential allergens that you should try to eliminate from your home before the baby arrives, such as pet allergens (see p. 245).

Pregnancy

First and foremost—don't smoke while you are pregnant, or afterward (see box on p. 107). Any other smokers in the household should smoke outdoors.

What about your diet during pregnancy? Should you be careful about certain foods? Food allergens, such as those from cow's milk, do reach the fetus, passed from the mother's blood to the baby's blood via the placenta. And a few babies are born already capable of making IgE against food allergens. On the basis of these findings, some doctors have suggested that avoiding potentially allergenic foods (such as eggs, cow's milk, and peanuts) during pregnancy might help to reduce the risk of food allergy. However, evidence from research trials in which pregnant women followed a restricted diet and their children were later studied for allergies, does not show any convincing benefit. And in some studies, the women on restricted diets did not gain as much weight as they should have, so their babies were slightly below average weight at birth. Most doctors now think that dietary restrictions during pregnancy are not worthwhile—it is more important to eat well and get enough nutrients.

It does seem sensible not to overeat any particular food during pregnancy, although there is no scientific evidence on this point (simply because researchers have not yet looked for such evidence). In particular, don't overdo it with milk and milk products. Make sure you get enough calcium, obviously, but don't force yourself to drink huge amounts of milk, especially if you have any distaste for it. Talk to your doctor or midwife about the possibility of a calcium supplement, if you dislike milk.

Breast-feeding

"The cornerstone of allergy prevention is breast-feeding," according to Dr. Erika Isolauri of Tampere University Hospital in Finland.

At one time, this would have been a controversial statement, but there is now a substantial body of scientific evidence to support the breast-is-best idea in relation to allergy prevention. A number of different studies have shown that exclusive breast-feeding, up to at least four months of age, reduces the risk of developing food allergy or atopic eczema (or both) in the early years of life.

Exclusive means exactly that—no solids at all until after four months, and no supplementary feeds with infant formula (which is made from cow's milk, and therefore contains cow's milk allergens). Unfortunately, it is sometimes far from easy to ensure that your newborn won't be given formula in the hospital nursery just after birth. Given what we now know about the immune system of the newborn, this is the worst possible time to be delivering an onslaught of potentially allergenic cow's milk proteins.

Quite apart from the immediate effect of introducing cow's milk allergens to the baby, a bottle can disrupt the development of a good breast-feeding relationship between mother and child, and may lead to the early abandonment of breast-feeding.

Why should this happen? First the baby does not have to suck as hard on a bottle as on a real nipple, and he or she may never develop the knack if given bottles at an early stage. Second, allaying the baby's hunger with a bottle can also mean that he or she takes less at the next breast-feed—and since the mother's milk supply is partly influenced by the level of demand, this reduced intake can be detrimental. Some experts believe that occasional bottle feeds can start a downward spiral of ever-diminishing supply from the mother.

Dr. Arne Høst of the Department of Pediatrics at Odense University Hospital in Denmark, who has made a special study of breast-feeding, recommends giving boiled water as a supplement during the first three to four days of life if the breast milk supply is inadequate. After that time, the mother's own supply should increase to meet the needs of her baby. Introducing bottle feeds at an early stage can prevent this delicate balance of supply-and-demand from ever being achieved. Talk to your doctor about how much water your baby needs.

Sometimes, despite everything being done just right, a mother's supply of milk never quite matches her infant's appetite. When this happens in an allergy-prone family, the breast milk should be supplemented with an ultrasafe type of formula feed called a hydrolysate (see box on p. 66).

Hydrolysates should also be used for infants at high risk of allergy who, for whatever reason, cannot be breast-fed. Note that there are two categories of hydrolysate—**extensively hydrolysed formula** and **partially hydrolysed formula**. Using an extensively hydrolyzed formula can reduce the risk of milk allergy. However, partially hydrolyzed formulas have been widely studied as supplements to breast milk or for exclusive feeding. The results from many studies indicate that whey hydrolysate formulas are comparable to breast milk in significantly reducing the risk of atopic disease, especially eczema, compared to babies fed soy or regular milk formulas. Whey hydrolysate formulas may also reduce the chance of milk allergy in the first 1–2 years of life. Whether they reduce the risk of asthma in later life remains controversial, although a few long-term studies have shown a reduction in asthma as well.

Preparing to breast-feed

Because breast-feeding is natural, many first-time mothers just assume it will come naturally. Sadly, it often doesn't. Cracked nipples are a major obstacle – they are the equivalent of chapped hands, caused by the prolonged wetness and chafing on the nipple during breast-feeding. Because cracked nipples are so sore, breast-feeding can then become a major ordeal rather than the pleasurable experience it should be.

What is more, infectious bacteria can enter the breast through the cracks in the skin, causing mastitis, a painful condition that calls for immediate medical attention, and may require antibiotic treatment. Some of the antibiotic may pass into the milk, and this is not necessarily a good thing for the baby (see p. 247).

Fortunately, cracked nipples can easily be avoided. The trick is to make the skin on the nipples tougher and more resilient, so that it does not crack. Start during pregnancy, in about your fourth month. When you take a bath or shower, rub your nipples vigorously with your washcloth for a few minutes. After three weeks of washcloth friction, graduate to a soft toothbrush. Gently work the bristles over the nipples, increasing the pressure as they get tougher. Progress to a medium, and then a hard toothbrush. By your seventh month of pregnancy, you should be on to a nail-brush. "I followed this program with my first baby," reports Jane, a mother of two, "and I was the only mother in my postnatal group who didn't get cracked nipples."

Breast-feeding support groups like La Leche League (see p. 255) can be enormously helpful when you start breast-feeding, or when you feel things are not going right. Some groups have local advisers, all mothers themselves with first-hand experience of breast-feeding. Having such an adviser with you, watching you breast-feed your new baby and making suggestions, or pointing out where you are going wrong, can make all the difference. Look for such a group locally, and establish contact with them, well before your due date. You may be able to talk with an adviser before the birth, which can be useful.

Having prepared yourself, you then have to prepare the nursing staff in the hospital where you will give birth for the fact that you want to breast-feed exclusively. That means no supplementary feeds from the staff—not even one bottle. The risk that this practice will sensitize vulnerable babies to cow's milk is still not widely known, so you will probably need to be persistent and make your feelings very clear. If you have a midwife, talk to her about this well before your expected delivery date, and find out what policy the hospital has about supplementary feeds. Then see the relevant staff at the hospital.

The nurses are most likely to give the baby a bottle because he or she is crying while you are asleep, and they don't want to wake you. Staff change all the time, so you will probably need to put a notice on the crib or bassinet, to be certain that the baby is never bottle-fed while you are sleeping. If this seems excessive, consider the experience of British researchers investigating allergy prevention who wanted to ensure that a group of newborns were never given supplementary feeds. They put warning stickers on both the babies' bassinets and the mothers' beds, as well as asking the midwives and mothers to be very vigilant. Despite this effort, several of the babies being studied were given bottles.

Sometimes nurses give a bottle because they believe that the baby is not getting enough milk from the breast. It is entirely possible that your milk supply will not be quite adequate in the first few days, but it should increase rapidly. The best thing, if breast milk supply is inadequate, is to give boiled water as a supplement during the first 3–4 days of life (see p. 242).

Diet during breast-feeding

"When I was nursing Toby, if I had red wine with dinner, he would cry and cry the next day. At first I thought maybe it was just coincidence, but then I kept a careful note of when he was cranky, and what I'd had the night before, and the pattern was so clear— it was the wine, sure enough."

Judy is not the only mother to have noticed the effects of red wine on a breast-fed baby, but it comes as a surprise to most women to learn that pretty much *everything* they eat works its way into breast milk, though in very tiny amounts.

The food molecules that get through into breast milk can certainly affect babies who are already sensitized to a food. Cow's milk is the classic example—its proteins get into human milk if the mother consumes any milk, cheese, yogurt, or other milk products. Babies who have already been sensitized to cow's milk (by a supplementary bottle feed, for example, or even in the womb— see p. 241) react badly to the breast milk, unless the mother avoids all dairy products.

What is less certain is whether the traces of allergen in breast milk—cow's milk allergen or that from any other food—might be capable of *starting off* allergy or sensitivity. Are these minute traces enough to sensitize babies with a tendency to allergy? If they are, then mothers of high-risk infants might be well advised to avoid certain allergenic foods while breast-feeding. Some

studies suggest that there is a reduction in food allergy if breast-feeding mothers avoid cow's milk, eggs, nuts, fish, and soy. But if this restrictive diet makes life impossible, then it is better to breast-feed and eat what you like, than to not breast-feed at all.

Unfortunately, some babies get eczema anyway, in spite of being exclusively breast-fed. If this happens with your child, there are various steps you can take to deal with the problem (see box on p. 248).

Weaning—when and how

The key to reducing the allergy risk for babies is to turn the old expression "too little, too late" on its head. Research shows that, as far as weaning is concerned, it is "too much, too early" that increases the chance of allergic reactions developing. Suddenly presenting an infant of three months with a great variety of solid foods, including potent allergens such as eggs, peanuts, and fish, can increase the likelihood of food allergy and/or eczema developing. Weaning late, with a limited number of safe foods, should be your goal.

At least four months of exclusive breast-feeding is now the standard recommendation for allergy prevention, and it is well supported by scientific evidence. Weaning should begin some time between four and six months of age.

But how long should breast-feeding continue after weaning begins? There is little concrete evidence here, but there is a strong belief in the medical community that breast-feeding should go on for several more months if possible, allowing the weaning process to be very gradual. The idea is to introduce new foods one at a time, alongside breast milk.

As well as allowing the immune system lots of time to adjust to each new food, prolonged breast-feeding may help in another way as well. Recent research suggests that breast milk contains substances which influence the baby's immune system, nudging it in the right direction—away from any tendency to allergies.

Avoid ready-made baby food which often contains potent allergens such as milk, wheat, or soy. Making your own baby foods is easy, and ensures that your child gets only low-risk foods.

Nipple cream—with peanuts

If your nipples begin to feel sore during breast-feeding, and you need a nipple cream, check very carefully that the product you buy doesn't contain peanut oil (arachis oil). This very early exposure may be responsible for sensitizing some children to peanuts.

When children react to peanuts the very first time they eat them—as sometimes happens—this shows that some earlier exposure to peanut allergens must have occurred to produce the allergic sensitization. It is possible that sensitization occurred because peanut allergens from the mother reached the baby in the bloodstream before birth, or later via breast milk. Hidden sources, such as nipple creams containing peanut oil, are possible culprits as well.

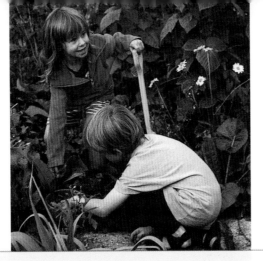

Other measures
TO PROTECT
AGAINST ALLERGY

No single factor lies behind the allergy epidemic—the causes are many and various (see p. 20). What this means for parents interested in allergy prevention is that there is no single measure to ensure that your children do not develop allergies. Instead, there are a great many different actions to take, each of which reduces the risk to some extent. The more of these things you do, the lower the risk becomes.

Avoiding allergens

If you want to reduce allergen exposure for your child starting before the birth is best (see p. 240). But if you have missed the boat with that one, don't despair—there is still a lot to be gained by reducing allergen exposure at a later stage.

If you are ridding your home of allergens after the child's birth, bear in mind that things will get worse before they get better—there will be a temporary surge in airborne allergen as a result of the cleanup operation, and you will need to protect the child from this. The best strategy is for the child to be away for a few days while the work is done, especially if you are taking out carpets, furniture, or mattresses. Remember to protect yourself as well, if you are allergy-prone (see p. 109).

One of the most important steps you can take to reduce allergen levels is to improve the ventilation of your home. This lowers the humidity (assuming you don't live in an extremely humid climate), which helps combat both molds and dust mites. Ventilation also flushes out allergens in the air, especially cat, dog, and mold allergens. Half the problem with modern houses is that the airtight seals around doors and windows, introduced to conserve heat and save energy, turn the indoor air into a rich stew of allergens and irritants.

Dust mites

Avoiding high levels of dust mites in the home is one of the most valuable things you can do to reduce the risk of allergies in your child. Not only are dust mites powerful allergens in their own right, they may also act as *agents provocateurs* as far as the immune system is concerned (see p. 12), and may help to initiate allergic reactions to *other* potential allergens—such as those from pets or indoor molds.

Even if you do nothing else to protect your new baby from mite allergen, at least buy a new firm infant mattress for the crib, with a ready-fitted allergen-proof cover. Do the same for the portable crib, if you have one. Choose anti-mite products that are designed for babies and are guaranteed safe—there is a risk of suffocation with loose mattress covers. To keep the baby warm it is best to use several lightweight blankets—not comforters—that you can add or remove according to room temperature. Buy blankets that can be washed at high temperature to kill dust mites.

You may want to eliminate dust mites from your own bed as well as the baby's, because there will probably be times when you take the baby into bed with you for a feed or a cuddle—and times when, as a toddler, he or she just barges in! It is good to know that your child is still breathing air free from dust-mite allergen in these circumstances.

Deal with your own bed as soon as you can. Some doctors believe that lowering your exposure to dust mites during pregnancy may reduce the risk of sensitizing your baby before birth (see p. 241).

When taking anti-mite measures with your own bed, make sure that there is no risk to the baby of suffocation from the allergen-proof materials used. Microporous membranes based on plastic could, if sucked onto the baby's face during sleep, cause suffocation. Loose covers on comforters are worrying in this respect. Buy a new comforter with a built-in allergen-proof cover, or a comforter that can be laundered at 131°F/55°C or above.

All the other measures for combating dust mites, described on pp. 114–17, will help to protect your child. Buy a good anti-allergen vacuum cleaner if you possibly can, and keep your baby out of the room while vacuuming if you can't (open the windows too). Make sure the baby has only new soft toys, preferably washable ones (see p. 116).

It is also an excellent idea to reduce dust-mite levels in carpets and soft furnishings (see p. 117), because children tend to have very close contact with these in their early years. A crawling baby, motoring enthusiastically around the living room floor, is stirring up the stockpile of dust-mite allergen that is found in any carpet, and inhaling it in full measure. An adult walking around the same room has a far lower exposure, because dust-mite allergen, being relatively heavy, stays near the ground.

The best possible option is to go for non-carpet flooring, which doesn't encourage dust mites. Parents tend to worry about the hardness of uncarpeted floors, for a baby or toddler. In fact, babies are far more robust than we generally believe, and a hard floor is actually no problem for a small child who has never known the luxury of carpeting.

If you really hate the idea of your baby having anything other than carpet to play on, the next best option is to get new carpet, so that you start with zero dust mites. You must then prevent dust-mite numbers from building up too much, by having good ventilation, or using a powerful dehumidifier (see p. 117).

Although the first year is the most vulnerable time for your baby, you mustn't let your guard drop too much as time passes. The moment when a toddler moves from a crib to a big bed is sometimes the beginning of allergy symptoms because, after carefully protecting their child from dust mites in infancy, parents then put him or her into a bed with a used mattress. This sudden exposure to a high dose of dust-mite allergen can be the start of asthma. Get a new mattress if you can, and put allergen-proof covers on it. Alternatively, put allergen-proof covers on the existing mattress.

Molds and pets

Mold spores are another potent allergen. If your child is vulnerable to allergies and you live in a damp house, a move may be advisable; molds grow abundantly in humid conditions. Even in a house that is not obviously damp, it is a good plan to reduce indoor humidity (see p. 119). Carpets and furnishings that are full of mold spores (see p. 122) should be replaced.

What about pet allergens—should you find another home for your cat or dog when you are expecting a baby? This is a difficult question because the latest research shows that pets are a double-edged sword as far as allergies are concerned.

As you might expect, a baby with allergic tendencies who is born into a house with a resident cat or dog is more likely to show allergic reactions to cats or dogs some years later. On the other hand, there is now research showing that having an animal in the house *reduces the risk of allergies overall*, especially for a child with no brothers or sisters. This is probably because the pet makes the environment less hygienic for the child, fulfilling the same anti-allergy role as brothers and sisters would in the early life of a child (see p. 246).

If you are planning to give your child the kind of grubby childhood that seems to protect against allergy (see p. 246), the additional protection provided by a pet is probably unnecessary. On the other hand, you could view your pet as having both pros and cons, and decide to keep it, while implementing all the other anti-allergy measures described here. If you do this, ensure the house is well ventilated (so pet allergens don't build up to very high levels indoors) and keep the pet out of the child's bedroom so that he or she is not inhaling huge amounts of pet allergen while asleep. You could also wash the pet regularly (see p. 125) to reduce allergen levels in the air.

Avoiding irritants

As well as increasing ventilation and eliminating cigarette smoke from the home completely, it may be worth evicting certain specific items that produce irritant gases.

The main ones are:

- gas stoves (if you can't afford to switch to an electric stove, at least improve the ventilation in your kitchen as much as possible)
- easy-clean plastic wall coverings and flooring
- materials such as chipboard and medium density fiberboard (MDF), which give off formaldehyde

The evidence regarding the possible role of these in increasing the risk of allergies and asthma is described on pp. 128–9. In addition, although there is no evidence on this point, common sense would suggest getting rid of any plastic or laquered items that have a powerful smell.

Generally speaking, although traffic pollution can act as an irritant, it seems to play a lesser role in *causing* allergies and asthma than most people imagine. However, it may sometimes play a part, especially if there are high levels of diesel fumes in the air (see p. 131).

Infections—friend or foe?

A large group of Italian military cadets were recently studied by doctors interested in the causes of allergy. By taking blood samples and testing them for antibodies to common infections, the doctors could see what diseases the men had been exposed to early in life. At the same time, the young conscripts were assessed for allergies.

Allergies were least frequent among the young men with antibodies against three common infections that are dispersed via food and feces—Hepatitis A, *Toxoplasma gondii* and *Helicobacter pylori*. Only one in 12 of the cadets in this group had allergies.

Among the men with no antibodies against any of these infections, the rate of allergy was nearly three times as high—one in five of these cadets had allergies.

The doctors carrying out this experiment believe that these three infections are not necessarily important in themselves, but that they identify individuals who were "reared in an environment that provides a higher exposure to many other orofecal or food-borne microbes." In other words, they grew up in the kind of household where washing your hands before meals wasn't considered too important.

This study adds to the growing body of evidence (see p. 21) which shows that an over-clean environment during childhood encourages the development of an allergic disposition.

Those with lower rates of allergy include:

- Children raised on farms with livestock. The more exposure the children have to farm animals, the less the likelihood of them developing allergies.
- Children from homes with high levels of bacterial toxins in the household dust (see p. 21).
- Children who have fewer baths, and wash their hands less often (see p. 21).
- Children with brothers and sisters, especially those with older siblings. One study showed that having brothers provided more protection against allergies than having sisters, possibly because boys tend to get dirtier than girls.
- Children who go into nursery school or daycare with other children at an early age, for example, under 12 months of age—this is only valuable for children without brothers and sisters.
- Children with pets at home—the benefits are much more pronounced for children without brothers and sisters.

The Italian study is especially important because, for the first time, it gives detailed information about *the kinds of* infections that make a difference in allergy prevention. The military cadets were also checked out for antibodies to measles, mumps, rubella, chicken pox, and herpes. None of these infections give protection against allergies—only infections carried in food and feces do.

Exactly what practical use you make of these discoveries is up to you. For most of us, the importance of hygiene was so firmly instilled during our own childhood that it is quite hard to suddenly become more relaxed about it. But do let your children play in the backyard, if you have one, and don't worry so much about how dirty they get. Encourage them to do some gardening—medical researchers believe that harmless bacteria in the soil may be particularly important in directing the immune system away from allergies (see p. 21). Let them play with pets, as long as the animals are not carrying harmful parasitic worms (talk to your vet about whether pets should be treated for parasites). Ease up on hand-washing and, if this is your first baby, make sure he or she plays with other children as early in life as possible.

A few chest infections do seem to increase the risk of asthma, notably respiratory syncytial virus (RSV). If this infects babies, it provokes an IgE-reaction (see box on p. 12), which may encourage the development of allergies. Unfortunately, there is very little you can do to protect your child from this common virus, but it makes sense not to take the baby to a hospital for unnecessary trips (visiting relatives, for example) because RSV infections are often picked up in hospitals.

Taking care with antibiotics

The possible role of antibiotics in making allergies more likely to develop is an exceedingly controversial topic. **Before making any practical decisions in this respect, you must consult your doctor. Never go against your doctor's advice if he or she thinks that antibiotics are necessary for your child**.

Several different studies have now produced evidence of a link between antibiotic use before the age of one or two and the later development of allergies, asthma, or both. The best of these studies was carried out by doctors in Oxford, England, who followed 1,900 children up to the age of 16. Among children at risk of allergy (because their mothers had allergies), taking antibiotics before the age of 2 was linked with an increase in the rate of allergy from 32 percent to 54 percent. The more courses of antibiotics a child received, the greater the risk.

The type of infection for which the drugs were prescribed was not important, as far as the risk of allergy was concerned, but the type of antibiotic did make a difference. Broad-spectrum antibiotics, which kill a wide range of bacteria, were more risky— suggesting that the depletion of friendly bacteria in the gut (see p. 204) could be responsible for increasing the allergy risk. Penicillins seemed less likely to promote allergies than erythromycin or cephalosporins.

This research is not widely known as yet. And because, in many parts of the world, there still exists an assumption that giving an antibiotic can do no harm, even if it is unnecessary, antibiotics are sometimes prescribed when they serve no purpose. In particular, antibiotics are often given for viral (virus) infections, especially in childhood, despite the fact that antibiotics are of no value whatever against viruses. Research shows that doctors are sometimes responding to pressure from anxious parents when they prescribe antibiotics—it is difficult for some parents to accept that a viral infection cannot easily be treated and just has to "run its course." (Although there are drugs that combat viruses, these are expensive and produce unpleasant side effects—they are reserved for very serious viral infections such as hepatitis.)

Obviously, when a child needs antibiotics to deal with a serious infection, there can be no question about giving them. This is why you should always follow your doctor's advice. But it is also worth asking the doctor the following questions before giving antibiotics to your child:

- is this likely to be a bacterial infection and not a viral infection?
- would it be possible to do tests and check that it is a bacterial infection, before prescribing antibiotics?
- what is the chance of the child overcoming the infection without antibiotics?
- would it be dangerous to wait and see if the infection clears up naturally?

Vaccination

The same Oxford research team that investigated antibiotics (see left) also looked at the question of vaccination and allergy. They found a link between vaccination for pertussis (whooping cough) and increases in asthma, eczema, and hay fever. However, the increases were not large, and a study from Sweden found that whooping cough vaccination did not have any effect on rates of allergy and asthma. And researchers in Ethiopia have found that whooping cough vaccination actually *reduces* the risk of allergy in their country.

This is clearly a complex issue. The contradictory results from different parts of the world suggest that the "big picture" is what counts here—the overall combination of childhood infections, antibiotic treatment, and exposure to harmless bacteria such as those in the soil or from animals. Depending on this big picture, vaccination against whooping cough may push the allergy risk one way or the other.

In addition, the current whooping cough vaccine is different from that used a few years ago, producing better immunity with less risk of serious side effects. How the new vaccine might affect allergy risk is unknown, but studies using the old vaccine are unlikely to be relevant in assessing the risk.

There are many other arguments both for and against vaccination and, given our current state of ignorance about the possible effect on allergy, these other considerations are probably more relevant. Discuss the matter in detail with your doctor before making a decision.

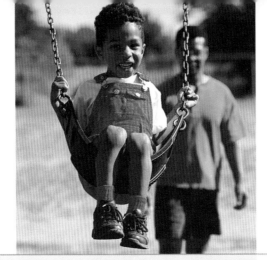

Protecting children

WHO ALREADY HAVE ALLERGIES

Doctors in Japan recently tried a very simple experiment in allergy prevention. They chose babies suffering from atopic eczema who were allergic to foods, but not allergic to dust mites. Dividing the babies into two groups, the doctors put special allergen-proof covers, designed to protect against dust mites (see p. 115), on the mattresses of all the babies in the first group. Babies in the second group were given ordinary cotton covers.

When the babies were one year old, they were tested again for allergy to dust mites. Two out of three children in the second group now gave a positive skin test to dust mites.

By comparison, only one in three of the children from the first group gave a positive skin test. In other words, using the anti-allergy covers for these high-risk children cut by half the number who developed an allergic reaction to dust mites.

As this experiment shows, even if a child has already developed allergies, it is not too late to bring protective measures into play. Indeed, an allergy problem in infancy, such as atopic eczema, can be seen as a warning sign to parents, telling them that they should reduce the child's exposure to allergens as much as possible.

As well as reducing dust-mite levels, you should minimize your child's exposure to molds at home by limiting indoor humidity (see p. 119) and cleaning up any existing mold growth (see pp. 122–3). This will lessen the chance of mold allergy developing.

Try to avoid staying, even temporarily, in any house that is damp or has old carpets and mattresses. When you are moving, or carrying out any kind of renovation work, remember that this will stir up a lot of dust-mite and mold allergens. Protect your child by arranging for a stay away from home during the disruption.

This proactive approach should apply not only to airborne allergens, but also to food, in the opinion of some experts. They suggest that any child with a true allergy to cow's milk or egg should not be given peanuts, tree nuts, fish, or shellfish until three years of age, to avoid sensitization.

Pets are a more difficult issue, with both pros and cons with regard to allergy-prone children (see p. 245). If you decide to keep your cat or dog, always ventilate the house well, and wash the animal regularly if you can (see p. 125). Be alert for signs that your child is developing an allergic reaction to your pet—don't turn a blind eye to the symptoms, as parents sometimes do because they are reluctant to accept that the child has become allergic to the family's much-loved pet. If your child does develop an allergy to the pet, the best option is to find the animal another home (see p. 124).

Breast-fed babies with atopic eczema

Although breast-feeding is a good way of protecting children against atopic eczema, it is no guarantee. Sometimes babies become sensitized to food, in spite of being breast-fed, and then they may react to traces of that same food, eaten by the mother and passed on through breast milk. Prick-puncture tests (see p. 91) may help to identify the foods responsible for the eczema. Otherwise, a simple elimination diet by the mother, as used for colic (see p. 203), may pinpoint the offending food. Keeping that food out of the mother's diet will often clear the baby's eczema.

Sometimes a breast-fed child's eczema remains severe, despite the elimination of suspect foods from the mother's diet. In this case, what should be done? New research from Dr. Erika Isolauri—a staunch advocate of breast-feeding—suggests that the best option at this point is to stop breast-feeding. Her research team found that breast-fed children with persistent eczema had a slower growth rate, either due to the disease itself, or to the restricted diet followed by their mothers. When these babies were switched to an artificial amino-acid formula (see box on p. 66), their eczema symptoms subsided, and their growth picked up.

Is vaccination safe for children with egg allergy?

The influenza vaccine and a few others (for example, yellow fever) are grown in eggs and can contain egg allergen. These are not usually given to people with egg allergy. The measles vaccine is grown in cells taken from eggs, and may contain a minute trace of egg allergen. Allergic reactions to measles vaccine have been reported among individuals with egg allergy—but only those who are extremely sensitive. New studies suggest that the risk from measles vaccine is very small, and children with egg allergy can be safely immunized. However, there should be resuscitation equipment available when the vaccine is given to children who have suffered a severe anaphylactic reaction to egg in the past, and those with severe asthma as well as egg allergy.

Never too late?

The role of modern ultraclean lifestyles in promoting allergies is now well established (see p. 21). If your child already has allergies, it may seem as if these discoveries have come too late to help—but that is not the case. Some research suggests that the battle for supremacy between Th1 and Th2 cells (see p. 11)—the unseen power struggle that decides whether a child will be allergy-prone—is not really settled until some time between the ages of 5 and 7 years. So there is still some potential for intervening up to this age. Some studies suggest that the immune system can be pushed away from an allergic disposition at an even later age, right up to adolescence.

Several research groups are working on vaccination strategies (for example, using extracts of soil bacteria) that might be able to achieve this. The initial results are promising and suggest that these vaccines can even help adults with allergies. Unfortunately, such treatments will not be available for many years. In the meantime, you can probably reduce your child's chance of developing new allergies, and perhaps make the existing ones less severe, by easing up on hygiene (see p. 246).

Fresh air and exercise

With the boom in watching TV and videos, and playing computer games, some modern children hardly go outdoors at all. As far as allergies and asthma are concerned, there are two big disadvantages to being a juvenile couch potato. For a start, the couch is also home to dust mites in their millions, and the child who spends most of the day slumped on it is breathing in more than his or her fair share of mite allergens.

The other drawback is that the child is not running about and using his or her lungs to the fullest. Airways that are never stretched (because the child never gets out of breath) lose their youthful flexibility in time. Once this has happened, the airways can never again be stretched to their full capacity. Some doctors believe that this may make asthma more likely to develop, or help to make it more severe once it has developed. Inactivity also encourages obesity, which increases the risk of asthma developing.

Getting outside and running around, or engaging in other vigorous exercise, should be encouraged for any child with allergies. Obviously, you should balance this against the need to protect the child from pollution peaks and (if your child has hay fever) pollen peaks. Children with exercise-induced asthma should use their reliever inhalers to allow them to take exercise (see p. 41).

Keep the air at home free from irritants such as nitrogen dioxide (see p. 128) which may encourage new allergies to develop, and can make existing asthma worse.

Medical treatments

Antihistamines may have a preventive role in very young children with allergies. A study of 1- to 2-year-olds with atopic eczema found that the antihistamine cetirizine, taken daily for 18 months, halved the chances of the children developing asthma later.

The children who benefited in this study were those with several risk factors for becoming asthmatic. They had moderate to severe atopic eczema, at least one close relative with allergies, and allergic sensitization to pollen or dust mite, as shown by prick-puncture tests (see p. 91).

The cetirizine was taken at fairly low doses and had no bad effects on the children in this study. What is more, it benefited their skin as well as reducing the risk of asthma: those taking the drug had less need of high-strength steroid creams. Unfortunately, these excellent results have not yet become widely known among doctors, so few children with atopic eczema are receiving antihistamines at present.

Currently, no one knows if other antihistamines have the same effect as cetirizine. Only ketotifen, which is an atypical antihistamine (see p. 159) has been studied. It too protected some children with allergies from developing asthma.

Immunotherapy may also have a protective effect. One study, involving children suffering from nasal allergies, found that those given immunotherapy were less likely to develop asthma (see p. 164). Another study shows that allergy shots for children with mite allergy halves the risk of their developing new allergic reactions to other allergens.

Index

Numbers shown in **bold type** indicate either definitions of technical terms or the main entry on a topic

Useful addresses

GENERAL

Asthma and Allergy Foundation of America (AAFA)
1233 20th Street, NW, Suite 402
Washington, DC 20036

Toll-free help line: 1-800-7-ASTHMA
(727-8462)
Fax: 202-466-8940
Web site: www.aafa.org
This organization can advise you if you need help in establishing your child's rights to equal treatment. Their Web site provides access to the latest information on asthma and allergies.

Allergy/Asthma Information Association (AAIA)
424–130 Bridgeland Avenue
Toronto, ON M6A 1Z4

Tel: 416-783-8944
Fax: 416-783-7538
E-mail:
www.aaia.national@sympatico.ca
The central office can put you in touch with the office for your region.

Web site: Allallergy.net
The most complete gateway to all asthma, allergy, and intolerance information on the Web.

Canadian Society of Allergy and Clinical Immunology
Web site: csaci.medical.org

American Academy of Allergy, Asthma and Immunology
Web site: aaaai.org

American Board of Medical Specialties
Toll-free number: 1-800-776-CERT
(2378)
Web site: abms.org
Provides information about physicians' certification status.

La Leche League International
Tel: 847-519-7730 (U.S.)
1-800-665-4342 (Canada)
Web site: www.lalecheleague.org

National Committee for Quality Assurance (NCQA)
Web site: NCQA.org

FOOD ALLERGY AND ANAPHYLAXIS

The Food Allergy Network (FAN)
10400 Eaton Place, Suite 107
Fairfax, VA 22030-2208

Tel: 703-691-3179
Toll-free number: 1-800-929-4040
Fax: 703-691-2713
Web site: www.foodallergy.org
FAN deals with classic IgE-mediated food allergies.

Anaphylaxis Network of Canada
P.O. Box 57524
2500 Royal York Road
Etobicoke (Toronto), ON M9P 3B6

Tel: 416-785-5666
Fax: 416-243-7733
Web site: www.anaphylaxis.org
E-mail: network@anaphylaxis.org

FOOD LABELING ERROR ALERTS

The **Food Allergy Network** (see above) provides a valuable service for those with food allergy in the U.S., issuing emergency alerts to members when a packaged food is found to have an allergenic ingredient such as peanut, milk, or egg not listed on the label.

In Canada, this kind of information can be obtained from **The Canadian Food Inspection Agency**

Web site: www.cfia-acia.agr.ca

ATOPIC DERMATITIS

National Eczema Association for Science and Education (NEASE)
1220 SW Morrison, Suite 433
Portland, OR 97205

Tel: 503-228-4430
Toll-free number: 1-800-818-7546
Fax: 503-224-3363
Web site: www.eczema-assn.org
E-mail: nease@teleport.com
An organization whose leaflets and Web site offer useful and very detailed advice about eczema. NEASE also runs a doctor referral system. This can help you find a regional doctor experienced in treating eczema who has been recommended by other eczema sufferers (or their parents).

ASTHMA

The Asthma Society of Canada
130 Bridgeland Avenue
Suite 425
Toronto, ON M6A 1Z4
Tel: 416-787-4050
Fax: 416-787-5807
Asthma Infoline: 1-800-787-3880
Web site: www.asthmasociety.com
E-mail: info@asthma.ca

Canadian Lung Association
Toll-free number: 1-888-566-LUNG
(5864)
Fax: 613-569-8860
Web site: www.lung.ca
E-mail: info@lung.ca
This organization does not provide educational materials, but will direct callers to the nearest regional lung association.

Allergy and Asthma Network • Mothers of Asthmatics, Inc. (AAN • MA)
2751 Prosperity Avenue, Suite 150
Fairfax, VA 22031

Tel: 703-641-9595
Fax: 703-573-7794
Toll-free help line: 1-800-878-4403
E-mail: aanma@aol.com
Web site: www.aanma.org

Asthma Education and Resource Council
5 Bon Air Road
Suite 110
Larkspur, CA 94977

Tel: 415-924-3647
Fax: 415-927-7387

National Jewish Medical and Research Center
Lung line
1400 Jackson Street
Denver, CO 80206

Toll-free help line: 1-800-222-LUNG
(5864) or (outside the U.S.)
303-388-4461
Web site: www.njc.org
E-mail: lungline@njc.org
A medical and research center devoted to respiratory, allergic, and immune system diseases. A good source of information for asthmatics.

EMERGENCY ALERT BRACELETS

These are sold by a nonprofit company, MedicAlert. Key medical information is engraved on the bracelet or necklace, and printed on the wallet card, plus a telephone number that gives medical staff access to a computer database that stores your essential medical data.
Web site: www.medicalert.org

MedicAlert Foundation
2323 Colorado Avenue
Turlock, CA 95382-2018

Tel: 1-800-IDALERT (1-800-432-5378)
Fax: 209-669-2495

Canadian MedicAlert Foundation
250 Ferrand Drive
Suite 301
Toronto, ON M3C 3G8

Toll-free number: 1-800-668-1507
(English) or
1-800-668-6381 (French)
Fax: 416-696-0156
Web site: www.medicalert.ca

ALLERGY-INTOLERANCE WEB SITE

For further information on topics covered in this book, and a comprehensive list of patient support organizations, medical associations, specialist allergy suppliers, sources of recipes, and more, log on to:

www.allergy-intolerance.com

From there, you can go directly to the Web sites of support organizations, suppliers, and so on. Or, if you have limited access to the Internet (for example, in a public library), you can print out the details found there and contact groups that interest you by mail or telephone.

Allergy news updates are also available on the Allergy-Intolerance Web site, and you can pose questions there on any of the subjects covered by this book. Questions can't usually be answered with a personal letter or message, but those that are of general interest will be answered on the Web site.

ACKNOWLEDGMENTS

Linda Gamlin would like to thank Professor Jonathan Brostoff and Dr. Anthony Ham Pong for their many helpful comments on the text, Dr. Michael Tettenborn for his advice about atopic eczema, Dr. Michel Joffres and Brenda Sabo for their observations on provocation-neutralization, and Dr. Grady Paden for his advice on the U.S. medical system. Thanks also to Professor John Warner for some very useful discussions, to David Reading of the Anaphylaxis Campaign for answering innumerable queries about food allergy and food labeling, and to Dr. Hedda Kraker von Schwarzenfeld, Dr. David Stern, Scott Adams of Celiac Support, and Dr. Maurice Smith of Unilever for help with specific questions. All the other doctors, medical researchers, and other health professionals whose work is described here, either directly or indirectly, are also gratefully acknowledged. Thanks are also due to Chris Allan, Denise Curwen, Janet Davies, Dee Gill, Ruth Simmons, Vicki Young, and the many other allergy sufferers whose stories are told in these pages, and to Hilary Mandleberg, Charlotte Harvey, and Elizabeth Stubbs for sharing their experiences as parents. Finally, special thanks are due to Dr. John Hart for his immense help during the final stages of the book.

PICTURE CREDITS

2 left Bubbles/Anthony Dawton; 2 center & right Patrick McLeavey; 3 robertharding.com/N A Callow; 4 NHPA/Stephen Dalton; 6 left Gettyone Stone/Peter Cade; 6 center The Image Bank/Joe Devenney; 6 right Gettyone Stone/Laurence Monneret; 8 The Image Bank; 10 Science Photo Library; 14 Anthony Blake Photo Library/Maximilian Stock Ltd; 16 Gettyone Stone/Laurence Monneret; 20 The Image Bank/Joe Devenney; 22 Gettyone Stone/Peter Cade; 24 left Bubbles/Loisjoy Thurston; 24 center Gettyone Stone/James Darrell; 24 right Anthony Blake Photo Library/Maximilian Stock Ltd; 26 NHPA/Stephen Dalton; 28 Gettyone Stone/James Darrell; 30 robertharding.com/Ydav Levy; 33 Bubbles/Loisjoy Thurston; 36 Gettyone Stone/Ralph H Wetmore; 41 The Image Bank/Paola Curto; 42 Bubbles/Loisjoy Thurston; 47 Collections/Sandra Lousada; 50 Elizabeth Whiting & Associates/Midgley; 54 The Stock Market/Mauro Panci; 58 robertharding.com/Mitch Diamond; 60 Science Photo Library/Claude Nuridsany; 62 Anthony Blake Photo Library/Martin Brigdale; 64 Anthony Blake Photo Library/Kieran Scott; 67 Anthony Blake Photo Library/Tim Hill; 68 Gettyone Stone/Jon Gray; 70 Anthony Blake Photo Library/Maximilian Stock Ltd; 72 Gettyone Stone/Laurence Monneret; 74 Anthony Blake Photo Library; 76 robertharding.com/John Miller; 80 Gettyone Stone/P Cade; 82 Science Photo Library; 84 Gettyone Stone/Roy Botterell; 86 left Gettyone Stone/Tony Latham; 86 center Science Photo Library/BSIP, Jolyot; 86 right The Image Bank/Ross Whitaker; 88 Gettyone Stone/Tony Latham; 90 Science Photo Library/BSIP, Taulin; 94 Science Photo Library/BSIP, Jolyot; 98 Linda Gamlin; 102 The Image Bank/Ross Whitaker; 106 Bubbles/Loisjoy Thurston; 108 left Bubbles/Jennie Woodcock; 108 center robertharding.com/Nelly Boyd; 108 right The Image Bank/Stephen Wilkes; 110 Anthony Blake Photo Library; 112 robertharding.com/N A Callow; 114 Gettyone Stone/Ian Shaw; 120 Gettyone Stone/Pal Hermansen; 124 Bubbles/Jennie Woodcock; 126 The Image Bank/Stephen Wilkes; 128 robertharding.com/Nelly Boyd; 132 DIAF/J C Gerard; 136 left Patrick McLeavey; 136 center Bubbles/Ian West; 136 right Linda Gamlin; 138 Patrick McLeavey; 140 Linda Gamlin; 148 John Walmsley; 152 Bubbles/Ian West; 164 The Image Bank/Noah Cross; 170 Patrick McLeavey; 172 Gettyone Stone/Joe Polillio; 176–192 Patrick McLeavey; 194 Bubbles/Loisjoy Thurston; 202 Gettyone Stone /Laurence Monneret; 204 Patrick McLeavey; 206 Katz Pictures/Adrian Kool; 208 Gettyone Stone/Andy Whale; 208 left robertharding.com/Scott Campbell; 208 center John Walmsley; 208 right Rex Features; 210 Retna/Philip Reeson; 214 Gettyone Stone/Andy Whale; 216 Rex Features; 218 John Walmsley; 222 robertharding.com /Scott Campbell; 226 Gettyone Stone/Zugy Kaluzny; 232 Gettyone Stone/Jon Bradley; 240 Bubbles/Anthony Dawton; 244 Linda Gamlin; 248 Powerstock Zefa.